COGNITIVE REHABILITATION FOR PERSONS WITH TRAUMATIC BRAIN INJURY

COGNITIVE REHABILITATION FOR PERSONS WITH TRAUMATIC BRAIN INJURY

A FUNCTIONAL APPROACH

edited by

JEFFREY S. KREUTZER, PH.D.
ASSOCIATE PROFESSOR
DEPARTMENTS OF REHABILITATION MEDICINE AND NEUROLOGICAL SURGERY
MEDICAL COLLEGE OF VIRGINIA
VIRGINIA COMMONWEALTH UNIVERSITY
RICHMOND

and

PAUL H. WEHMAN, PH.D.
PROFESSOR
DEPARTMENT OF PHYSICAL MEDICINE AND REHABILITATION
MEDICAL COLLEGE OF VIRGINIA
VIRGINIA COMMONWEALTH UNIVERSITY
RICHMOND

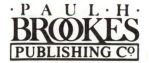
·PAUL·H·
BROOKES
PUBLISHING CO

Baltimore • London • Toronto • Sydney

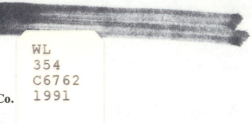
Paul H. Brookes Publishing Co.
P.O. Box 10624
Baltimore, Maryland 21285-0624

Typeset by Brushwood Graphics, Inc., Baltimore, Maryland.
Manufactured in the United States of America by
The Maple Press Company, York, Pennsylvania.

Permission to reprint the following quotations is gratefully acknowledged:
Pages 44, 45, 46, and 48:   Quotations from Sork, T. (1990). Theoretical
foundations of education program planning. *Journal of Continuing
Education in the Health Professions, 10*(1), pp. 73–83. Reprinted by
permission.

Library of Congress Cataloging-in-Publication Data
Cognitive rehabilitation for persons with traumatic brain injury : a functional
  approach / edited by Jeffrey S. Kreutzer and Paul H. Wehman.
    p.   cm.
Includes bibliographical references and index.
ISBN 1-55766-071-9 :
  1. Brain—Wounds and injuries—Patients—Rehabilitation.   2. Cognition
disorders—Treatment.   3. Brain—Wounds and injuries—Complications and
sequelae.   I. Kreutzer, Jeffrey S., 1953—   .   II. Wehman, Paul.
  [DNLM: 1. Brain Injuries—complications.   2. Brain Injuries—
rehabilitation.   3. Cognition Disorders—rehabilitation.   WL 354 C676]
RD594.C64   1991
616.8′043—dc20
DNLM/DLC
for Library of Congress   91-8287
                                                                        CIP

Contents

CONTRIBUTORS

Brenda L.B. Adamovich, Ph.D.
Director of Rehabilitation Services
Associate Professor
Albany Medical Center
Department of Physical Medicine and Rehabilitation
New Scotland Avenue (A79)
Albany, New York 12208

Michael S. Alberts, Ph.D.
Department of Medical Psychology
Oregon Health Sciences University
Portland, Oregon 97201

Peggy P. Barco, M.S., OTR
Head Injury Resource Center
St. John's Mercy Rehabilitation Center
755 South New Ballas Road
St. Louis, Missouri 63141

Laurence M. Binder, Ph.D.
Psychology Service 116 B (P)
Veterans Administration Medical Center
P.O. Box 1034
Portland, Oregon 97207

Jean L. Blosser, Ed.D.
Department of Communicative Disorders
West Hall
University of Akron
Akron, Ohio 44325

Corwin Boake, Ph.D.
The Institute for Rehabilitation and Research
1333 Moursund Avenue
Houston, Texas 77030

M. Melinda Bolesta, M.S., CCC-Sp/L
Head Injury Resource Center
St. John's Mercy Rehabilitation Center
755 South New Ballas Road
St. Louis, Missouri 63141

Lorraine F. Camenzuli, Ph.D.
Private Practice
3536 Front Street
San Diego, California 92103

Bruce Crosson, Ph.D.
Department of Clinical and Health Psychology
Box J-165, Health Sciences Center
University of Florida
Gainesville, Florida 32610

Ann V. Deaton, Ph.D.
Supervisor, Rehabilitation Psychology and
    Neuropsychology Services
Sheltering Arms Day Rehabilitation Center
9210 Forest Hill Avenue
Richmond, Virginia 23235

Roberta DePompei, M.A., CCC SLP/A
Department of Communicative Disorders
West Hall
University of Akron
Akron, Ohio 44325

Catherine W. Devany, M.S.
Department of Rehabilitation Medicine
Medical College of Virginia
Box 677, MCV Station
Richmond, Virginia 23298-0677

Anthony DiCesare, Ph.D.
Assistant Professor of Psychology
Towson State University
Towson, Maryland 21204

Wayne A. Gordon, Ph.D.
Mount Sinai Medical Center
School of Medicine
Department of Rehabilitation Medicine
Box 1240
One Gustave Levy Place
New York, New York 10029

Mary R. Hibbard, Ph.D.
Mount Sinai Medical Center
School of Medicine
Department of Rehabilitation Medicine
Box 1240
One Gustave Levy Place
New York, New York 10029

Sally Kneipp, Ph.D., C.R.C.
Director, Community Skills Program
1616 Walnut Street, #800
Philadelphia, Pennsylvania 19103

Jeffrey S. Kreutzer, Ph.D.
Associate Professor
Departments of Rehabilitation Medicine and
    Neurological Surgery
Medical College of Virginia
Box 677, MCV Station
Richmond, Virginia 23298-0677

Will Levin, Ph.D.
Oregon Rehabilitation Center
1255 Hilyard
Eugene, Oregon 97401

Kathleen O'Kane Martin, M.Ed.
Instructor
Continuing Education in Medicine and Allied Health
   Professions
Medical College of Virginia
Box 48, MCV Station
Richmond, Virginia 23298-0048

Jennifer Harris Marwitz, M.A.
Department of Rehabilitation Medicine
Medical College of Virginia
Box 677, MCV Station
Richmond, Virginia 23298-0677

Catherine A. Mateer, Ph.D., ABPP/ABCN
Neuropsychological Services
1322 Third Street, S.E.
Suite 250
Puyallup, Washington 98372

Paul E. Mazmanian, Ph.D.
Associate Professor
Department of Preventive Medicine
Director, Continuing Education in Medicine and
   Allied Health Professions
Box 48, MCV Station
Richmond, Virginia 23298-0048

Stefanie L. Myers, B.S.
Department of Rehabilitation Medicine
Medical College of Virginia
Box 677, MCV Station
Richmond, Virginia 23298-0677

Rick Parenté, Ph.D.
1212 Brookview Road
Towson, Maryland 21204

Ronald M. Ruff, Ph.D.
Director
Neurobehavioral Rehabilitation Services
St. Mary's Hospital and Medical Center
Rehabilitation Services
450 Stanyan Street
San Francisco, California 94117-1079

Robert J. Sbordone, Ph.D., ABCN
Private Practice
7700 Irvine Center Drive
Suite 750
Irvine, California 92718

Tamara B. Story, M.A., CCC-SLD
President and Clinical Director
Head Injury Therapy Services, Inc.
2707 Ashman Street
Midland, Michigan 48640

Robert Stout, B.S., OTR
Head Injury Resource Center
St. John's Mercy Rehabilitation Center
755 South New Ballas Road
St. Louis, Missouri 63141

Paul H. Wehman, Ph.D.
Professor
Department of Physical Medicine and Rehabilitation
Medical College of Virginia
Virginia Commonwealth University
Box 677, MCV Station
Richmond, Virginia 23298-0677

Diane Werts, M.A., CRC, LPC
Premiercare Neurorehabilitation Program
Bethesda General Hospital
3655 Vista Avenue
St. Louis, Missouri 63110

Dennis Williams, Ph.D.
Neuropsychological Services
1322 Third Street, S.E.
Suite 250
Puyallup, Washington 98372

Nathan D. Zasler, M.D.
Director, Brain Injury Rehabilitation Services
Medical College of Virginia
Box 677, MCV Station
Richmond, Virginia 23298-0677

PREFACE

Research has established the certainty of long-term adverse sequelae following traumatic brain injury. Especially for persons with more severe injuries, neurological impairment is relatively permanent. As a consequence of brain dysfunction, memory, attention, perception, motor speed, intelligence, and other areas of cognitive ability are affected. Ultimately, the ability to perform activities of daily living is impaired. Evidence of academic failure, employment difficulties, and social isolation has accumulated.

Despite the apparent permanence of neurological dysfunction, there is evidence that functional improvements can occur for decades following injury. Improvements are inevitable, given the commitment of persons with brain injury, their families, and professionals. Virtually all persons with brain injury retain the ability to learn. The capacity to learn ensures opportunities for improvement of existing skills and for acquisition of new skills. Furthermore, improved functioning can undoubtedly occur as a consequence of developing compensatory strategies and restructuring environments.

Cognitive rehabilitation is a set of strategies designed to improve the perceptual, intellectual psychomotor, and behavioral skills of persons with brain dysfunction.[1] The ultimate goal of therapy is to enhance the individual's ability to perform activities of daily living in home, academic, vocational, and community settings. The field of cognitive rehabilitation has arisen from the hopes of persons who see a better future for individuals with brain injury.

This book is intended to provide practical information about cognitive rehabilitation. Exemplary practice requires knowledge of diverse issues including research findings, cognitive theory, evaluation methods, therapy planning, and computer technology as well as group and individual intervention formats. Practitioners must also understand factors that potentially influence therapy outcome including prescribed medications, psychosocial and behavioral difficulties, limited motivation, poor self-awareness, and substance abuse.

This volume is organized into four sections. The first section provides information on the evolution of cognitive rehabilitation as a field. Details regarding research, underlying theory, practice, and training issues are discussed. The second section describes the consequences of brain injury along with interactive factors that influence overall outcome. The remaining sections of the book provide practical information on techniques of assessment and intervention. A wide variety of approaches intended to be useful within medical centers, outpatient clinics, and real-world settings are presented.

Realistically, we feel that professionals have just begun to address the many important issues confronting the practice of cognitive rehabilitation. Nevertheless, clinical and research efforts have yielded important conclusions that will guide practice. We know that cognitive rehabilitation requires interdisciplinary involvement and teamwork. We know that the ultimate goal of therapy is improvement in the ability of persons to carry out day-to-day activities within the community. Finally, we know that there is not a single rehabilitation approach that is appropriate for every client. Therapists must have a wide variety of tools available, and the choice of tools is dependent on a diversity of factors related to individual and environmental characteristics.

Despite remaining questions about "What works best for whom in which environments?" we are optimistic about continued progress in the field. In concert with advances in technology, the creativity of professionals and the motivation of persons with brain injury and their families will ensure continued progress.

---

[1]For purposes of clarification, readers should note that the terms *cognitive remediation* and *cognitive rehabilitation* have both been used in this book, often interchangeably. The term cognitive remediation was used by some professionals in the early 1980s, partly due to concerns that cognitive rehabilitation might be confused with other forms of rehabilitation or with cognitive therapy, a form of psychotherapy. Such concerns about confusion of terms have since subsided. Today, most professionals use the term cognitive rehabilitation.

ACKNOWLEDGMENTS

We are pleased to recognize the contributions of the individuals and organizations that made the publication of this book possible. Appreciation is expressed to Stephen Ayres, R.B. Young, Karen Rucker, Bruce Leininger, Margie Rigsbee, Sung Choi, and Doug Simmons, our colleagues at the Medical College of Virginia. Their support and guidance were valuable and essential. Much of our own research was funded through the National Institute on Disability and Rehabilitation Research (NIDRR), within the United States Department of Education. Within NIDRR, Paul Thomas and Toby Lawrence especially have provided timely advice and encouragement. Gratitude is also expressed to International Business Machines Corporation and Bruce Mahaffey for their supportive efforts.

We are grateful to Susan Hughes Gray, Melissa Behm, and Roslyn Udris, our colleagues at Paul H. Brookes Publishing Company, for their tireless assistance and encouragement. We are especially thankful to the authors of the individual chapters. The time they have taken away from their busy clinical and research activities is kindly appreciated. Appreciation is also expressed to Mitchell Rosenthal and Muriel Lezak for their wisdom and guidance. Finally, we are thankful to Henry Stonnington, a seer and eternal optimist, who has been a continuing source of inspiration.

We dedicate this book to our children. They have helped us understand the meaning and value of life. In doing so, they have given us hope and inspired our efforts to help others.

Cognitive Rehabilitation
for Persons with
Traumatic Brain Injury

FOUNDATIONS OF COGNITIVE REHABILITATION

Although cognitive rehabilitation efforts predate the 1980s, it was then that the field began to receive increasing attention. The number of practitioners and organized therapy programs grew rapidly. This growth was a consequence of at least two factors. First, improved medical care had yielded an increasing number of persons who survived brain injury. Second, there was mounting evidence that the quality of life for these individuals was relatively poor. Residual sequelae, including memory, intellectual, sensory, motor, and perceptual problems, prevented many persons from achieving life satisfaction. Furthermore, long-term follow-up research suggested that many brain injury sequelae were permanent. Professionals struggled to develop and provide therapeutic services to ameliorate cognitive problems. An immediate response to the need for services was made more urgent by pressures exerted by individuals with brain injury, family members, and advocacy organizations.

This rapid growth in the field of cognitive rehabilitation allowed little opportunity for reflection on underlying theory, professional training and development, empirical foundations, and long-term planning. Thus, this section of the book is intended to help readers achieve a better understanding of the evolution and foundations of cognitive rehabilitation.

Progress in developing efficacious therapies will be limited by research and integration of theory. Furthermore, an understanding of historical development, theory, and research will provide a framework for building expertise and training new cognitive rehabilitation professionals.

History of Cognitive Rehabilitation Following Head Injury

CORWIN BOAKE

Although cognitive treatment of persons with brain injury has existed since World War I, the term *cognitive rehabilitation* did not appear until the 1970s. (The reader is referred to Chapters 2 and 18, this volume, for a discussion of various definitions of cognitive rehabilitation/remediation.) The association between head injury and cognitive rehabilitation has remained a constant in the history of cognitive rehabilitation ever since. In fact, the history of cognitive rehabilitation and that of head injury rehabilitation are nearly identical.

WORLD WAR I

World War I marked the first time in medical history that there was appreciable survival from severe brain trauma due to changes in neurosurgical care of head injury. According to one estimate (Gurdjian, 1973), the mortality rate from severe brain injury among American servicemen fell from over 50% to 35%. Introduction of the new neurosurgical techniques is partly credited to Harvey Cushing, who is regarded as a founder of neurosurgery.

Most of our information about brain injury rehabilitation and cognitive rehabilitation during World War I comes from Germany and the United States. The history of cognitive rehabilitation in other countries during this time is less well known.

Germany

Major innovations in cognitive rehabilitation during the first world war occurred primarily in Germany, probably because Germany was a world center of clinical neuroscience (Howard & Hatfield, 1987). The many neurologists and psychiatrists interested in cognitive and behavioral disorders secondary to brain injury quickly became aware of the large number of persons with head injury produced by the war. A group of rehabilitation centers for members of the military with head injury was begun with locations in both Germany (Cologne, Frankfurt, and Munich) and Austria (Graz) ("Schools for soldiers," 1916). The directors of these centers were neurologists well known for their research in neurobehavioral disorders, particularly in aphasia. For example, the Munich center was directed by Max Isserlin, who is noted for describing the syndrome of agrammatism.

The center in Frankfurt became the best known because of its director, the neurologist Kurt Goldstein (Figure 1.1). Goldstein, who is probably the main creator of the field of brain injury rehabilitation, was a prominent neurology researcher at the University of Frankfurt (Simmel, 1968). Many of Goldstein's conclusions and recommendations from World War I were presented in a book, later published in English under the title *After-effects of Brain Injury in War* (Goldstein, 1942).

Goldstein designed his center to include a hospital, a psychological laboratory, and a school that provided rehabilitation therapies. The psychologist Adhemar Gelb directed the psychological laboratory and coauthored with Goldstein a series of case studies of patients treated at the center (Simmel, 1968). The plan of rehabilitation called for patients to undergo detailed psychological evaluations to reveal their strengths and

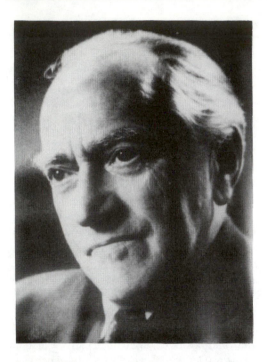

Figure 1.1. Kurt Goldstein, 1875–1965. (From Simmel, M.L. [Ed.]. [1968]. *The reach of mind: Essays in honor of Kurt Goldstein* [p. 2]. New York: Springer Publishing Company, Inc., New York 10012; used by permission.)

nicians were aware that choice reaction time was a more sensitive measure of cognitive impairment than simple reaction time. This dissociation was rediscovered by neuropsychologists in the 1970s (Levin, Benton, & Grossman, 1982).

The nature of cognitive rehabilitation as it was practiced in the German head injury centers is unclear because little documentation is available regarding therapy programming and techniques. According to Goldstein (1942, 1948) many of the therapists were actually school-teachers who had been recruited to work with head-injured patients. It is likely that the therapy programming focused primarily on speech and language disorders, because most centers were directed by neurologists interested in aphasia. In addition, most of the men probably suffered from penetrating brain injuries due to missile wounds. Goldstein (1942, 1948) was intensely concerned with aphasia therapy and described therapy techniques used in cases of impairments of speech articulation, word finding, reading, and writing. He was aware of both restorative and compensatory approaches to therapy, but felt that a compensatory approach was generally more appropriate. The therapeutic techniques he recommended followed a compensatory approach in which patients were trained to use different strategies to perform tasks (e.g., whole-word reading) or to relearn lost functions (e.g., shaping speech sounds from mouth movements). In contrast to current approaches to cognitive rehabilitation, Goldstein (1942, 1948) did not describe any therapies for attention, memory, and visual perception.

Goldstein (1942) regarded the prediction of vocational potential as a special assessment problem and he described two complementary but potentially opposed assessment approaches. The first approach, termed *abstract performance testing,* used laboratory psychological techniques, such as reaction time measurement, to identify patients' basic cognitive deficits. This differed from the type of psychological testing mentioned earlier in that this was testing for vocational purposes, focused on the patient's ability to initiate and maintain work activity. Goldstein (1942) felt the major advantages of this approach were that the tests were standardized and free

deficits, and then to receive therapies under medical and psychological guidance. Later, a vocational workshop was added to assess potential for different occupations. Goldstein was aware of the difficulties facing patients after discharge, noting that "when left to their own resources, many of these men will be utterly helpless" and recommending that "no man should be discharged before a decision is made about his future, his residence, his social care" (1942, p. 221).

The theoretical outlook of the German rehabilitationists was also quite advanced. Their knowledge of neuropsychological syndromes included not only different aphasic syndromes, but also visuoperceptual and frontal lobe syndromes. (Apparently, they were less knowledgeable regarding syndromes of closed head injury [e.g., amnesia] or syndromes of visuospatial disorientation and visual neglect, which were better characterized in the next world war.) One mark of sophistication was their use of specialized psychological tests in order to assess cognitive impairments. Further, the German cli-

from individual differences due to preinjury skills. He noted that "the main disadvantage of abstract testing is that the performances and the situation in general are remote from the working conditions in real labor; therefore the conclusions from the results as concerns actual capacity for work are vague" (1942, p. 106).

The second assessment approach, which Goldstein (1942) termed *concrete labor testing,* used real work that was performed in the vocational workshops attached to the hospital. The work tasks were chosen to have market value and patients were paid on a piecework basis, so that trends in productivity could be measured objectively. In addition to using realistic tasks, Goldstein believed it was essential that "the psychological conditions under which the man is working must be regulated as nearly as possible to conform with those of regular labor" (1942, p. 137). He felt the weakness of this approach, if used alone, was that patients' performances might be affected if they suspected that their disability compensation payments would be determined by their test results. He was critical of clinicians, such as Walther Poppelreuter of the Cologne head injury center, who used work tasks as a "practical procedure" to directly determine patients' vocational potential. Goldstein (1942) felt it was necessary to combine both assessment approaches in order to make an accurate assessment of patients' work potential.

Finally, one of the most important contributions of the German head injury rehabilitation centers during World War I was in long-term follow-up of patients, both for research and clinical service. For example, the Munich head injury rehabilitation center continued follow-up of World War I veterans until after World War II. The follow-up data from this center, which may be the world's oldest head injury data base, have been used to study the impact of seizures and other complications of the longevity of persons with head injury (Weiss, Caveness, Einsiedel-Lechtape, & McNeel, 1982).

Tragically, the Jewish rehabilitationists who worked in these centers were either killed or forced to flee the Holocaust. Goldstein himself was briefly jailed in Germany and then expelled to the Netherlands. He later fled to the United States, where he worked at universities in Boston and New York until his death in 1965 (Simmel, 1968).

United States

Because of the lack of rehabilitation models and the limited tradition of clinical neuroscience, head injury rehabilitation in the United States was far less advanced than that in Germany. In fact, before World War I, occupational therapy and physical therapy were not recognized therapy disciplines in the United States, and physical medicine and rehabilitation was not a recognized medical specialty. The development of general medical rehabilitation in the United States was obstructed by an interdisciplinary conflict between orthopedic surgeons and vocational educators. The surgeons proposed the establishment of a national network of specialized rehabilitation hospitals for wounded servicemen, with the stipulation that the physicians in charge of hospital-based rehabilitation should also have authority over vocational rehabilitation. Vocational educators opposed this control, and the specialized hospital system was never realized (Gritzer & Arluke, 1985). It is interesting to speculate how such a rehabilitation hospital system would have affected the later development of rehabilitation in the United States.

In the end, rehabilitation in the United States was implemented through special sections of general military hospitals. Records show that rehabilitation sections operated in 16 hospitals in 1918, increasing to a peak of 46 in 1919, after which most of the hospitals were closed (Crane, 1927). This rapid growth may have overextended the available physical and personnel resources (Figure 1.2). The organizational models and treatment methods in the military rehabilitation system were detailed in contemporary publications (Crane, 1927; Weed, 1923). In general, the clinical approach used in these hospitals was a practical one that emphasized prevention of psychological complications and preparation of patients to return to work. Recovering patients were engaged in a routine activity schedule, beginning with occupational therapy in their hospital wards and progressing to vocational training in workshops attached to the hospitals. To en-

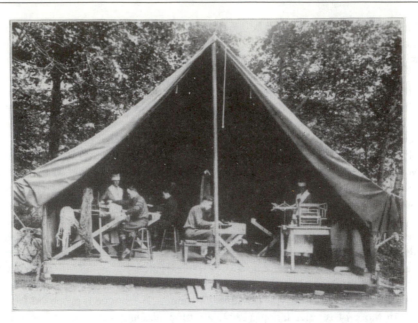

Figure 1.2. World War I occupational therapy unit in a military hospital in the United States of America. (From Crane, A.G. [1927]. *The Medical Department of the United States Army in the World War: Vol. 13. Physical reconstruction and vocational education, Pt. 1* [p. 80]. Washington, DC: U.S. Government Printing Office.)

courage activity and improve morale, patients were involved in recreational events, competitions, associations, and newsletters. The rehabilitation system provided the foundations for therapy specialties that evolved into occupational therapy and physical therapy.

For patients with head injury, the disadvantage of the American military rehabilitation system was that their special needs, except for strictly medical differences, were not generally addressed. One exception was General Hospital No. 11 (Hospital for Head Surgery) in Cape May, New Jersey (Figure 1.3), which specialized in the surgical care of patients with head wounds (Frazier & Ingham, 1920; Weed, 1923). Although the hospital's mission was primarily surgical, rather than rehabilitative, the problem was recognized that many patients exhibited speech and language deficits, and the hospital recruited 10 speech-reading and three speech-correction teachers to form a Section of Defects of Hearing and Speech. Probably fewer than 50 patients with head injury were treated while the unit was in operation from 1918 to 1919 (Carhart, 1943). Therapy of patients with head injury was primarily aimed at aphasic syndromes, with "daily in-

dividual instruction and exercise in conversation, reading and writing adapted to the needs of the patient and the character of his language disturbance" (Frazier & Ingham, 1920, p. 31). It is unknown what therapy services were provided to nonaphasic head-injured patients, aside from therapy for physical deficits.

The major theoretical statement about rehabilitation to come out of the United States after World War I was the book *Nervous and Mental Re-education,* by the psychologist Shepherd I. Franz (1923). His book describes rehabilitation methods for patients with physical disabilities, including those with brain injury, as well as psychiatric patients. Franz, who was probably the first clinical neuropsychologist in the United States, had established a psychological laboratory at St. Elizabeth's Hospital in Washington, D.C. He had a longstanding interest in clinical neuroscience and had written on cognitive assessment and on rehabilitation of aphasia and hemiplegia (Franz, 1930). During the war, he attempted to organize a rehabilitation research institute through an interdisciplinary committee representing neurology, psychiatry, and other medical specialties. However, the committee,

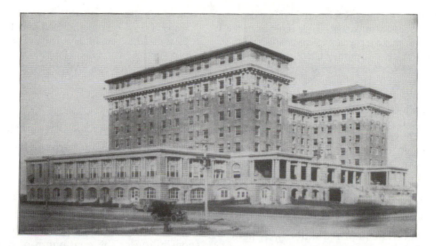

Figure 1.3.   General Hospital No. 11 (Hospital for Head Surgery), Cape May, New Jersey, which provided medical care and rehabilitation for patients with head injury during World War I. (From Weed, F.W. [1923]. *The Medical Department of the United States Army in the World War: Vol. 5. Military hospitals in the United States* [p. 526]. Washington, DC: U.S. Government Printing Office.)

which Franz had organized through the fledgling American Psychologicial Association, failed to obtain government support and the research institute never came about.

WORLD WAR II

There is little information in the literature regarding cognitive rehabilitation between the two world wars, and this may reflect a decline of interest in brain injury rehabilitation during this period. Cognitive rehabilitation was essentially reborn during World War II, with the development of head injury treatment centers in the United States, the Soviet Union, Great Britain, and other nations. The major difference from the previous war was that patients with head injury were segregated into special neurosurgical centers, creating the basis for dedicated rehabilitation programs similar to the German centers in World War I. Work at the rehabilitation centers was more carefully documented than in the previous war, however, and thus had a formative influence on modern brain injury rehabilitation, including neuropsychology, aphasia therapy, and vocational rehabilitation of persons with brain injury. In fact, many leading figures in brain injury rehabilitation during World War II became prominent in neuropsychology and speech-language pathology after the war.

Soviet Union

Soon after the invasion of the Soviet Union, the physician-psychologist Alexander Luria was appointed to organize a head injury rehabilitation hospital, partly in recognition of his research in neuropsychology. Patients with head injury received neurosurgical care in Moscow and were then transferred to the Neurosurgical Rehabilitation Hospital, which was located in the Urals (Luria, 1979). By early 1943, approximately 800 patients with penetrating head injuries had been treated at the hospital (Luria, 1947/1970). After 3 years at this hospital, Luria's group was transferred to Moscow to continue their work. Luria's experiences in head injury rehabilitation during World War II formed the basis for his influential theory of functional systems, which he discussed in his books *Traumatic Aphasia* (1947/1970) and *Restoration of Function after Brain Injury* (1948/1963).

As in Goldstein's center during World War I, Luria's approach called for in-depth neuropsychological assessment to plan each patient's rehabilitation. The details of Luria's (1947/1970) assessment methods have had a long-lasting influence on neuropsychology. An additional point of similarity was the use of special sections for vocational assessment and training. Luria explained the role of the vocational workshop as follows:

In order to make a more precise study of the course of work processes in patients with injuries to the brain, and to make a psychological analysis of the principal ways in which they adapt themselves to work, special workshops were set up at the Rehabilitation Hospital where patients were trained in certain work operations to help them compensate their disabilities resulting from wounding, and to facilitate their return to useful working life. The patients were greatly attracted by this dual task to the systematic work in these workshops, and many of the wounded thereby gained additional qualifications. (1948/1963, pp. 243–244)

Luria's most important contribution to cognitive rehabilitation was his finding that patients could relearn certain impaired skills by changing to a strategy that would rely only on intact functions. This reorganization concept had been discussed earlier by Goldstein (1942, 1948), whom Luria credited as the "investigator who has contributed perhaps more than any other to our understanding of the restoration of speech functions after focal brain damage" (1947/1970, p. 373). However, this concept was expressed in a more fully developed form by Luria:

This training begins with the transfer of the defective operation to the level of the patient's consciousness, which formerly it never completely reached; the patient begins to introduce new methods into this process, while remaining aware all the time of the system of methods used. Only after a long period (sometimes many months) of training does a newly-formed method begin to become automatic, and full automatization frequently never occurs. (1948/1963, p. 73)

Finally, Luria and his colleagues described various neurobehavioral problems presented by patients with frontal lobe injuries, such as decreased motivation and poor planning, and commented that such patients often gained less benefit from rehabilitation than other patients with head injury. Luria (1948/1963) recognized that such patients may require long-term living and working arrangements extending beyond the medical rehabilitation system:

The main condition for the resettlement of the patients of this group is the creation of a special environment, constantly directing their behaviour, inhibiting unwanted and distracting factors, and greatly simplifying the demands made on the patient. . . . The patient can cope with tasks in an environment that is simple and so organized that all his actions are determined by suitable external conditions, irrespective of his internal activity. It is perfectly clear that these conditions demand the organization of a special environment (special residential factories or sheltered employment). (pp. 261–262)

Great Britain

Plans for a head injury neurosurgical hospital had been discussed before World War II by British neurologists and neurosurgeons. With Great Britain's entry into the war, these plans were expanded to establish a group of head injury neurosurgical units in England and Scotland (Denny-Brown, 1942). The British centers, like their counterparts in the Soviet Union, took responsibility for the continuum of rehabilitation from acute stages to community reentry. The problem of managing agitated and disoriented patients was discussed by McKissock (1942), who recommended that "a room be provided where the individual may enjoy peace and quiet [instead of] the noise and bustle of a large or busy ward [that] often induce a restlessness and irritability in recovering head injuries" (p. 79).

Work at the Military Hospital for Head Injuries in Oxford and at the Brain Injuries Unit in Edinburgh is well documented. The Oxford center is known primarily because of the research carried out by the neurologist W. Ritchie Russell (1971) on post-traumatic amnesia and determinants of outcome from head injury. Also, a data base of patients with penetrating injuries was used to study localized cognitive deficits (Newcombe, 1969). Hugh Cairns, the neurosurgeon who directed the Oxford center, advocated a multidisciplinary approach to head injury rehabilitation and described its application to several case studies (1942a, 1942b). In one case example, "impaired memory and loss of learning capacity, combined with some lack of insight, demanded a down-grading of occupation in an able young man . . . who was reluctant to give up his earlier ambitions" (Cairns, 1942b, p. 85). Cairns noted that "this type of patient is much more difficult to rehabilitate than those in whom a gross permanent disability makes it clear from the outset that change of occupation is inevitable" (1942b, p. 86).

The Edinburgh center is known for its research in aphasia therapy and in cognitive assessment and training (Pentland, Boake, & McKinlay, 1989). From the center's clinical staff, the speech therapist Edna Butfield and the psychologist Oliver Zangwill completed the first systematic evaluation study of aphasia therapy, concluding that therapy was generally effective and that the most improved patients were those with milder, expressive syndromes (Butfield & Zangwill, 1946).

In an important theoretical paper published in 1947, Zangwill distinguished between two general approaches to the "re-education" of patients with brain injury. He defined the *substitution* approach as "the building up of a new method of response to replace one damaged irreparably by a cerebral lesion" (1947, p. 63), and contrasted this to the *direct training* approach, which attempted to restore impairments. Zangwill (1947) favored the substitution approach because he was skeptical of the assumption, underlying the direct approach, that damaged abilities could be newly acquired by other brain regions. However, he did not rule out the usefulness of direct training in all cases and concluded that "direct, as opposed to substitutive, training has a real, though limited, part to play in re-education " (Zangwill, 1947, p. 66).

Zangwill, who was later a founder of the International Neuropsychological Society, was particularly concerned with neuropsychological assessment and carried out several studies of memory disorders and visuoperceptual disorders (Zangwill, 1945). Like Goldstein and Luria, he addressed the issue of predicting employment potential from cognitive testing, noting that "an assessment based on a single short psychological examination may give a most misleading impression of a brain-injured patient's capacity to cope with protracted work" (Zangwill, 1945, p. 249). As a solution to this problem, he stated that:

> [We] check our findings at frequent intervals against the patient's work record in the occupational therapy department. In special cases we have even arranged to give a patient an extended practical trial in a line of work akin to his own and under realistic conditions. (Zangwill, 1945, p. 249)

Rowbotham (1945), a neurosurgeon working at the head injury unit in Manchester, described a residential rehabilitation center used for patients with head injury to continue in rehabilitation after hospital discharge. The center, which was located in a rural castle and named simply the Rehabilitation Centre, provided a therapy program based largely on physical exercise and reconditioning. This center can be regarded as a forerunner of current transitional living centers.

United States

In contrast to the previous world war, American patients with head injury were treated separately from patients with other injuries, in a system of neurosurgical units located across the United States (Figure 1.4) (Spurling & Woodhall, 1958). Although this reorganization was originally dictated by the requirements of specialized medical and surgical services, and not by the need for specialized rehabilitation, the neurosurgical centers quickly developed rehabilitation programs aimed specifically at patients with head injury. The lead in head injury rehabilitation was taken by the field of speech-language pathology, beginning with the establishment of the first speech disorders unit in May 1943 at Brooke General Hospital in Fort Sam Houston, San Antonio, Texas. Over the next 2 years, approximately 13 such units were established, each in association with a neurosurgical unit and usually directed by a speech-language pathologist, psychologist, or neurologist (Peacher, 1947).

Therapy programming in these centers followed different orientations. For example, the program directed by the psychologist Louis Granich (1947) at England General Hospital in Atlantic City was based on a factor analysis of cognitive abilities and on training techniques recommended by Goldstein (1942, 1948). The program of the unit at Letterman General Hospital in San Francisco was directed by the psychologist–speech-language pathologist Joseph Wepman, and was described in his book *Recovery from Aphasia* (1951); it influenced the development of aphasia therapy in the United States. In their general form, these rehabilitation programs resembled current head injury units with interdisciplinary teams including physical therapy, occupational therapy, psychotherapy, and vocational services as well as speech-language therapy.

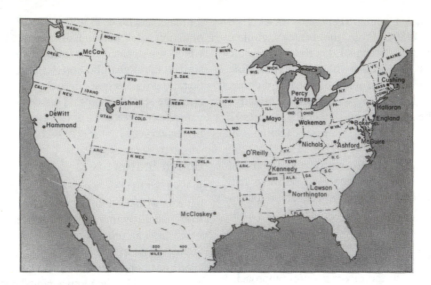

Figure 1.4.   Military hospitals with neurosurgical units in April 1945. (From Spurling, R.G., & Woodhall, B. [Eds.]. [1958]. *Medical Department, United States Army, surgery in World War II: Neurosurgery* [Vol. 1, p. 19]. Washington, DC: Office of the Surgeon General.)

POSTWAR PERIOD TO PRESENT

With the end of World War II and the abrupt drop in incidence of head injury, there was a concomitant decline of interest in head injury rehabilitation. Ironically, the segregation of patients with head injury from general rehabilitation during the war may have contributed to this decline, despite the period of rapid growth in general rehabilitation and the development of physiatry as a medical specialty.

The 1950s, 1960s, and 1970s were mostly quiet decades for cognitive rehabilitation and head injury rehabilitation, although considerable advances were made in stroke rehabilitation, aphasia therapy, and neuropsychological research. The major exceptions were Luria's writings (1948/1963, 1947/1970, 1979) and Leonard Diller's research studies at the New York University Medical Center on cognitive retraining of visuoperceptual disorders in stroke patients (Diller, Ben-Yishay, Weinberg, Goodkin, & Gordon, 1974).

The first major signs of renewed interest in head injury rehabilitation were international conferences held in 1969 (Walker, Caveness, & Critchley, 1969) and 1971 (Hook, 1972). During the same period, medical rehabilitation units dedicated to patients with head injury were es-

tablished at Loewenstein Rehabilitation Hospital near Tel Aviv, Israel (Najenson et al., 1974), Rancho Los Amigos Hospital near Los Angeles, California (Malkmus, Booth, & Kodimer, 1980), and the Royal Air Force Medical Rehabilitation Unit in Chessington, Scotland (Evans, 1981). The assessment and treatment protocols developed at Rancho Los Amigos Hospital have been extremely influential, and are the standard of practice in many American rehabilitation units. From this beginning, the number of inpatient head injury rehabilitation programs has multiplied several times and continues to increase (National Head Injury Foundation, 1990).

However, the very rapid growth of medical rehabilitation units did not address the long-term adjustment of patients with head injury, who were generally unable to return to work or function as full members of society. This problem was noted in several countries, but especially in Israel, due to the large number of persons who sustained head injuries during the 1973 Yom Kippur war. In a joint project of the Rehabilitation Department of the Israeli Ministry of Defense and the New York University Institute of Rehabilitation Medicine, the neuropsychologists Yehuda Ben-Yishay and Leonard Diller established a day treatment program for patients with head injury in 1975 near Tel Aviv. The program marked a turning point in the history of cognitive rehabilitation as the first program to focus primarily on patients' cognitive and behavioral deficits. Therapy programming consisted of individual exercises to improve cognitive functioning, group exercises to improve awareness and social behavior, and family counseling, culminating in placement in volunteer job trials.

The new field of postacute head injury rehabilitation grew rapidly from this point. In 1978, Ben-Yishay established a day program on the same model at the New York University Medical Center and similar programs were later founded at several locations in the United States. The first postacute residential treatment center, the Center for Comprehensive Services, was established in 1977 in Carbondale, Illinois. The next year, residential programs were started at Ashby House

in Toronto, Canada, and at Tangram Ranch (later renamed Tangram Rehabilitation Network) in San Marcos, Texas.

In the years since, many treatment models for day and residential cognitive rehabilitation have been introduced. However, the key problem remains that many severely injured individuals need long-term supports, which cannot be provided by time-limited treatment programs; in recent years, a small number of supported employment and independent living programs have been established. Assuming continued economic and social support for rehabilitation, the next stage of the history of cognitive rehabilitation may feature the development of long-term services. It would certainly be fitting for the concerns of the founders of the field 70 years ago to be addressed at last.

REFERENCES

Ben-Yishay, Y., Ben-Nachum, Z., Cohen, A., Gross, Y., Hoofien, D., Rattok, J., & Diller, L. (1978). Digest of a two-year comprehensive clinical rehabilitation research program for out-patient head injured Israeli veterans (Oct. 1975 to Oct. 1977). In Y. Ben-Yishay (Ed.), *Working approaches to remediation of cognitive deficits in brain damaged persons* (Rehabilitation Monograph No. 59). New York: New York University Medical Center, Institute of Rehabilitation Medicine.

Butfield, E., & Zangwill, O.L. (1946). Re-education in aphasia: A review of 70 cases. *Journal of Neurology, Neurosurgery, and Psychiatry, 9*, 217–222.

Cairns, H. (1942a). Discussion on rehabilitation after injuries of the central nervous system. *Proceedings of the Royal Society of Medicine, 35*, 299–302.

Cairns, H. (1942b). Rehabilitation after head injuries. *British Journal of Physical Medicine and Industrial Hygiene, 5*, 84–88.

Carhart, R. (1943). Some notes on official statistics of speech disorders encountered during World War I. *Journal of Speech Disorders, 8*, 97–107.

Crane, A.G. (1927). *The Medical Department of the United States Army in the World War: Vol. 13. Physical reconstruction and vocational education, Pt. 1.* Washington, DC: U.S. Government Printing Office.

Denny-Brown, D. (1942). The sequelae of war head injuries. *New England Journal of Medicine, 227,* 771–780, 814–821.

Diller, L., Ben-Yishay, Y., Weinberg, J., Goodkin, R., & Gordon, W. (1974). *Studies in cognition and rehabilitation in hemiplegia* (Rehabilitation Monograph No. 50). New York: New York University, Institute for Rehabilitation Medicine.

Evans, C.D. (Ed.). (1981). *Rehabilitation following severe head injury.* Edinburgh, Scotland: Churchill-Livingstone.

Franz, S.I. (1923). *Nervous and mental re-education.* New York: Macmillan.

Franz, S.I. (1930). Shepherd Ivory Franz. In C. Murchison (Ed.), *A history of psychology in autobiography* (Vol. 2, pp. 89–113). Worcester, MA: Clark University Press.

Frazier, C.H., & Ingham, S.D. (1920). A review of the effects of gunshot wounds of the head. Based on the observation of two hundred cases at U.S. General Hospital No. 11, Cape May, N.J. *Archives of Neurology and Psychiatry, 3,* 17–41.

Goldstein, K. (1942). *After-effects of brain injuries in war.* New York: Grune & Stratton.

Goldstein, K. (1948). *Language and language disturbances.* New York: Grune & Stratton.

Granich, L. (1947). *Aphasia: A guide to retraining.* New York: Grune & Stratton.

Gritzer, G., & Arluke, A. (1985). *The making of rehabilitation: A political economy of medical specialization, 1890–1980.* Berkeley: University of California Press.

Gurdjian, E.S. (1973). *Head injury from antiquity to the present with special references to penetrating head wounds.* Springfield, IL: Charles C Thomas.

Hook, O. (Ed.). (1972). International symposium on rehabilitation in head injury, Goteborg 1971 [Special issue]. *Scandinavian Journal of Rehabilitation Medicine, 4*(1).

Howard, D., & Hatfield, F.M. (1987). *Aphasia therapy: Historical and contemporary issues.* Hillsdale, NJ: Lawrence Erlbaum Associates.

Levin, H.S., Benton, A.L., & Grossman, R.G. (1982). *Neurobehavioral consequences of closed head injury*. New York: Oxford University Press.

Luria, A.R. (1963). *Restoration of function after brain injury* (B. Haigh, Trans.). London: Pergamon Press. (Original work published 1948)

Luria, A.R. (1970). *Traumatic aphasia: Its syndromes, psychology and treatment* (D. Bowden, Trans.). The Hague, Netherlands: Mouton. (Original work published 1947)

Luria, A.R. (1979). *The making of mind: A personal account of Soviet psychology* (M. Cole & S. Cole, Eds.). Cambridge, MA: Harvard University Press.

Malkmus, D., Booth, B.J., & Kodimer, C. (1980). *Rehabilitation of the head injured adult: Comprehensive cognitive management*. Downey, CA: Professional Staff Association of Rancho Los Amigos Hospital.

McKissock, W. (1942). Rehabilitation of head injuries. *Practitioner, 149*, 75–80.

Najenson, T., Mendelson, L., Schecter, I., David, C., Mintz, N., & Groswasser, Z. (1974). Rehabilitation after severe head injury. *Scandinavian Journal of Rehabilitation Medicine, 6*, 5–14.

National Head Injury Foundation. (1990). *National directory of head injury rehabilitation services*. Southborough, MA: Author.

Newcombe, F. (1969). *Missile wounds of the brain*. Oxford, England: Oxford University Press.

Peacher, W.G. (1947). Speech disorders in World War II: VI. Survey of speech clinics in the U.S. and British armies. *Journal of Nervous and Mental Disease, 106*, 52–65.

Pentland, B., Boake, C., & McKinlay, W. (1989). Scottish head injury rehabilitation: An historical account. *Scottish Medical Journal, 34*, 411–412.

Rowbotham, G.F. (1945). *Acute injuries of the head: Their diagnosis, treatment, complications and sequels* (2nd ed.). Baltimore: Williams & Wilkins.

Russell, W.R. (1971). *The traumatic amnesias*. London: Oxford University Press.

Schools for soldiers with brain injuries. MEDICAL NEWS, Berlin Letter. (1916). *Journal of the American Medical Association, 66*, 969.

Simmel, M.L. (1968). Kurt Goldstein, 1878–1965. In M.L. Simmel (Ed.), *The reach of mind: Essays in honor of Kurt Goldstein* (pp. 3–11). New York: Springer.

Spurling, R.G., & Woodhall, B. (Eds.). (1958). *Medical Department, United States Army, surgery in World War II: Neurosurgery* (Vol. 1). Washington, DC: Office of the Surgeon General.

Walker, A.E., Caveness, W.F., & Critchley, M. (Eds.). (1969). *The late effects of head injury*. Springfield, IL: Charles C Thomas.

Weed, F.W. (1923). *The Medical Department of the United States Army in the World War: Vol. 5. Military hospitals in the United States*. Washington, DC: U.S. Government Printing Office.

Weiss, G.H., Caveness, W.F., Einsiedel-Lechtape, H., & McNeel, M.L. (1982). Life expectancy and causes of death in a group of head-injured veterans of World War I. *Archives of Neurology, 39*, 741–743.

Wepman, J.M. (1951). *Recovery from aphasia*. New York: Ronald Press.

Zangwill, O.L. (1945). A review of psychological work at the Brain Injuries Unit, Edinburgh, 1941–5. *British Medical Journal, 2*, 248–250.

Zangwill, O.L. (1947). Psychological aspects of rehabilitation in cases of brain injury. *British Journal of Psychology, 37*, 60–69.

CHAPTER 2

The Theory and Practice of Cognitive Remediation

WAYNE A. GORDON AND MARY R. HIBBARD

Cognitive deficits are the basis of many of the day-to-day difficulties experienced by individuals with traumatic brain injury. Cognitive deficits such as memory loss, reduced organizational skills, concrete thinking, slowed information processing, and attentional problems often underlie the individual's inability to shop, count change, balance a checkbook, understand what is read, travel independently in the community, return to work, and so on. In designing intervention programs for individuals with these cognitive difficulties, there is little agreement as to the level at which the treatment of cognitive dysfunction should commence. On the one hand, there are those who believe that interventions should be focused on the direct modification of aberrant behaviors (Butler & Namerow, 1988). On the other hand, there are those who argue in favor of an approach to intervention that is hierarchically organized in terms of the cognitive demands that are placed on the learner (Diller & Gordon, 1981a, 1981b; Gordon, Hibbard, & Kreutzer, 1989).

Whyte (1986) provided a hierarchical schema for conceptualizing cognitive activity that is useful in delineating the distinctions between the level at which cognitive remediation and other types of interventions are focused in order to promote behavioral change. At the base of this hierarchy of cognitive activity are *cognitive operations,* which according to Whyte are the most basic mental activities (e.g., looking) that may be common to many different skills or tasks. *Cognitive processes* are more complex than cognitive operations and are usually at the level of mental activities typically assessed by neuropsychological tests. Cognitive processes comprise many different cognitive operations and include mental activities such as naming ability, visual scanning, and motor speed. A *skill* (e.g., reading) is a more complex level of function than is a cognitive process, and requires the coordinated action of many different cognitive processes. More complex behaviors or *metaskills* result from the linking of multiple skills and the generalization of learning across skills. The highest level of activity is a *global function* (e.g., working), which requires the integration of all aspects of the person's cognitive function.

Using this hierarchical model, defective performance of a skill or metaskill may result from impairments of underlying cognitive functions. Thus, treating the faulty behavior, in and of itself, will have little impact on the cognitive impairments that are the foundations for skilled behavior.

COGNITIVE PROCESS MODEL OF REMEDIATION

Cognitive remediation (Diller & Gordon, 1981a, 1981b; Gordon, 1987) is a form of intervention in which a constellation of procedures are applied by a trained practitioner (usually a neuropsychologist, speech-language pathologist, or occupational therapist) to provide brain-injured individuals with the skills and strategies needed to perform tasks that are difficult or impossible for them, due to the presence of underlying cognitive deficits. A key premise of cognitive remediation is that impaired cognitive processes are treated before skills. It is believed that an improvement in basic cognitive functions will

The preparation of this manuscript was supported in part by Grant #G0087C0218 from NIDRR, United States Department of Education.

effect greater behavioral gains than the direct modification of the individual's behavioral repertoire—because learning will generalize to the range of skills to which the relevant cognitive process relates.

Support for a cognitive process model can be derived from both developmental psychology and learning theory. Developmental psychology has taught us that simple behaviors are the prerequisites for the learning of more complex behaviors (Piaget, 1950). Learning theorists (e.g., Gagne, 1965; Singley & Anderson, 1989) have argued that learning is indeed a hierarchical process in which skills and more complex behaviors are learned only when underlying basic cognitive processes are intact. Implicit in this approach is the view that cognitive processes are the foundations that support skilled behavior. The learning of skilled behavior without first building on adequate foundations results in superficial situation-specific learning. This type of learning fails to generalize to new situations, has limited heuristic value, and has little practical utility to the individual.

CRITICISMS OF COGNITIVE REMEDIATION

Cognitive remediation is a relatively new field, and has therefore been the subject of few well-designed systematic outcome studies (Butler & Namerow, 1988). While several studies have documented the efficacy of cognitive remediation (Ben-Yishay & Diller, 1983; Prigatano et al., 1984), critics have typically cited the lack of generalization, the slow pace of learning, and/or the finding of improved test scores, rather than improved behavioral outcomes, as proof of the futility of this form of rehabilitation therapy (Glisky & Schacter, 1986, 1988; Glisky, Schacter, & Tulving, 1986a, 1986b; Schacter & Glisky, 1986).

Rather than accept a nihilistic view of the utility of cognitive remediation, it is more fruitful to examine the methodological flaws of some of the research in the area so that more rigorous evaluations can be undertaken. More specifically, the deficits to be treated and the outcomes sought require more precise definition. Simi-

larly, experimental designs need to be applied with appropriate comparison groups, and measurement tools used to assess change need to be both sensitive and appropriate. For example, memory remediation studies have been problematic because: 1) the specific nature of the posttraumatic brain injury memory impairments have not been adequately isolated, and 2) there is little agreement about how to define a memory deficit. When there is little clarity about the nature of a memory impairment, it is not surprising that approaches to intervention are similarly muddled. For example, a memory impairment could be defined in any of the following manners: 1) a discrepancy between current test performance and premorbid ability; 2) a discrepancy between current intelligence (e.g., Wechsler Adult Intelligence Scale–Revised [WAIS-R] [Wechsler, 1981] Verbal IQ) and performance on a global test of memory function (e.g., Wechsler Memory Scale Revised [WMS-R] [Wechsler, 1987]); 3) a discrepancy between current performance on a global test of memory function and performance on a test of functional memory abilities (e.g., Rivermead Behavioral Memory Test [Wilson, Cockburn, & Baddeley, 1985]); or 4) a specific deficit in episodic, implicit, or semantic memory. Thus, there is ambiguity about the specific deficit to be treated and how it is to be operationalized from both a psychometric and diagnostic perspective. In sum, the negative outcomes of memory retraining could easily be associated either with studies that were inadequately conceptualized, designed, or implemented, or with deficits that indeed were intractable to intervention.

Omnibus day treatment programs have been criticized for not adequately evaluating program efficacy using a dismantling design (i.e., systematically examining the effects of each intervention in order to determine what aspects of the intervention are associated with the improvements that have been observed) (e.g., Butler & Namerow, 1988). While this criticism is pertinent, given the number of issues that require study and the well-documented positive outcomes of these types of programs (e.g., Ben-Yishay & Diller, 1983; Prigatano et al., 1986; Scherzer, 1986), this is not of high priority. Indeed, Ben-Yishay, Piasetsky, and Ezrachi (1984) compared the effects of three combinations of interventions on the outcomes of their day treatment program. The three components of the program that were provided to participants were: attention training, cognitive remediation, and social skills training. One group of participants received all three subprograms; a second group received attention training and social skills training; and a third group received attention training and cognitive remediation. Thus, attention training was common to all three groups. It was found that the same changes (i.e., improvements on neuropsychological tests, ratings of interpersonal behaviors, and vocational outcomes) were exhibited by the participants, no matter which combination of interventions they received. All subcomponents of the programs resulted in generalized nontreatment-specific improvements that were positively related to successful vocational outcome.

There are those who believe that the conceptual foundations of cognitive remediation are weak and contend that the premise behind cognitive remediation is not supported by the research on functional recovery following brain injury (e.g., Butler & Namerow, 1988). More specifically, the point has been made that there is no reason to believe that structural/anatomical changes occur in the brain other than those that are produced by spontaneous recovery following injury. This position sets up and then destroys a straw man, however, because nowhere in the literature has the claim been made that cognitive remediation has a structural impact on the brain. The only claim that has been made for cognitive remediation is that learning has taken place as evidenced by altered behavior. Clearly, claims can be made for the efficacy of interventions with brain-injured individuals based on improved performance, without documenting any alterations (i.e., improvements) in neuropathology. For example, there are not only reports of improved cognitive functioning following cognitive remediation, but improved ability to walk and take care of basic needs following physical and occupational therapy and improved language functioning following speech-language therapy. This criticism, then, appears to be directed

at all rehabilitation efforts—not just cognitive remediation.

ESSENTIAL CHARACTERISTICS OF COGNITIVE REMEDIATION PROGRAMS

Reviews of treatment successes (e.g., Ben-Yishay & Diller, 1983; Prigatano et al., 1986) as well as treatment failures (e.g., Batchelor, Shores, Marosszeky, Sandanam, & Lovarini, 1988) suggest several characteristics that are associated with positive outcomes of cognitive remediation programs. These characteristics are discussed next.

Training Must Be Based in Theory

Training must be theoretically based on a clear understanding of the neuropsychological nature of the dysfunction, as well as grounded in both learning theory and sound pedagogy (Diller, 1976; Mateer & Sohlberg, 1988). A program that is conceptually based provides an opportunity to understand better the nature of the deficit, how best to treat it, and why training either succeeds or fails. In addition, an understanding of how learning takes place and how learning abilities become impaired following brain injury is crucial to any successful cognitive remediation program. A program that is neither conceptually based nor pedagogically grounded is more likely to fail, and will add little to our understanding of the nature of learning in individuals with brain injury.

Training Must Be Multimodal in Nature

Diller and Gordon (1981b) and Diller and Weinberg (1977) made the point that diagnosing a cognitive deficit is often like peeling an onion: The presence of one deficit reveals another that, upon first blush, was not readily apparent. Therefore, the source of cognitive failure is often multidetermined. For example, a short-term memory deficit may be the result of impaired mnemonic skill, an attentional disorder, or both. Similarly, Gordon et al. (1985); Weinberg et al. (1977, 1979); and Weinberg, Piasetsky, Diller, and Gordon (1982), in their work on the treatment of visual scanning disorders of persons who had had a stroke, conceptualized what initially appeared as a simple cognitive deficit (i.e., visual neglect) as one that actually involved a variety of visual information processing skills (i.e., scanning, visual synthesis and analysis, and somatosensory perception). Their intervention program evolved to reflect this complexity by incorporating specific protocols designed to remediate the diverse facets of this visual information processing deficit. Similarly, Sohlberg and Mateer (1987) proposed a multimodal remediation program for attentional disorders that incorporates aspects of focused attention, sustained attention, and divided attention. Thus, to achieve maximum impact (i.e., generalization), training must address all elements that are believed to be nested within the specific cognitive disorder.

Intervention Must Integrate Both Cognitive and Skills Training

Despite the evidence that cognitive remediation is an effective intervention for those with traumatic brain injury, there are those who believe that direct training of skills is a more direct and efficient method of treating the cognitive difficulties of brain-injured individuals. This impression of efficiency comes from the notion that if one can successfully modify the targeted behavior without having to alter the substrate, then time and energy are saved. As other investigators have extensively discussed the benefits of skill training (Gross & Schutz, 1986; Hart & Hayden, 1986; Mayer, Keating, & Rapp, 1986) and behavior modification (Eames & Wood, 1985; Wood, 1986, 1987), they are not examined here. However, no data exist to support the assertion that one approach is better than the other.

The most ambitious application of a skills training approach is the supported employment model of vocational rehabilitation (Wehman et al., 1989; Wehman et al., 1988). While outcome studies have supported a skills-based approach, Wehman and his colleagues (1988) noted that when compared to other populations on whom this skills training model has been applied, individuals with traumatic brain injury require more counselor contacts and time than do those with other disabling conditions. One could posit several reasons for these findings. The counselors

may not have been adequately trained to understand the functional implications of an often diverse array of cognitive deficits seen in clients with traumatic brain injury. Conversely, the brain-injured individuals participating in this program may have had greater learning impairments than other groups studied. An alternative explanation from a cognitive process approach is equally likely; that is, faulty underlying cognitive processes were not adequately retrained prior to the learning of new work skills, hence skills learning could be neither adequately supported nor efficiently assimilated.

In sum, more appears to be needed than purely "in vivo" skills training if intervention is to be maximally effective for individuals with traumatic brain injury. Rather than assuming a dichotomous view of either cognitive remediation or functional skills training, it is the authors' belief that the most efficacious approach to the retraining of complex behavior is one that includes retraining of *both* cognitive processes and skills. Training of cognitive processes provides the necessary foundation for the more complex task of learning new skills and behaviors. Learning must occur hierarchically to ensure maximal generalization of what is learned. In this way, new learning can be incorporated and assimilated into formerly intact learning paradigms. In implementing programs of remediation, the issue, then, is to develop integrated methods of intervention that are hierarchically arranged such that the band of behaviors being taught is constantly being expanded while resting on a foundation of either intact or remediated cognitive processes.

Training Must Generalize To Be Ecologically Valid

Training must be relevant to the individual's life and must generalize to actual real-world functioning (Hart & Hayden, 1986). Gordon (1987) described the following three-level hierarchy of generalization:

Level 1: Ability to demonstrate behavioral change on alternate forms of the training materials both within session and between sessions

Level II: Ability to demonstrate changes on tests that tap behaviors that are similar but one step removed from the actual task demands being trained

Level III: Ability to demonstrate transfer of learning to the tasks of day-to-day living

Based on this conceptualization of generalization, it is clear that improvements in neuropsychological test scores (i.e., Level II) have some heuristic value. However, from the standpoint of justifying an intervention or improving the functioning of an individual, test score changes provide insufficient evidence of generalization. Indeed, one can argue that what passes under the guise of cognitive remediation is actually training to improve test scores, rather than retraining of cognitive processes that underlie dysfunctional behavior. Level III generalization represents the true test of the effectiveness of a cognitive remediation program. Yet criteria with which to evaluate changes in functioning are woefully lacking. Tools that systematically assess the functional analogs of the cognitive skills need to be developed. An excellent model of such a functional assessment tool is the Rivermead Behavior Memory Test (Wilson et al., 1985), which serves as a functional analog to areas evaluated in the traditional neuropsychological memory assessment.

Despite the absence of adequate assessment tools, there are examples of training programs that have documented Level III generalization effects. The visual-scanning programs of Gordon et al. (1985), Weinberg et al. (1977, 1979), and Weinberg et al. (1982) generalized to all three levels; that is, they resulted in improved performance on a test of basic scanning (Level I), improved reading test scores (Level II), and an increased proportion of time that clients spent at home reading (Level III). A similar form of visual-scanning training was also found to generalize to driving behavior and wheelchair navigation skills (Sivak et al., 1984; Sivak, Olson, Kewman, Won, & Henson, 1981). Thus, these data suggest that: 1) scanning difficulties are often the root of difficulties with diverse functional skills such as reading, driving, and wheelchair navigation in individuals with brain injury; and

2) the effects of comprehensive training programs were found to generalize to real-life behaviors. These training programs provide excellent models for future research demonstrating the impact of cognitive remediation on everyday functioning.

Intervention Requires Sufficient Time To Effect Behavioral Change

Cognitive remediation is often belittled as being based merely on overlearning and practice (e.g., Butler & Namerow, 1988). Learning *is* based on practice and repetition. Since learning is known to be impaired in persons with traumatic brain injury, extensive practice is required for individuals to learn a new skill. Learning is usually a time-consuming process even under the best of circumstances. When it is attempted with a brain-injured individual, the speed of the processing is further reduced because the brain, the organ that mediates all learning, has been impaired. Therapists are often overwhelmed by the amount of time needed to effect improvement in even the most basic aspects of behavior in individuals with brain injury. For example, the clients included in the studies by Gordon et al. (1985), Weinberg et al. (1977, 1979), and Weinberg et al. (1982) received at least 35 hours of individual training; those in the Sohlberg and Mateer (1987) study received between 28 and 72 sessions of individual training. The positive outcomes attained by those in Ben-Yishay and Diller's (1983) program required a minimum of 20 weeks of intervention, 4 days a week, 5 hours per day (a total of at least 400 hours). The extent of time needed for successful intervention becomes more clear when one considers that most individuals with traumatic brain injury have multiple cognitive deficits, each requiring a different type of intervention. Thus, in order to obtain maximal benefits from cognitive remediation, the client, the family, and the therapist must be willing to commit the necessary resources (i.e., time, patience, and money) to achieve a successful outcome.

Cognitive remediation is not just practice for the sake of practice. Effective learning in cognitive remediation programs is associated both with the way in which materials are presented and practiced by the clients and with the structure of the training program per se. For example, Ben-Yishay, Diller, Gerstman, and Gordon (1970) coined the phrase "saturation cuing" to describe a form of training that was found to be an effective method of teaching clients with brain injury. In this approach, cues were systematically removed so that the client learned via repetition to complete a task independently. This type of learning paradigm, when performed in reverse, has been called a system of "vanishing cues" (Glisky et al., 1986a, 1986b) and has been successfully applied to teach visual scanning skills to persons with brain injury resulting from stroke (Gordon et al., 1985; Weinberg et al., 1977, 1979; Weinberg et al., 1982) as well as to teach computer skills to persons with amnesia (Glisky & Schacter, 1988; Glisky et al., 1986a, 1986b; Schacter & Glisky, 1986). Learning to respond to a situation within a specific hierarchy of cuing is not a method that was introduced to psychology or rehabilitation by those practicing cognitive remediation, but rather is a method of teaching based on sound pedagogy (Gagne, 1965; Skinner, 1953). Thus, cognitive remediation involves neither the presentation of materials in a haphazard manner nor practice for practice's sake. When implemented appropriately, there is a sound theoretical rationale behind the materials that are used, the methods of presentation, and the frequency of stimulus repetition.

Time Since Injury Does Not Preclude Effective Intervention

The length of time postinjury appears to have little effect on a client's ability to profit from cognitive remediation. The benefits of early intervention are obvious in terms of maximizing cognitive gains that are obtained during the period of spontaneous recovery. Recent work by Diller, Kay, and Goodgold (1988) indicated that spontaneous recovery is in itself a process that is subject to individual differences. In this study, the amount of recovery, as defined as psychometric changes over time, was far from uniform. Some individuals with traumatic brain injury failed to make positive change, some improved, and others got worse during their initial 1-year "recovery" period. Thus, no single pattern of change was found to be associated with sponta-

neous recovery. Some individuals continue to recover for years, as they continue to learn. For example, those individuals participating in studies by Ben-Yishay and Diller (1983), Prigatano et al. (1984, 1986), and Scherzer (1986) were all at least 1 year postinjury. Thus, spontaneous recovery did not limit these clients' abilities to learn at later points in time.

Intervention Approaches May Vary in Locus

The locus of training has varied in the models of cognitive remediation that have been developed. Diller (1976) advocated the systematic manipulation of either the stimulus materials or the responses to be elicited from the individual. Materials can be altered by changing either the nature or the complexity of the stimulus (e.g., from letters to numbers or shapes), or by making the tasks more difficult. The individual's response can be altered by increasing the cognitive load of the task or by altering the pace at which information is processed. Others have advocated the shaping of the individual's responses (i.e., behavior) either by using behavior modification or by changing the way in which those in the individual's environment respond to the individual (Eames & Wood, 1985; Wood, 1986, 1987). An equally important consideration is the consistency of the intervention, for individuals benefit from interventions only when continuity is provided on a day-to-day basis. Sudden changes in the intervention without adequate explanation usually result in regression.

Evaluation of Intervention Requires Appropriately Standardized Measurement

The tools used to evaluate program efficacy have often been standardized on populations with other disabling conditions. For example, Blair and Lanyon (1987) used the Adaptive Behavior Scale (Nihira, Foster, Shellhaas, & Leland, 1975) to evaluate the effectiveness of their cognitive remediated program. The choice of this instrument can be questioned as it was developed for use with mentally retarded individuals. Thus, the scoring criteria, the specific behaviors being observed, and the available normative data were derived from individuals whose aberrant behavior is of different etiology. The implicit assumption in using this scale with brain-injured individuals (i.e., the maladaptive behaviors of those with mental retardation and those with traumatic brain injury are the same) has not been empirically validated. Although the behaviors being observed may be similar, their frequency of occurrence, the reason why they are being emitted, and their potential for modification may be different. In contrast, Mateer, Sohlberg, and Crinean (1987) developed a self-report memory questionnaire based on the responses of a large group of individuals with traumatic brain injury. Factor analysis of the scale revealed that it tapped four discrete clusters of memory difficulties common to brain-injured persons and therefore suggests that it would be a useful tool in evaluating the efficacy of memory retraining in individuals with traumatic brain injury.

An Individual's Awareness of Cognitive Deficits Is Crucial to Successful Intervention

Lack of awareness is often viewed as one of the hallmarks of brain injury (e.g., Stuss & Benson, 1986). A key to the success of cognitive remediation is the individual's becoming aware of the nature of his or her cognitive deficits, and their impact on his or her functioning in daily activities. Lack of awareness results in the individual's inability to understand the need for cognitive remediation, infringes upon the individual's participation in therapy, and may doom the intervention to failure. Crosson et al. (1989) suggested three different levels of awareness that can be observed in brain-injured persons: intellectual awareness, emergent awareness, and anticipatory awareness (see also Chapter 11, this volume). The presence or absence of awareness, as well as the level of awareness of an individual during the process of remediation, will dictate both the clinical approach used by the therapist, and the types of compensatory mechanisms that can be successfully utilized by the individual. Consequently, the level of the individual's awareness of his or her cognitive deficits must be carefully assessed as part of an initial neuropsychological evaluation and reexamined during the process of therapy. While rarely documented, improvement in a individual's awareness is, in itself, an important measure of therapeutic success.

Psychotherapy Is an Important Component of Cognitive Remediation

Cognitive deficits have a profound impact on the personality structure of individuals with traumatic brain injury. The way that individuals with brain injury experience and perceive their environment is often altered by an impaired ability to process accurately the onslaught of information from the world around them. Multiple cognitive deficits further limit an individual's ability to respond flexibly to both the emotional and intellectual demands of daily life. Ways of responding to situations that were once effective (i.e., prior to the injury) may become dysfunctional. Premorbid personality traits can become exaggerated or even blunted to the point that they are no longer adaptive. A discrepancy or chasm typically develops between who the person was before the injury, and who the person is now. The larger the perceived discrepancy, the greater the potential for affective distress. Many individuals with traumatic brain injury become prone to profound mood swings, seemingly unprovoked outbursts of anger or crying, and distorted thinking. At times, paranoid or psychotic thought processes may be observed. These changes in the client's affect state and personality structure cannot be ignored by the therapist; supportive intervention must be integrated into ongoing remediation sessions. Frequently, psychotropic medications are needed to stabilize the client's mood or irrational ideational state. Following traumatic brain injury, an individual's response to medication is often quite variable and unpredictable. Dosage requirements are often different from that of non-brain-injured individuals or individuals with psychiatric disorders. Therefore, the use of psychotropic medications needs to be carefully monitored by a psychiatrist familiar with the management of organically based disorders. (For further discussion of the use of medications, the reader is referred to Chapter 7, this volume.)

Verbal Self-Regulation Is an Effective Intervention Tool

Verbal self-regulation (self-talk) has been shown to be effective in teaching individuals to control previously automatic functions. For example, Stuss, Delgado, and Guzman (1987) found that the performance of individuals on a motor impersistence task could be improved through the use of self-talk. Three important points can be learned from this study. First, training that took place on one task (e.g., "Close your eyes") was found to generalize to other tasks (e.g., "Hold your breath," "Tap your finger"). Second, since impaired motor impersistence performance has been related to damage to the frontal system (Stuss & Benson, 1986), this study provides support for the belief that higher cortical functions regulated by the frontal system may be amenable to treatment. Third, verbal self-regulation is similar to the verbal labeling interventions used in cognitive-behavioral psychotherapy (Beck, Rush, Shaw, & Emery, 1979; Meichenbaum, 1977) in which "self-talk" has been used as a means of promoting cognitive restructuring and behavioral change. Since many individuals with traumatic brain injury have lost the ability to sequence activities, plan ahead, or modulate their emotional responses to others and to their environment, self-talk can be a powerful intervention. Teaching individuals to talk their way through situations, anticipate responses, and so forth provides them with a way of taking control of actions that previously were automatic. Here again, systematic evaluation of self-regulatory technique is essential in future research.

Computerized Training Must Be Used Judiciously

Clinical applications of the use of computers in cognitive remediation suggest that this approach has limited utility with traumatically brain-injured clients. There are several potential reasons for this finding. Most striking is the fact that the theoretical rationale behind the choice of given software programs is often lacking: It often appears as if the programs used are simply chosen out of one of the many software catalogs that are available (e.g., Gianutsos & Klitzer, 1981; Kreutzer, Hill, & Morrison, 1987). Much of the software available for use in cognitive remediation was developed for use in either early childhood education or special education and was not designed specifically for individuals with traumatic brain injury (Kreutzer et al., 1987). Computerized programs thus lack sufficient

flexibility for use with brain-injured individuals. For example, lack of key elements such as the variable speed of presentation of stimuli, and variable length of the interstimulus interval and adequate gradations of learning make the software difficult to use with traumatically brain-injured individuals. In addition, the software often lacks the sophistication needed to engage adults in computer programs; clients are often offended by activities that appear to them to be "child's play."

Limitations of computer-assisted cognitive retraining do not rest solely with the software. The skills being taught using computerized programming usually bear little relationship to real-world behaviors. What is often being trained is a "splinter" skill. When used as a sole intervention tool, this approach makes generalization difficult. However, when carefully chosen, computer programs can serve as an adjunct to remediation, and are useful in reinforcing the cognitive skills learned during individual therapy sessions. For example, if categorization skills are being taught to enhance encoding for a memory-impaired individual, computerized categorization games may be useful vehicles with which to practice the newly acquired skills, teach independent follow through on tasks, and provide external feedback about an individual's performance. (For a different view of the potential use of computers in the cognitive rehabilitation of persons with traumatic brain injury, the reader is referred to Chapter 13, this volume.)

SUMMARY AND CONCLUSIONS

This chapter has provided an overview of basic issues in cognitive remediation research. It is hoped that this discussion will provide a firmer basis for rational decision making with regard to choice of intervention approaches in the development of cognitive remediation programs.

Systematic interventions are needed for the rehabilitation of cognitive deficits resulting from traumatic brain injury. Cognitive remediation is a new form of intervention that is being applied by rehabilitation practitioners (e.g., neuropsychologists, speech-language pathologists, occupational therapists). While the final verdict on the efficacy of cognitive remediation awaits sustained programmatic research, there are sufficient available data to justify the application of this intervention to those in need.

REFERENCES

Batchelor, J., Shores, E.A., Marosszeky, J.E., Sandanam, J., & Lovarini, M. (1988). Cognitive rehabilitation of severely head-injured patients using computer-assisted and noncomputerized treatment techniques. *Journal of Head Trauma Rehabilitation, 3,* 78–83.

Beck, A.T., Rush, A.J., Shaw, B.F., & Emery, G. (1979). *Cognitive therapy of depression.* New York: Guilford Press.

Ben-Yishay, Y., & Diller, L. (1983). Cognitive remediation. In M. Rosenthal, E.R. Griffith, M.R. Bond, & J.D. Miller (Eds.), *Rehabilitation of the head injured adult* (pp. 367–378). Philadelphia: F.A. Davis.

Ben-Yishay, Y., Diller, L., Gerstman, L.J., & Gordon, W.A. (1970). Relationship between initial competence and ability to profit from cues in brain damaged individuals. *Journal of Abnormal Psychology, 75,* 248–259.

Ben-Yishay, Y., Piasetsky, E., & Ezrachi, O. (1984). Rehabilitation of cognitive and perceptual deficits in persons with chronic brain damage—a comparative study. In L.A. Diller, W.A. Gordon, & M. Brown (Eds.), *Second annual progress report, NIDRR grant #G008300039.* New York: New York University Medical Center.

Blair, C.D., & Lanyon, R.I. (1987). Retraining social and adaptive skills in severely head injured adults. *Archives of Clinical Neuropsychology, 2,* 33–43.

Butler, R.W., & Namerow, N.S. (1988). Cognitive retraining in brain-injury rehabilitation: A critical review. *Journal of Neurological Rehabilitation, 2,* 97–101.

Crosson, B., Barco, P., Velozo, C., Bolesta, M., Cooper, P., Warts, D., & Brobeck, T. (1989). Awareness and compensation in post acute head injury rehabilitation. *Journal of Head Trauma Rehabilitation, 4,* 46–54.

Diller, L. (1976). A model for cognitive retraining in rehabilitation. *Clinical Psychologist, 29,* 13–16.

Diller, L., & Gordon, W.A. (1981a). Interventions for cognitive deficits in brain injured adults. *Journal of Consulting and Clinical Psychology, 49,* 822–834.

Diller, L., & Gordon, W.A. (1981b). Rehabilitation and clinical neuropsychology. In S. Filskov & T. Boll (Eds.), *Handbook of clinical neuropsychology* (Vol. I, pp. 702–733). New York: John Wiley & Sons.

Diller, L., Kay, T., & Goodgold, J. (1988). *Final report, NIDRR grant #G008300039.* New York: New York University Medical Center.

Diller, L., & Weinberg, J. (1977). Hemi-inattention in rehabilitation: The evolution of a rational remediation program. In E. Weinstein & R. Friedland (Eds.), *Advances in neurology* (pp. 63–82). New York: Raven Press.

Eames, P., & Wood, R. (1985). Rehabilitation after severe brain injury: A follow-up study of a behavior modification approach. *Journal of Neurology, Neurosurgery, and Psychiatry, 48,* 613–619.

Gagne, R. (1965). *The condition of learning.* New York: Holt, Rinehart & Winston.

Gianutsos, R., & Klitzer, C. (1981). *Computer programs for cognitive rehabilitation.* Bayport, NY: Life Sciences Associates.

Glisky, E.L., & Schacter, D.A. (1986). Remediation of organic memory disorder: Current status and future prospects. *Journal of Head Trauma Rehabilitation, 3,* 54–63.

Glisky, E.L., & Schacter, D.A. (1988). Long-term retention of computer learning by patients with memory disorders. *Neuropsychologia, 26,* 173–178.

Glisky, E.L., Schacter, D.A., & Tulving, E. (1986a). Computer learning by memory-impaired patients: Acquisition and retention of complex knowledge. *Neuropsychologia, 24,* 313–328.

Glisky, E.L., Schacter, D.A., & Tulving, E. (1986b). Learning and retention of computer-related vocabulary in memory-impaired patients: Method of vanishing cues. *Journal of Clinical and Experimental Neuropsychology, 8,* 292–312.

Gordon, W.A. (1987). Methodological issues in cognitive remediation. In M. Meir, A.L. Benton, & L. Diller (Eds.), *Neuropsychological rehabilitation* (pp. 111–131). London: Churchill Livingston.

Gordon, W.A., Hibbard, M.R., & Kreutzer, J.S. (1989). Cognitive remediation: Issues in research and practice. *Journal of Head Trauma Rehabilitation, 4,* 76–84.

Gordon, W.A., Ruckdeschel-Hibbard, M., Egelko, S., Diller, L., Scotzin-Shaver, M., Lieberman, A., & Ragnarsson, K.T. (1985). Impact of a comprehensive perceptual remediation program on right brain damaged stroke patients. *Archives of Physical Medicine and Rehabilitation, 66,* 353–359.

Gross, Y., & Schutz, L.E. (1986). Intervention models in neuropsychology. In B. Uzzell & Y. Gross (Eds.), *Clinical neuropsychology of intervention* (pp. 179–204). Boston: Martinus Nijhoff.

Hart, T., & Hayden, M.E. (1986). The ecological validity of neuropsychological assessment and remediation. In B. Uzzell & Y. Gross (Eds.), *Clinical neuropsychology of intervention* (pp. 21–71). Boston: Martinus Nijhoff.

Kreutzer, J.S., Hill, M., & Morrison, K. (1987). *Cognitive rehabilitation resources for the Apple II computer.* Indianapolis, IN: NeuroScience.

Mateer, C.A., & Sohlberg, M.M. (1988). A paradigm shift in memory rehabilitation. In H.A. Whitaker (Ed.), *Neuropsychological studies of nonfocal brain damage: Dementia and trauma* (pp. 202–225). New York: Springer-Verlag.

Mateer, C., Sohlberg, M., & Crinean, J. (1987). Focus on clinical research: Perceptions of memory function in individuals with closed-head injury. *Journal of Head Trauma Rehabilitation, 2,* 74–84.

Mayer, N.H., Keating, D.J., & Rapp, D. (1986). Skills, routines and activity patterns of daily living: A functional nested approach. In B. Uzzell & Y. Gross (Eds.), *Clinical neuropsychology of intervention* (pp. 205–222). Boston: Martinus Nijhoff.

Meichenbaum, D. (1977). *Cognitive-behavior modification: An integrated approach.* New York: Plenum.

Nihira, K., Foster, R., Shellhaas, M., & Leland, H. (1975). *Manual: AAMD Adaptive Behavior Scale, 1975 Revision.* Washington, DC: American Association on Mental Deficiency.

Piaget, J. (1950). *The psychology of intelligence.* New York: Harcourt Brace.

Prigatano, G.P., Fordyce, D.J., Zeiner, H.K., Roueche, J.R., Pepping, M., & Wood, B.C. (1984). Neuropsychological rehabilitation after closed head injury in young adults. *Journal of Neurology, Neurosurgery and Psychiatry, 47,* 505–513.

Prigatano, G.P., Fordyce, D.J., Zeiner, H.K., Roueche, J.R., Pepping, M., & Wood, B.C. (Eds.). (1986). *Neuropsychological rehabilitation after brain injury.* Baltimore: Johns Hopkins University Press.

Schacter, D.A., & Glisky, E.L. (1986). Memory remediation: Restoration, alleviation and the acquisition of domain specific knowledge. In B. Uzzell & Y. Gross (Eds.), *Clinical neuropsychology of intervention* (pp. 257–282). Boston: Martinus Nijhoff.

Scherzer, B.P. (1986). Rehabilitation following severe head trauma: Results of a three-year program. *Archives of Physical Medicine and Rehabilitation, 67,* 366–374.

Singley, N.K., & Anderson, J.R. (1989). *The transfer of cognitive skill.* Boston: Harvard University Press.

Sivak, M., Hill, C.S., Henson, D.L., Butler, B.P., Silber, S.M., & Olson, P.L. (1984). Improved driving performance following perceptual training in persons with brain damage. *Archives of Physical Medicine and Rehabilitation, 65,* 163–168.

Sivak, M., Olson, P.L., Kewman, D.G., Won, D., & Henson, D.L. (1981). Driving and perceptual/cognitive skills: Behavioral consequences of brain damage. *Archives of Physical Medicine and Rehabilitation, 62,* 476–483.

Skinner, B.F. (1953). *Science and human behavior.* New York: Macmillan.

Sohlberg, M.M., & Mateer, C.A. (1987). Effectiveness of an attention-training program. *Journal of Clinical and Experimental Neuropsychology, 9,* 117–130.

Stuss, D.T., & Benson, D.F. (1986). *The frontal lobes.* New York: Raven Press.

Stuss, D.T., Delgado, M., & Guzman, D.A. (1987). Verbal regulation in the control of motor impersistence: A proposed rehabilitation procedure. *Journal of Neurological Rehabilitation, 1,* 19–24.

Wechsler, D. (1981). *The Wechsler Adult Intelligence Scale–Revised.* New York: Psychological Corporation.

Wechsler, D. (1987). *The Wechsler Memory Scale–Revised.* New York: Psychological Corporation.

Wehman, P., Kreutzer, J., Sale, P., West, M., Morton, M.V., & Diambra, J. (1989). Cognitive impairment and remediation: Implications for employment following traumatic brain injury. *Journal of Head Trauma Rehabilitation, 4,* 66–75.

Wehman, P., Kreutzer, J., Stonnington, H., Wood, W., Sherron, P., Diambra, J., Fry, R., & Groah, C. (1988). Supported employment for persons with traumatic brain injury: A preliminary report. *Journal of Head Trauma Rehabilitation, 3,* 82–93.

Weinberg, J., Diller, L., Gordon, W.A., Gerstman, L.J., Lieberman, A., Lakin, P., Hodges, G., & Ezrachi, O. (1977). Visual scanning training effect on reading-related tasks in acquired right brain damage. *Archives of Physical Medicine and Rehabilitation, 58,* 479–486.

Weinberg, J., Diller, L., Gordon, W.A., Gerstman, L.J., Lieberman, A., Lakin, P., Hodges, G., & Ezrachi, O. (1979). Training sensory awareness and spatial organization in people with right brain damage. *Archives of Physical Medicine and Rehabilitation, 60,* 491–496.

Weinberg, J., Piasetsky, E., Diller, L., & Gordon, W.A. (1982). Treating perceptual organization deficits in non-neglecting RBD stroke patients. *Journal of Clinical Neuropsychology, 4,* 59–75.

Whyte, J. (1986). Outcome evaluation in the remediation of attention and memory deficits. *Journal of Head Trauma Rehabilitation, 1,* 64–71.

Wilson, B., Cockburn, T., & Baddeley, A. (1985). *The Rivermead Behavioral Memory Test.* Reading, England: Thames Valley.

Wood, R.L.I. (1986). Rehabilitation of patients with disorders of attention. *Journal of Head Trauma Rehabilitation, 1,* 43–53.

Wood, R. (1987). *Brain injury rehabilitation: A neurobehavioral approach.* Rockville, MD: Aspen.

CHAPTER 3

Research Challenges for Behavioral Rehabilitation

Searching for Solutions

RONALD M. RUFF AND LORRAINE F. CAMENZULI

Every clinician wants to achieve progress for his or her clients, but in the absence of progress, a question arises as to the underlying reasons. In the search for those reasons, the clinician must make sure that it is neither the technology nor the measurement of the gains that is at fault. Similarly, when clients do improve, clinicians would like to be certain which factors were most contributory to that success. Research is ideally suited for the systematic assessment of improvements or the lack thereof.

Systematic research may also improve communication between and among key players in the rehabilitation process, including the client, family, and treatment team, by clarifying and specifying the goals and procedures relevant to successful intervention outcomes. Additionally, research can most convincingly demonstrate to individuals and agencies funding these interventions that their dollars are well spent, in that the quality of life of head injury survivors is significantly improved. The need for optimal intervention technologies and measurement techniques, in turn, gives rise to the need for empirical studies in the field of rehabilitation. In short, the scientific study of rehabilitation serves the practical purpose of securing its progress and future.

This chapter is intended for the clinician who, despite being well versed in the folklore of what constitutes "success" in therapy, must creatively reformulate goals, procedures, and outcomes on a daily basis for individual clients who do not fit the lore. It is intended for the administrator who does the planning in support of such interventions and who wants to be assured of maximum utilization of the resources assembled. Finally, it is intended for the researcher who seeks practical solutions for some of the thorniest problems yet to arise in rehabilitation outcome.

This chapter identifies the major hurdles and challenges that complicate research in behavioral rehabilitation. The term *behavioral rehabilitation* is used here in its broadest sense, and is meant to include cognitive, physical, emotional, and social components. Moreover, the chapter focuses on behavioral rehabilitation as it affects those individuals who have sustained traumatic brain injuries.

HETEROGENEITY OF PERSONS WITH TRAUMATIC BRAIN INJURY

Problem

Individual differences between brain-injured clients occur not only as a result of varying preinjury characteristics, but of extensive variability in the brain trauma in itself. Since the introduction of the Glasgow Coma Scale (Teasdale & Jennett, 1974), the emphasis has been on classifying severity according to three levels: severe, moderate, and mild. (The reader is referred to Chapter 5, this volume, for further discussion of the Glasgow Coma Scale.) But while severity is an important dimension, it is only one dimension in a complex array of factors that delineate brain damage. Among these are the size and location of the lesions and the extent of the axonal shearing, as well as the presence of intracranial pressure, vascular changes, and/or hypoxia (e.g., Bigler, 1990; Ruff, Cullum, & Luerssen, 1989).

Moreover, the duration of coma and the duration of post-traumatic amnesia have been identified as important markers for outcome (Levin, Benton, & Grossman, 1982). Other bodily traumas occurring at the time of the head injury, such as spinal cord injuries, for example, need to be considered, as does the preinjury history of physical (Morris, MacKenzie, & Edelstein, 1990), psychiatric, or neurological disorders. Age, sex, time of onset, education, socioeconomic status, vocation, ethnicity, and cerebral dominance have also been recognized as influencing recovery (Meier, Benton, & Diller, 1987). In short, the heterogeneity in persons with traumatic brain injury arises due to the complex array of neurological and medical factors that needs to be quantified and integrated with an equally complex array of emotional, cognitive, psychosocial, vocational, and financial factors.

Searching for Solutions

For research as well as intervention purposes, the diagnostic classifications of traumatic brain injury need to be expanded to incorporate this heterogeneity. No doubt it is most important to have the severity of the brain injury rated along the lines of the Glasgow Coma Scale (Teasdale & Jennett, 1974) as mild, moderate, or severe. However, the severity classification should also include the duration of the coma, the duration of the post-traumatic amnesia, and the location of the brain lesions. Finally, other medical complications or physical injuries should be considered.

However, even a severity index as comprehensive as this still only refers to the initial extent of the damage and would not be sufficient to describe the status of individuals months and years postinjury. An analogy to psychiatry illustrates the limitations of such a classification system: It would be as if an individual diagnosed with affective disorder or schizophrenia were then classified as mild, moderate, and severe, and generalized interventions were devised accordingly. Obviously, therapy, whether psychiatric or rehabilitative, should be responsive to the changing needs across time and stages of recovery. It is essential, therefore, that an assessment be made of preinjury functioning and that the individual's present status be carefully evaluated at multiple levels and various stages over time.

To date, the Rancho Los Amigos Scale of Cognitive Function provides the most useful classification schema of the individual's present state and capacity to function in a specific "stage" (Hagen, 1982; Hagen & Malkmus, 1979) (see Table 19.1, this volume, for a description of the various levels of the Rancho Scale). Medical, psychological, cognitive, and psychosocial issues are evaluated and incorporated into the classification. However, the scale is more or less unidimensional since it was not designed to describe or account for the progress that is typically achieved following a course of rehabilitation or, for that matter, for the persistence of deficits.

To resolve the quantification of these many components, a multidimensional schema is proposed similar to that of the *Diagnostic and Statistical Manual of Mental Disorders* (third edition, revised) (*DSM-III-R*) (American Psychiatric Association, 1987), which provides the nosology for psychiatric patients. Similar to the *DSM-III-R,* such a diagnostic manual would require multidisciplinary teamwork to identify and classify the major symptoms of acquired brain injury. This schema would include evaluations of the individual's present status analogous to the Rancho Los Amigos Scale (Hagen & Malkmus, 1979) and the severity of the brain damage analogous to the Glasgow Coma Scale (Teasdale & Jennett, 1974). However, in addition, it would take chronicity into consideration; or, more specifically, it would evaluate therapy gains that have been made in the various areas between the onset and the present evaluation. Moreover, it would seem helpful to note the highest level of functioning achieved with respect to level of needed supervision. Finally, it seems essential that the premorbid status be woven into this classification schema. The proposed framework for such a multiaxial system is presented in Table 3.1.

The proposed multiaxial diagnosis could enhance the precision with which we classify individuals and, in turn, facilitate communication among the disciplines. Subsequently, a diligent and creative approach to matching individuals to their most appropriate interventions could provide road maps for successful outcomes and po-

Table 3.1. Multiaxial classification of acquired brain injury

I. Present status
1. Physical-medical
2. Emotional-psychological
3. Mental-neuropsychological
4. Psychosocial
5. Vocational-financial

II. Severity (e.g., for the traumatic brain injury)
1. Duration of coma
2. Duration of post-traumatic amnesia
3. Glasgow Coma Scale score
4. Location of lesion
5. Other physical injuries

III. Chronicity: period between accident and present evaluation
1. Intervention for physical ailments
2. Intervention for emotional instability
3. Intervention for mental or cognitive remediation
4. Intervention for pyschosocial adjustment
5. Intervention for vocational and financial aspects

IV. Highest level of functioning achieved
1. Level of independence
2. Need for supervision

V. Premorbid status
1. Physical-medical
2. Emotional-psychological
3. Mental-neuropsychological
4. Psychosocial
5. Vocational-financial

tentially decrease rehabilitation costs. However, the correlations between diagnostic subtypes and intervention approaches must not become a preoccupation, since the essence in therapy is to change the behavior of a unique individual. The field of rehabilitation could lose its broader focus if we rigidly attempt to match up different global classification schemata with global intervention directions. Rehabilitation practice would be better served by combining these multiaxial data bases with a focus on changing specific sets of behaviors in individual clients.

With regard to research with persons with traumatic brain injury, the issue of heterogeneity can lead to some pitfalls in sample selection. The decision about who should be included for study can be decisive for intervention success or failure, and may contribute to conflicting findings

reported in the literature. For example, in some studies, cognitive remediation techniques have been employed without controlling for chronicity (i.e., time between onset of the brain injury and therapy). Obviously, it is misleading to claim a certain level of success—for example, that of returning clients with traumatic brain injury back to gainful employment—if the cases accepted for intervention are selected without taking into account the multiple dimensions outlined above. Significant confounding factors typically include etiology (e.g., traumatic brain injury versus stroke) and the nature of neuropathology, which, if not controlled for or specifically manipulated, can influence the potential for outcome independent of the behavioral techniques introduced. To date, our understanding of factors crucial for intervention planning is limited, and, therefore, predictor variables for outcome are very restricted. Employing the multiaxial system outlined in Table 3.1 could help reduce, if not eliminate, such dilemmas in sample selection for future research.

SPONTANEOUS RECOVERY VERSUS RELEARNING

Problem

Although a tremendous benefit for almost every client, spontaneous recovery presents a major challenge for researchers. Spontaneous recovery or healing can be influenced by demographic features such as age and gender, as well as by the nature, site, and severity of the lesion. With respect to traumatic brain injury, healing can take place not only within the anatomical structures (e.g., reduction of edema, brain distortions shifts, hernias), but also on neurophysiological levels (e.g., reduction of intracranial pressure, normalization of hyper- or hypotension) and on various neurochemical levels (e.g., balance can be established among neurotransmitters) (Miller, Pentland, & Berrol, 1990; Whyte, 1990). Prototypically, the greatest spontaneous recovery takes place during the first 6–12 months (Goldstein, 1984; Rubens, 1977).

The improvements achieved during spontaneous recovery typically occur without any special effort on the part of the client or any training by the rehabilitation team. Although it is presumed that intervention undertaken during this period may enhance overall gains, there is a problem with attempting to separate the contributions of the spontaneous versus relearning components. The obvious strategy to study their relative influence is, of course, to withhold therapy during this phase of recovery and to compare improvements here with those from specific interventions later on. However, even under the auspices of research, this strategy raises troubling ethical issues, despite the fact that many of these interventions have not yet been well documented. The challenge for behavioral rehabilitation, therefore, is to differentiate the gains to be attributed to spontaneous recovery versus the gains to be attributed to the interventions based on relearning. Table 3.2 highlights some of the differentiations between healing and relearning.

Searching for Solutions

One attempt to meet this challenge in the past has been to study only those individuals who have been 1 or more years postinjury (e.g., Ben-Yishay, Piasetsky, & Rattok, 1987). Although with this strategy spontaneous recovery is controlled for in describing intervention effects at later recovery stages, significant early changes are missed. This type of research design safeguard, therefore, does not resolve the clinical dilemma of needing to treat individuals at the earliest time periods and throughout the recovery process.

Another solution has been group comparison studies, which have enjoyed the greatest recognition in peer review journals. In this approach, the effects of both spontaneous recovery and repeated testing can be controlled for through randomization of subjects. However, soliciting clients who consent to being randomly assigned into either an experimental or control therapy condition can be most challenging. Once again, individuals in need of help are being asked to forego that help. One option for resolving this issue is to provide the control group with some potential benefits (e.g., receiving the experimental intervention at a later date). Even if recruitment can be achieved, however, the matching of the experimental and control group for not only demographic but neurological features is virtually impossible; thus, randomized group assignment is the procedure of choice.

To minimize the effects of spontaneous recovery or different durations of chronicity, two techniques have been introduced. In one of the first studies conducted to evaluate the efficacy of cognitive remediation, Ruff, Baser, et al. (1989) conducted a randomized group comparison, utilizing an additional waiting period. Table 3.3 demonstrates an example of introducing a comparable time period prior to the experimental intervention in order to evaluate the effects of spontaneous recovery within a group design.

A second acceptable technique is to utilize single-case designs. Multiple behavioral or cognitive domains can be divided into intervention-specific versus nonspecific domains (i.e., areas that clearly fall outside of expected intervention effects). Thus, spontaneous recovery can be analyzed by comparing the slope of gains made in either domain (i.e., contrasting measurements of intervention-nonspecific versus intervention-specific domains). Numerous examples

Table 3.2.   Spontaneous recovery versus relearning

Factor	Spontaneous recovery (healing)	Relearning
Mechanism	Automatic without conscious effort	Work intensive result of conscious effort
Role of motivation	Minimal or none	Essential for gains to be possible
Time course	Disproportionate, greatest gains in first 6–12 months postonset	Proportionate, gains are related to effort relatively independent of time course
Time limitations	First 24 months are primary	None, possible on lifetime basis

Table 3.3. Experimental design

Group	Baseline testing 1	8 weeks	Baseline testing 2	8 weeks	Post-treatment testing
Group C_1	Test forms A	Waiting period	Test forms B	Day treatment	Test forms A
Group E_1	Test forms B	Waiting period	Test forms A	Neuropsychological intervention	Test forms B
Group E_2	Test forms A	Waiting period	Test forms B	Neuropsychological intervention	Test forms A
Group C_2	Test forms B	Waiting period	Test forms A	Day treatment	Test forms B

Each group included 10 subjects: C = control, E = experimental.

Two different versions of the memory and learning measures, forms A and B, were used to test each group, as shown. In addition, the groups were counterbalanced for the order of form administration.

of single-case designs have been studied in the literature (e.g., Moore-Sohlberg & Mateer, 1987). Barlow and Hersen (1984) presented an excellent review of different single-case designs.

Niemann, Ruff, and Baser (1990) juxtaposed the single-case design with a group design. Group comparisons typically do not allow for individualized tracking across different intervention phases. A combination of designs can thus be recommended, because it provides the benefit of identifying for each individual case the specific intervention benefits. However, multiple cases can be analyzed as subgroups. Niemann et al. contrasted a computer-assisted attention training with a memory training in two separate groups. The effects of either training on both attentional and memory measures were delineated for each subject according to a single-case design. At the same time, pre- and post-therapy comparisons were made for both groups. The experimental design is shown in Table 3.4.

Although group comparisons are extremely expensive, granting agencies need to be convinced to finance comprehensive rehabilitation programs for experimental purposes. Behavioral rehabilitation is weakened if it is based exclusively on single-case studies. Thus, creative alternatives need to be found to establish meaningful group comparisons, and it is essential that random group assignment be employed when possible. Without comparing groups, spontaneous recovery cannot be rigorously separated from the effects of relearning. Thus, without demonstrating that the interventions have, on the basis of scientifically rigorous methodologies,

been proven efficacious, behavioral rehabilitation will not achieve full acceptance.

CONTROL GROUP

Problem

Most clinicians have accumulated over the years a substantial archival data base. However, the quantifications of these data are drastically limited, since as a rule neither time nor financial incentives exist to compare intervention "success" to a control condition. Without adequate controls, any reported intervention gain is limited. For example, if the rehabilitation team reports that it has returned 90% of its clients with traumatic brain injury back to competitive employment versus another program that returns 30%, no valid comparison can be made. If, for example, the former group (i.e., 90% success rate) were compared to a randomized control group from which 85% of subjects also return to work, then the success rate of the experimental group would be unimpressive. Similarly, if the latter group (i.e., 30% success rate) were drawn from a subject pool of individuals who otherwise would not have been able to return to competitive employment and contrasted with a control group who failed to return to work, the 30% success rate would be very impressive. In summary, in the absence of appropriate controls, success rates are anecdotal and without scientific validity.

Searching for Solutions

Given the need for an adequate control group, the next question that arises is: What are accept-

Table 3.4. Experimental design

Dependent variables	Weeks														
	(1)	(2)	(3)	(4)	(5)	(6)	(7)	(8)	(9)	(10)	(11)	(12)	(13)	(14)	(15)
Experimental group							--- Attention training ---								
Set One	X	X				X	X	X	X	X	X	X		X	X
Set Two			X										X		
Control group							--- Memory training ---								
Set One	X	X				X	X	X	X	X	X	X		X	X
Set Two			X										X		

Set One refers to the multiple baseline measures and Set Two refers to selected tests of the San Diego Neuropsychological Battery (Baser & Ruff, 1987). For Set One, the testings were administered at 7- to 9-day intervals: three times prior to, six times throughout, and two times after completion of the training.

able ways to establish a nonintervention control group? As already discussed, it is imperative that both experimental and control subjects continue to receive traditionally practiced or standard acceptable care. Experimental designs, therefore, should contain both standard care and new experimental interventions. Furthermore, since group assignment must be random, it is not ideal to solicit those subjects as controls who have not previously entered therapy due to lack of motivation, family support, or financial resources.

One acceptable way of establishing a control group is to provide a placebo or alternate therapy. For example, in their study designed to evaluate the benefits of cognitive remediation, Ruff, Baser, et al. (1989) had the control group participate in an alternate intervention. However, even in the absence of an alternate intervention, control subjects may experience gains as a result of the attention they receive from professionals conducting the research. If, for example, the controls lead relatively inactive lives or if they are generally neglected and receive little stimulation in the home environment, any attention may serve as a placebo therapy.

Setting up alternative therapy paradigms is expensive and would necessitate outside funding. Often the granting agencies need to be convinced that the expense is justified, which is difficult to do prior to completing the research. If funding is not available, an alternate approach would be to use the subject as his or her own control and compare performance on two or more experimental interventions (e.g., comparing different types of attention training or attention versus memory training).

QUANTIFICATION AND STANDARDIZATION OF THERAPY

Problem

A fundamental principle in science is that the experiment (i.e., the specific intervention) can be duplicated with similar results. If a client with traumatic brain injury is enrolled in a 3–6-month program, it is essential, yet still very challenging, to document the intervention regimen in such a standardized fashion as to be able to repli-

cate earlier findings. Otherwise, the outsider can neither have a full appreciation for the intervention strategies employed, nor differentiate to what extent success was dependent upon extraneous variables versus the therapy in question. Without this objective delineation of intervention approaches, the substantial gains reported by behavioral rehabilitation programs must be called into question.

Another major challenge to investigators is to quantify the differential effects of the experimental intervention from other concurrent intervention. For example, in studies where specific memory training is introduced, investigators often ignore what role other interventions such as speech therapy, physical therapy, or individual or group psychotherapy play.

Finally, there is one aspect of the therapeutic process that has defied quantification, yet clinically appears to be a critical factor in successful outcome: the clinician variables. It has been demonstrated in the psychotherapeutic literature that the experience of the clinician is a significant predictor of success (Auerbach & Johnson, 1977; Bergin & Lambert, 1978). This appears to be the result of having developed certain skills, such as empathy. Although this would no doubt hold true for rehabilitation specialists as well, little has been documented about the process of interacting with the brain-injured individual and his or her family. For specific therapy regimens to be effective, the therapist, for example, must possess not only a knowledge of behavioral learning principles and neuropathology but an awareness of cuing hierarchies, motivational issues, physical limitations, and premorbid personality functioning of the particular client. Interpersonal skills such as empathy, self-awareness, and conflict resolution are also essential for achieving therapeutic goals. It is, therefore, not only *what* we do with the client and his or her family, but *how* we do it. This is often highly individualized, and obviously difficult to count.

Searching for Solutions

Standardization is relatively simple if the intervention approach is narrow or reduced to a *micro* level. Examples of such a micro approach include the improvement of procedural memory, range of motion, or cooking a meal. A systematic structuring of therapeutic sessions can manipulate or control for aspects of training such as time spent on each task per session, level of task difficulty, and criteria for advancement to the next level of difficulty, as well as the nature and schedule of reinforcements and contingencies. Essentially, with this approach, behaviors can be shaped according to rigorous and objective learning principles, and clearly documented. The challenge here then is to create techniques that are tailored to an individual, yet at the same time allow for quantification across subjects.

Although it is valuable to have micro studies conducted, every effort needs to be made to integrate these into the overall therapy direction or systems approach, referred to in the following as the *macro* approach. In training attention, for example, it is critical not only to evaluate the behavior under training in daily life circumstances, but also to monitor the generalization of that training to those environments when training is completed.

Jepson Wulff, together with his colleagues at Learning Services Corporation, has designed a system for a macro intervention approach for traumatically brain-injured individuals, with the following specifications: 1) intervention outcome must be individually determined for each client, 2) the disciplines involved in providing the intervention must be integrated, and 3) ongoing reassessments are required to evaluate how the individual responds to the various intervention efforts.

According to this system, each client is evaluated according to a conceptually integrated framework derived from an interdisciplinary assessment. Out of this orchestrated initial data collection, specific problems are formulated according to A:B statements. That is, "A" refers to undesired state and "B" refers to desired state. These A:B statements are formulated on a behavioral level and must allow quantification, so that if the desired outcome is reached it can be objectively measured. Based on a series of A:B statements generated for each individual, a case manager is then assigned the task of placing these into a hierarchy. Subsequently, the A:B

statements are contracted out to the rehabilitation team, which is then accountable for achieving the desired outcome. The case manager coordinates the team's efforts and facilitates an effective partnership on behalf of the individual client, the financial resources, and the family members. Although such models have been implemented for years, no empirical validation is available at this time. However, such a model does begin to meet the challenge of treating individuals in a quantifiable manner, while also providing an avenue for collecting and evaluating data from groups of clients with traumatic brain injury.

More attention needs to be paid to evaluation of the therapists. While there are not as yet any standardized evaluations of clinician style or performance during therapy, informal evaluations are routinely conducted in rehabilitation settings, if only as a management tool to document performance for salary increases. Behavioral observations might easily be made either by outside observers, such as a manager or peer, or by the clinician's indicating what "extra" interventions were necessary during a particular session in order to complete the therapy task at the desired criterion levels. For example, did the clients have to be comforted and encouraged when they experienced failure? Did they have to be counseled regarding perfectionist traits? Did the clinician have to defuse the client's belligerence or deal with resistance to therapy? And, if so, how was this handled? For that matter, how does the clinician handle the sometimes conflicting interactions with the client's family?

The literature (e.g., Adler, 1972) has suggested that the therapist's own sense of helplessness or confidence can have a significant influence on the client's capacity to withstand the stress of therapy. However, more objective instruments regarding these "clinician variables" need to be devised so as to expand our understanding of the therapeutic process and to supplement our client data with such behavioral descriptions of clinical interactions. At minimum, the specification of the treating clinician's age, gender, and level of experience would also provide significant information toward identifying the relevant clinician variables.

The second problem raised with respect to quantification is how the effects of one intervention can be separated out from the effects of concurrent interventions. One way in which this separation can be achieved is by setting up therapy schedules where the sample of subjects is randomly assigned into one of two groups. The first group receives the experimental intervention in conjunction with all concurrent interventions, while the second group receives only the concurrent interventions. After a designated period of time, the schedules are switched and the first group now receives only the concurrent therapies, while the second receives all available therapies. A comparison of their relative gains during each condition will extract the desired variable.

ASSESSMENT TECHNIQUES AND LEVEL OF GENERALIZATION

Problem

The generalization of newly learned behaviors to settings other than the therapy session has long been recognized as the principal goal of any intervention; in fact, it defines successful outcome. For a specific behavioral change to have a lasting impact on an individual's life, it must be available across various situations, with various people, and over time. Furthermore, it is hoped that the change would spread to other related behaviors in the individual (Stokes & Baer, 1977). However, generalization is still often regarded as a phenomenon that happens without any special intervention, as a natural consequence of traditional therapy paradigms. Some authors have suggested that this is indeed not the case and that generalization requires a specific programming and technology of its own (e.g., Stokes & Baer, 1977). Furthermore, given the limitations in attention, memory, abstraction, and flexibility of thinking in persons with brain injury, it is highly unlikely that new learning will transfer "naturally."

Even when specific therapy tasks are structured to enhance generalization, they are not often adequately assessed or monitored. As mentioned earlier, in much of the literature the focus has been on the micro approach, and a somewhat naive assumption has been made to define outcome in statistical terms. That is, successful outcome was thought to be achieved when there was a statistically significant therapy effect, which was operationalized as an improvement of two standard deviations. Behavioral rehabilitation, however, may benefit from a more individualized approach, particularly if it is to take into account generalization effects. Thus, for some clients, therapy success may be an improvement of 30%; for others, a 15% gain may indicate success. Clinically sensitive goals that include aspects of generalization to the living environments need to replace the traditional—but blind—statistical definitions.

Searching for Solutions

When implementing either pre- or post-therapy comparisons or single-case designs, the psychometric measures should have gender, age, and educational norms available. Furthermore, test-retest reliability coefficients are needed to identify the degree of practice effects in the normal as well as the client population. Appropriate parallel test forms are critical to achieving this. In addition, efforts should be directed toward the development of self- and expert-ratings if feasible, based on the client's videotaped behavior. Other possibilities for more relevant descriptions of behavior include taking frequency counts of target behaviors and evaluating direct, real-life performances of, for example, driving or work-related tasks.

The challenge remains to measure the generalization of the therapy successes, three major levels of which are discussed in the following paragraphs.

Gains Measured According to Training Materials In this approach, subjects are typically exposed to baseline assessments; then, subsequent to the intervention, the gains that have been made on the therapy materials are evaluated. Problems with this technique arise, of course, when the same materials are used for both therapy and outcome measures, since generalization cannot be addressed.

Psychometrically Captured Therapy Gains In this approach, a specific behavioral intervention is evaluated according to psycho-metric tools that are close, but not identical, to the therapy materials. For example, a specific memory training program may be introduced, but separate standardized memory measures are used to quantify success. At this level of general-ization, the behavioral remediation can be quan-tified in a more objective fashion.

As a client's progress is followed over time and tests are repeated, it also becomes necessary to differentiate the learning from repeated test-ing versus that from therapy. Alternate versions of specific tests can eliminate that problem. However, at the present time, few measures with alternate versions are readily available that in-clude standardized error of measurement and ad-equate norms for age, gender, and educational stratifications. Moreover, there exists a sparsity of measures that quantify for the emotional, psy-chosocial, and quality of life domains for indi-viduals with neurological impairment. Although the techniques to develop these types of mea-surements are available, few sophisticated psy-chometric measures exist that can be applied for this research. Even if such techniques are de-veloped, it would be necessary to integrate the various psychometric measures into a frame-work that allows for valid predictions of every-day-life behavior.

Measurements of Everyday-Life Func-tioning The essential characteristic of any be-havioral intervention is that an individual can change in a meaningful fashion in his or her ev-eryday life. However, while it is acknowledged that this ecological validity needs to be built into the research design, there is no universal method by which to accomplish it. Individual needs in separate settings must be addressed indepen-dently, with an appreciation for behaviorally de-fined goals and outcomes.

CONCEPTUALIZATION OF OUTCOME

Problem

No intervention should be introduced without a clear conceptualization of the expected outcome. If a successful outcome is not defined, there is no way to chart the individual's progress, and

the ultimate goal of generalization of learning to daily life may be jeopardized. Some clinicians and therapies deal exclusively with everyday-life skills such as providing training for driving, washing clothes, preparing meals, and so on. Although this approach uses a clear statement of goals and outcomes, it is too narrowly conceived and again threatens the overall goal of general-ization to other learning situations. More specifi-cally, this approach fails to provide the client with an underlying principle that can be effec-tively applied in different environments (e.g., driving different vehicles, washing clothes in a variety of ways, preparing a variety of meals in different kitchens). Rehabilitation also fails, therefore, if it only trains someone in overt skills: Underlying cognitive principles must be taught, too.

Searching for Solutions

It is somewhat surprising that definitions of out-come receive such sparse attention in the litera-ture. One way of defining a successful outcome for behavioral rehabilitation that emphasizes generalization encompasses the following three dimensions: 1) meeting the basic needs, 2) se-lecting the appropriate living arrangement, and 3) self-management.

While basic needs (see Table 3.5) are more or less the same for all individuals, the needs have to be met at a satisfactory level, and the level of satisfaction is directly related to an indi-vidual's socioeconomic background. In defining outcome, the client's ability to meet these spe-cific needs must be carefully delineated on an in-dividual basis.

Any good outcome is related to selecting the appropriate living arrangment (i.e., the se-lection of a rural versus an urban environment, based upon the individual's social and vocational goals). Access to certain services such as shops, medical care, recreation, and public transporta-tion must also be taken into consideration in the selection process. Optimally, any chosen living arrangements should not create a problem that could be resolved by selecting a different living arrangement.

Self-management is pivotal in creating a successful outcome. This viewpoint is anchored

Table 3.5. Basic needs to be evaluated as part of outcome

Needs	Examples
Medical care	Monitoring of medications and physical status; availability of primary physician for flu, sprained ankle, and so on
Dental care	Regular checkups for prevention
Safety	Level of supervision needed; monitoring of judgment, avoiding substance abuse, safe sex, and so on
Feeding	Balance nutrition, weight control, economical food shopping
Physical fitness	Regular exercise
Goods and services	Purchasing clothes, appliances, and furniture; organizing banking, insurances, utilities, and so on
Education	Attending school, keeping up to date by reading newspapers
Employment	According to ability, ranging from competitive full- or part-time employment to volunteer jobs or sheltered workshops
Income	Breakdown of all sources of income from employment, insurances, state disability, savings, family support, and so on
Social interactions	Select appropriate interactions with friends, family, or clubs
Recreation/leisure	Plan activities around hobbies, socialization, physical exercise, and so on
Spiritual	Selected attendance of religious meetings and activities, reading, praying, meditation, and so on
Identity/self-worth	Balance needs to maintain healthy self-image and dignity, attempt to prevent mood swings, irritability, depression, and so on

in the philosophy that considers individual freedom a fundamental human right. Thus, in a democratic system, even an individual with brain injury must be allowed to select and determine how basic needs are to be met. For *each* of the needs listed in Table 3.5, it is essential to determine how much self-management is possible. For example, if an individual with brain injury is not considered capable of selecting an appropriate apartment independently, then at least he or she can make choices or have input on how his or her room should be furnished. Successful outcome, therefore, depends on providing an optimal level of self-determination integrated with conscientious risk management. The guiding principle must be to empower the individual to manage his or her own affairs to the greatest extent possible.

SUMMARY AND CONCLUSIONS

As a research clinician with a strong interest in rehabilitation, the senior author of this chapter began his career by developing specific computerized therapy modules in the areas of attention, memory, and problem solving. The authors are still convinced that there is some value to these types of programs.

However, after working in the field of rehabilitation and appreciating the complexities, the realization has grown that our research must integrate the micro with the macro approach. Thus, the individual's motivation, vocational interests, cultural backgrounds, and family support all play a crucial role in a clinician's ability to provide attention or memory training effectively. For these reasons, we have spent the last few years trying to investigate a *systems* approach for behavioral rehabilitation that is sensitive to the complexity of an individual's preinjury status and the level and type of neurological disorder, as well as setting realistic outcome goals.

Research needs to be conducted across all of these levels. However, in doing such research we must not focus on two-dimensional data collections, but rather we must weave our research interests into the complexities of three-dimensional life.

REFERENCES

Adler, G. (1972). Helplessness in the helpers. *British Journal of Medical Psychology, 45*, 315–326.

American Psychiatric Association. (1987). *Diagnostic and statistical manual of mental disorders* (3rd ed., rev.). Washington, DC: Author.

Auerbach, A., & Johnson, M. (1977). Research on the therapist's level of experience. In A. Gurman & A. Razin (Eds), *Effective psychotherapy* (pp. 84–102). New York: Pergamon Press.

Barlow, D.H., & Hersen, M. (1984). *Single case experimental designs: Strategies for studying behavior change* (2nd ed.). New York: Pergamon Press.

Baser, C.N., & Ruff, R.M. (1987). Construct validity of the San Diego Neuropsychological Test Battery. *Archives of Clinical Neuropsychology, 2*, 13–32.

Ben-Yishay, Y., Piasetsky, E.B., & Rattok, J. (1987). A systematic method for ameliorating disorders in basic attention. In M. Meier, A. Benton, & L. Diller (Eds.), *Neuropsychological rehabilitation* (pp. 163–181). New York: Guilford Press.

Bergin, A.E., & Lambert, M.J. (1978). The evaluation of therapeutic outcomes. In S.L. Garfield & A.E. Bergin (Eds.), *Handbook of psychotherapy and behavior change* (pp. 139–189). New York: John Wiley & Sons.

Bigler, E.D. (1990). Mechanisms of damage, assessment, intervention, and outcome. In E.D. Bigler (Ed.), *Traumatic brain injury* (pp. 13–49). Austin, TX: PRO-ED.

Goldstein, G. (Ed.). (1984). *Advances in clinical neuropsychology* (Vol. 1). New York: Plenum.

Hagen, C. (1982). Language-cognitive disorganization following closed head injury: A conceptualization. In L.E. Trexler (Ed.), *Cognitive rehabilitation* (pp. 131–151). New York: Plenum.

Hagen, C., & Malkmus, D. (1979, November). *Intervention strategies for language disorders secondary to head trauma.* Paper presented at the American Speech-Language-Hearing Association Convention, Atlanta.

Levin, H.S., Benton, A., & Grossman, R.G. (1982). *Neurobehavioral consequences of head injury.* New York: Oxford University Press.

Meier, M.J., Benton, A.L., & Diller, L. (1987). *Neuropsychological rehabilitation.* New York: Guilford Press.

Miller, J.D., Pentland, B., & Berrol, S. (1990). Early evaluation and management. In M. Rosenthal, M.R. Bond, E.R. Griffith, & J.D. Miller (Eds.), *Rehabilitation of the adult and child with traumatic brain injury* (2nd ed., pp. 21–49). Philadelphia: F.A. Davis.

Moore-Sohlberg, M., & Mateer, C.A. (1987). Effectiveness of an attention-training program. *Journal of Clinical and Experimental Neuropsychology, 9*, 117–130.

Morris, J.A., Jr., MacKenzie, E.J., & Edelstein, S.L. (1990). The effect of pre-existing conditions on mortality in trauma patients. *Journal of the American Medical Association, 263*, 1942–1946.

Niemann, H., Ruff, R.M., & Baser, C.A. (1990). Computer-assisted attention retraining in head injured individuals: A controlled efficacy study of an outpatient program. *Journal of Consulting and Clinical Psychology, 58*(6), 811–817.

Rubens, A. (1977). The role of changes within the central nervous system during recovery from aphasia. In M. Sullivan & M. Kommens (Eds.), *Rationale for adult aphasia therapy* (pp. 28–43). Omaha: University of Nebraska Press.

Ruff, R.M., Baser, C.A., Johnston, J.W., Marshall, L.F., Klauber, S.K., Klauber, M.R., & Minteer, M. (1989). Neuropsychological rehabilitation: An experimental study with head-injured patients. *Journal of Head Trauma Rehabilitation, 4*(3), 20–36.

Ruff, R.M., Cullum, C.M., & Luerssen, T.G. (1989). Brain imaging and neuropsychological outcome in traumatic head injury. In E.D. Bigler, R.A. Yeo, & E. Turkheimer (Eds.), *Neuropsychological function and brain imaging* (pp. 161–183). New York: Plenum.

Stokes, T.F., & Baer, D.M. (1977). An implicit technology of generalization. *Journal of Applied Behavior Analysis, 10*, 349–367.

Teasdale, G., & Jennett, B. (1974). Assessment of coma and impaired consciousness: A practical scale. *Lancet, 2*, 81–84.

Whyte, J. (1990). Mechanisms of recovery of function following CNS damage. In M. Rosenthal, M.R. Bond, E.R. Griffith, & J.D. Miller (Eds.), *Rehabilitation of the adult and child with traumatic brain injury* (pp. 79–87). Philadelphia: F.A. Davis.

CHAPTER 4

Professional Development and Educational Program Planning in Cognitive Rehabilitation

PAUL E. MAZMANIAN, KATHLEEN O'KANE MARTIN, AND JEFFREY S. KREUTZER

Planning and evaluating continuing education for health professionals involves a complex analysis of needs and a set of very practical decisions that must be made in order to implement successful programs of learning. This chapter fits selected observations into current theories regarding professional development, change, and learning. It explores the organizational context of continuing education for providers of cognitive rehabilitation therapy and offers a model for continuing education and training programs. It does not provide a detailed analysis of the organizational factors influencing the development of cognitive rehabilitation therapy, nor does it offer an exhaustive study of the cognitive and emotional factors that generate change and learning. Rather, the intent is to provide an overview, sorting out and defining some of the forces influencing the development of cognitive rehabilitation therapy and helping to identify implications for educational program planning. The theoretical frameworks applied in interpreting the authors' observations are highlighted for those who choose to study further the professional development and continuing education of those who provide cognitive rehabilitation services.

PROFESSIONAL DEVELOPMENT

Is the Practice of Cognitive Rehabilitation Therapy Prevalent?

Many believe that cognitive rehabilitation is a primary method of intervention in the rehabilitation of persons with head injury (Rosenthal & Berrol, 1989). To determine how widespread the practice of cognitive rehabilitation therapy might be, directors of 398 health care facilities providing rehabilitative services to adults or children with brain injury were surveyed by mail in 1989 (Mazmanian, Martin, & Kreutzer, 1991). One hundred four of the facilities were approved by the Commission on Accreditation of Rehabilitation Facilities (CARF). Two hundred ninety-four were not approved facilities (non-CARF). Seventy-one percent of the CARF facilities responded, as did 61% of the non-CARF group. A total of 252 facilities responded to the survey, a response rate of 63%.

The survey (Mazmanian et al., 1991) determined that 237 of the reporting facilities (94%) provide cognitive rehabilitation therapy. Nearly all (92%) of the facilities provide cognitive rehabilitation therapy services within their facilities, with well over half (60%) providing one-to-one therapy. These percentages equate roughly with the number of providers and format of therapy reported by Bracy in 1984. Clearly, the practice of cognitive rehabilitation therapy is commonplace among rehabilitation facilities offering care to persons with brain injury. Who provides these services? What qualifications do they bring to client care? Are providers of cognitive rehabilitation therapy professional?

Are Providers of Cognitive Rehabilitation Therapy Professional?

To find a meaningful answer to this question, it is important to set current observations against the-

oretical precepts that enable explanation and prediction. There is a basic educational pattern of
professional workers (Figure 4.1). Early in life,
and occasionally even at birth, a choice of occupation is made by an individual or by those
who control his or her destiny. The selection may
carry forward an ancestral tradition in a profession such as medicine, teaching, or ministry. It
may result from the conviction that the individual has been called for special service to God,
to the state, or to humanity. The selection may
be seen as a means of social or economic advancement. It may result from an awareness
of personal strengths, weaknesses, and special
characteristics, or it may result from a multitude
of other causes, either purposefully pursued or
resulting from chance (Houle, 1980).

> At some time after the choice is made, formal edu-
> cation for the occupation begins. Specialized study
> is usually prefaced by years of basic training and
> often by general or liberal education, which es-
> tablishes broad foundations of knowledge. Then
> comes a narrowing of focus. Occupational study
> may begin on a part-time basis, as when a college
> student is enrolled in a premedical or prelegal cur-
> riculum. At some point, the original choice of an
> occupation by an individual is ratified by his or her
> acceptance into a course of study that calls for deep
> immersion in a specialized content and the acquisi-
> tion of difficult skills and a complex value system.
> This formal process is reinforced by a differentiated
> life-style (perhaps in a hospital, a library, or a wel-
> fare agency), which separates the individual (psy-
> chologically if not always physically) from the gen-
> eral public and permeates his or her thought with a
> distinctive point of view. (Houle, 1980, pp. 2–3)

Having completed formal preparatory study
and reorientation of values, the acculturation of
professionals continues. Initial judgments regarding the competence of the individual are made,
first by those who guided the initial course of

study; then, in most cases, by some larger sanc-
tioning authority—the organized profession, the
state, or both. Subsequent learning activities
generally are regarded as continuing education.

Bracy (1984) and Parenté and Bennett (1989)
suggested that therapists come from a variety of
academic backgrounds. In describing the educational background of the person who bears the
major responsibility for cognitive rehabilitation
therapy, the results of Mazmanian et al. (1990)
tended to support those reported by Bracy. Mazmanian et al. found psychologists (20%) and
speech-language pathologists (18%) were named
with about equal frequency, with no significant
differences between CARF and non-CARF facilities. Occupational therapists were the next most
frequently named group (5%), followed by a
combined category of educators and special educators (2%). The largest categorical response
indicated that cognitive rehabilitation therapy is
a team effort, conducted by multiple providers
(35%). Twenty percent of the facilities did not
respond to the question of who provides cognitive rehabilitation therapy, with no significant
differences between CARF and non-CARF facilities. With such diversity in educational background, consideration of educational background
alone is inadequate to determine whether the
variety of persons practicing cognitive rehabilitation therapy are professional.

What Is a Professional?

In general, the lives of some men and women are
structurally shaped by their being deeply versed
in advanced and subtle bodies of knowledge,
which they apply with dedication in solving
complex practical problems. Such professionals,
Houle (1980) suggested, learn by study, appren-
ticeship, and experience, both by expanding

Selection or Admission	Certification of Competence		
General Education (often including higher education with emphasis on the basic content re-quired for specialization)	Preservice Specialized Education (often marked by grad-uate studies or profes-sional school studies)	Induction (sometimes marked by fellowships or other programs increasing specialization)	Continuing Education ⟶

Figure 4.1.   Classic model of professional education. (Adapted from Houle, 1980.)

their comprehension of formal disciplines and by finding new ways to achieve specific ends, constantly moving forward and backward from theory to practice so that each enriches the other.

Although there is no commonly held answer to the question of what constitutes a profession, there are three schools of thought with differing approaches to help bring understanding to the development of cognitive rehabilitation therapy. Each offers an alternative perspective to help interpret the work of those who provide cognitive rehabilitation therapy services.

The *static approach,* pioneered by Abraham Flexner (1915), asserted "there are certain objective standards that can be formulated" that distinguish professions from other occupations. He identified six characteristics as essential for an occupation to claim professional status. Professions must: 1) involve intellectual operations, 2) derive their material from science, 3) involve definite and practical ends, 4) possess an educationally communicable technique, 5) tend to self-organization, and 6) be altruistic. Many occupations striving for higher status apply these criteria to decide whether their occupation is a profession. This is called the static approach because objective criteria firmly discriminate between those occupations that are inherently professions and those that are not. Once this distinction is made, it is unlikely that those occupations that are not considered professional could ever develop into professions (Cervero, 1988).

Compared to the static approach, the *process approach* offers gradience. The question of whether an occupation absolutely is, or is not, a profession gives way to several questions, each relating to a valued characteristic of the occupation. Conceptually, two fundamental questions are applied: To what extent does the occupation possess this valued characteristic? How is the occupation working toward its further refinement? When asked of cognitive rehabilitation therapy, two such questions might be: To what degree do providers of cognitive rehabilitation therapy control their practice? What are they doing to increase that control?

The process approach differs from the "yes or no" determination required with the static approach, because all occupations are viewed as existing on a continuum of professionalization. The highest values of the occupations are championed, and the overriding question becomes: How professionalized is the occupation? Within the process approach, there are no clear-cut boundaries separating professions from other occupations. Developing professions may, in fact, deprofessionalize within the process approach (Cervero, 1988).

The *socioeconomic approach* contrasts with both static and process approaches. It assumes no such thing as an ideal profession and no criteria necessarily associated with it. An occupation is commonly regarded by the general public as a profession or it is not. The title "profession" is ascribed in honor. It is a collective symbol, suggesting its members are highly valued by a society. Having achieved status and privileges, the recognition of an occupation as a profession is both socially constructed and socially granted.

The socioeconomic approach emphasizes that social construction is not a random process but a political war (Schudson, 1980). Varyingly high degrees of social and economic rewards are accorded the winners of the war. Such people protect one another, Houle (1980) suggested, and are sometimes granted special protection by society, far beyond that granted to other citizens. The price of protection is vigilance against poor performance and unethical behavior. That vigilance is to be exercised by the privileged person, by others of similar specialization, and by society.

What Is the Role of Higher Education in Training and Credentialing? How Is Competence Assured?

What role do colleges and universities perform in supporting cognitive rehabilitation therapy? Frangicetto (1989) reported the experience of a community college in developing its associate degree program in cognitive retraining. In a paper reporting results of a survey of persons interested in cognitive rehabilitation therapy, Parenté (1989) found two institutions of higher learning providing degree programs in cognitive rehabilitation therapy: One offers a 2-year associate degree through a community college; the other offers a 4-year bachelor of science degree.

Despite the small number of training programs in higher education dedicated to the study of cognitive rehabilitation, there appears to be a growing body of knowledge and skills associated with the roles and responsibilities of the service provider. Although it is often stated that evidence of the scientific reliability and validity of cognitive rehabilitation therapy is inconclusive (Rosenthal & Berrol, 1989), the number of scientific articles and texts indicating principles and techniques for successful assessment or therapy of persons with head injury continues to grow, as does the number of texts positing principles and strategies for implementing cognitive rehabilitation therapy (Kreutzer, 1989; Sohlberg & Mateer, 1989; Uzzell & Gross, 1986). The Williamsburg Conference (*Proceedings,* 1988, 1989, 1990) and the annual meeting of the National Head Injury Foundation (1989) are two of several well-established conferences for health care professionals that have begun to offer education or training in cognitive rehabilitation therapy. Highly regarded journals across disciplines have begun to link new methods for supporting cognitive rehabilitation with procedures traditionally accepted as the domain of their individual professions (Abreu & Toglia, 1987; Alexandre, Columbo, Nertempi, & Benedetti, 1983; Bottcher, 1989). Also, an interdisciplinary association has been chartered to promote and foster the development and advancement of medical and scientific research and education in the field of cognitive rehabilitation (Society for Cognitive Rehabilitation, 1990).

These activities suggest a movement toward the professionalization of cognitive rehabilitation therapy. However, the varied educational backgrounds, preestablished professional relationships, biases, and socioeconomic caste of health care providers may result in a splintered advance. Each established discipline then will be left to adjust its perspective only enough to enhance its individual health care armamentarium or to train and assign technologists whose services might be supervised by the winners of the political wars.

In reviewing their personal background, training, and experience as cognitive rehabilitation specialists, experimental psychologists

Parenté and Bennett (1989) suggested the importance of training those who are already providing cognitive rehabilitation therapy to head-injured clients. They further suggested supporting diversity within university-grounded disciplines as an appropriate approach to the development of cognitive rehabilitation therapy:

> It may not be feasible to specify a sequence of courses that any body of professionals would ever agree was sufficient for ensuring adequate training. Rather than developing a new clinical major, it would be better to develop core content areas that the various disciplines could define for their students. (Parenté & Bennett, 1989, p. 20)

Cervero (1988) indicated that universities may be key to the establishment of a profession. For a professional market to exist, a distinctive commodity must be produced.

> Unlike industrial labor, most professions produce intangible goods in that their product is inextricably bound to the person who produces it. Therefore, the producers themselves have to be "produced" if their products are to be given a distinctive form. In other words, professionals must be adequately trained and socialized to provide recognizably distinct services. This process has been institutionalized in the modern university which gives professions the means to control their knowledge base as well as to award credentials certifying that practitioners possess this recognizably distinct type of knowledge. Therefore, an occupation's level of professionalization can be assessed by the extent to which public and political authorities accept its credentials as necessary to provide a specific type of service. (Cervero, 1988, pp. 9–10)

Credentialing is a way to help assure the competence of professionals. Credentials may include degrees of educational completion, licenses to practice, or certificates of specialization. Licenses are issued by governmental bodies, regulating (through legislation) the flow of who may or may not practice certain kinds of work. Educational completion might include an associate's, bachelor's, master's, or doctoral degree. Certificates suggest specialization and might include completion of degree work in a selected discipline such as a master of science in nursing with certification in gerontology. Certification may also include documented proficiency at predetermined tasks. For example, a speech-language pathologist who has completed graduate education may choose to earn a certificate of clinical competency (CCC-Sp).

For purposes of credentialing, competence is measured in several ways, including: achievement of a passing score on an examination, completion of an approved program of study, demonstration of satisfactory performance, and testimony from a recognized authority that the individual should have the right to practice. For some professions in some states, two or three of the basic methods are applied. For others, there may be no system of licensure or certification and the professional degree itself becomes the establishing credential. Kreutzer and Boake (1987) asserted that: 1) clinicians are already free to practice cognitive rehabilitation therapy professionally on the basis of certificates or licenses in related rehabilitation disciplines, and 2) there are few opportunities for training clinicians or students in cognitive rehabilitation. Accordingly, they suggested, "the most realistic of the available credentialing options is probably a multidisciplinary approach in which credentials for competence in cognitive rehabilitation are awarded separately by each rehabilitation discipline" (Kreutzer & Boake, 1987, p. 201).

What Is the Standard of Care in Cognitive Rehabilitation Therapy?

It is widely understood that most third-party payers of health care do not offer financial reimbursement for cognitive rehabilitation therapy. Health care providers often bill for such services under psychotherapy, occupational therapy, speech therapy, or other recognized rehabilitative services (Bracy, 1984). That much of cognitive rehabilitation therapy is conducted by multiple providers (Bracy, 1984; Mazmanian et al., 1991) may suggest the lack of accepted standards of care to which payers may refer in judging what is required for optimum provision and supervision of cognitive rehabilitation therapy.

The Neuropsychology Division (Division 40) of the American Psychological Association (APA) and the Committee on Interprofessional Relationships With Neuropsychology of the American Speech-Language-Hearing Associa-

tion (ASHA) issued a position statement (ASHA, 1990) aimed at delineating the scope of work associated with brain injury. The organizations agreed on the following:

1. Neuropsychology is the scientific study of the relationship between brain function and behavior.
2. Neuropsychology is an interdisciplinary knowledge area.
3. It is inappropriate that the knowledge base of neuropsychology be regarded as proprietary by any given discipline or profession.
4. Various techniques and applications of neuropsychology may not be mutually exclusive between professions.
5. All relevant disciplines and professions should contribute to the expanding knowledge base of neuropsychology and to its appropriate applications in client care.

Several agencies have moved toward issuance of standards associated with cognitive rehabilitation. The 1990 *Standards Manual* of the Commission on Accreditation of Rehabilitation Facilities indicated that the cognitive capacity of brain-injured persons should be assessed, and all services "should be delivered by registered, certified, licensed, or degreed personnel or should be performed substantially in their presence" (p. 56). An interdisciplinary special interest group of the American Congress on Rehabilitation Medicine (ACRM) in 1989 (Harley, 1989) presented "Standards for Cognitive Rehabilitation," describing who should provide cognitive rehabilitation therapy. These standards suggest that cognitive rehabilitation therapy should be provided by qualified personnel who have completed specific course work or formalized training.

> Since there is no formal mechanism to monitor the compliance of an individual's credentials as a qualified practitioner, it is the ultimate responsibility of the individual person to determine if he/she is sufficiently qualified. This determination should be made with consideration for both the welfare of the client and professional ethical standards. (Harley, 1989, p. 328)

The APA and other organizations have explored standards and a code of ethics regarding the use of computers in cognitive rehabilitation therapy (Harley, 1989), one of the methods sometimes applied in the assessment of and interventions designed for brain-injured persons (see also Chapter 13, this volume).

Is Cognitive Rehabilitation Therapy a Profession?

Wilensky (1964) argued strongly that there is a typical process by which producers of special services constitute and control the market for their services. In this process, occupations attempt to negotiate the boundaries of a market for their services and to establish their control over it.

> In sum, there is a typical process by which the established professions have arrived: men begin doing the work full time and stake out a jurisdiction; the early masters of the technique or adherents of the movement become concerned about standards of training and practice and set up a training school, which, if not lodged in universities at the outset, makes academic connection within two or three decades; the teachers and activists then achieve success in promoting more effective organization, first local, then national—through either transformation of an existing occupational association or the creation of a new one. Toward the end, legal protection of the monopoly of skills appears; at the end, a formal code of ethics is adopted. (Wilensky, 1964, pp. 145–146)

Measured against Wilensky's (1964) model, there is considerable evidence that the practice of cognitive rehabilitation therapy currently is widespread (Bracy, 1984; Mazmanian et al., 1991) and that health care workers maintain a long history of providing cognitive rehabilitation therapy for persons with head injury (Boake, 1989; Goldstein, 1942). That providers are concerned about standards of practice and training is evident from the ACRM (Harley, 1989), ASHA (ASHA, 1990), and CARF (CARF, 1990) position statements. That colleges and universities slowly are responding to an apparent need for training is clear from Parenté's (1989) survey of persons interested in cognitive rehabilitation. That formerly organized national associations are moving to accommodate the interests of cognitive rehabilitation therapy providers is clear from the establishment of special interest groups in ACRM, APA, and ASHA. In addition, a new

organization, the Society for Cognitive Rehabilitation (SCR) has been chartered, aiming to foster and promote the development of cognitive rehabilitation.

Missing from the formula is a cogent statement of the unique body of knowledge and skills offered by those who practice cognitive rehabilitation therapy. Missing, too, is a recognized credentialing process, legal protection, and an overarching code of ethics to inform ideal behavior.

The knowledge and skills practiced within cognitive rehabilitation therapy include such activities as comprehensive neuropsychological assessment, memory retraining, psychotherapeutic intervention, job coaching, and language development. Are providers of cognitive rehabilitation therapy professional? Some may be, by virtue of previous achievement. Others may be professionalizing. What is apparent, for the near future, is that those providing cognitive rehabilitation services will continue to act from identities associated with previous training and experience. Psychologists tend to see themselves as psychologists, speech-language pathologists tend to see themselves as speech-language pathologists, and occupational therapists tend to see themselves as occupational therapists. There will be continued difficulty in generating a common base of knowledge, resources, and techniques singularly and readily identified with cognitive rehabilitation therapy, and the associated entitlements of separate professional recognition are unlikely to be granted soon. The diverse practice of cognitive rehabilitation therapy will continue with increasing attention to developing the technical skills of practitioners. Although institutions of higher education may be interested in cognitive rehabilitation, they typically do not act as agents of change. Their programs may be expected to research and reflect cognitive rehabilitation therapy, as it is practiced.

PROGRAM PLANNING FOR CONTINUING EDUCATION

For those charged with providing continuing education or training for those who practice cognitive rehabilitation therapy, the wide range of knowledge and skills and the context in which cognitive rehabilitation therapy is applied pose interesting challenges. Most persons responsible for providing continuing education to cognitive rehabilitation practitioners have little or no formal training in adult education or program planning. Clarification of some terms may offer a helpful beginning.

The question of whether an instructional activity is adult education, continuing education, or staff training is sometimes debated by those who study such activities. Arguments often hinge upon whether the program imparts technical information, whether it is implemented primarily to advance corporate goals, or whether it bears undergraduate and graduate credits of an institution of higher learning. Subtle differences that might exist in planning for adult education, continuing education, and staff training are not addressed by the general model presented in the current discussion. The terms adult education, continuing education, and staff training are used interchangeably, with the understanding that the decisions and activities of program planning vary reasonably within the theoretical constructs of the model.

Much of the lifelong learning of adults involves participation in formal programs, designed and offered by persons whose intentions in providing the program may vary as much as the values, beliefs, and attitudes of those who participate in the planning process. The goal of most continuing education for health care workers is to enhance the knowledge, skills, and attitudes comprised by proficiencies that constitute the capability of the individual to perform satisfactorily, given the opportunity. The gaps or discrepancies between current and desired proficiencies can lead to high motivation and active participation of learners, if the gaps are not perceived as small and trivial or so large as to be overwhelming (Knox, 1985). Participation in formal continuing education is a major source of learning for providers of cognitive rehabilitation therapy (Mazmanian et al., 1991), but, as might be expected, some of the training programs are carefully planned, while others are literally just thrown together (Caffarella, 1988).

Program planning is of central interest to many who practice or study continuing educa-

tion and training. It is often seen as a decision-making process enacted to produce the outcome and design specifications for a systematic instructional activity that is expected to change adult capability in some respect (Sork, 1990). Rooted in Ralph W. Tyler's (1949) work in curriculum development, the classical model of adult education program planning includes four major sets of activities: 1) assess learning needs, 2) determine learning objectives, 3) develop instructional design to enable attainment, and 4) evaluate learners' progress in relation to objectives.

Oversight agencies sometimes are developed to monitor and to help improve the program planning process implemented by provider organizations. Such agencies have been established for general adult education (Council on the Continuing Education Unit), and for selected occupations such as medicine (Accreditation Council on Continuing Medical Education) and pharmacy (Accreditation Council for Pharmaceutical Education). Both the American Speech-Language-Hearing Association and the American Psychological Association have developed a network of approved continuing education provider organizations. Such providers must have demonstrated a continuing education mission, financial viability, and compliance with the fundamental planning activities generally as espoused by Tyler (1949). In the absence of a single oversight agency to help assure the quality of continuing education programs offered to practitioners of cognitive rehabilitation therapy, continuing education providers and trainers can help to assure high-quality programs through careful program planning.

Many academicians and researchers have offered theoretical formulations of program planning in continuing education. Most are prescriptive (Caffarella, 1988; Houle, 1972; Knowles, 1980; Nadler, 1982; Walker, 1971), either logically based in Tyler's (1949) classical work on curriculum development or suggesting how program planning should be practiced. Others are descriptive (Mazmanian, 1980; Pennington & Green, 1976), generated from studies examining how program planning is actually practiced.

In his review of theoretical foundations of educational program planning, Sork (1990) presented a six-step model to discuss the elements of educational planning as they relate to continuing education in the health professions. His model departs from many in the literature by beginning with an analysis of the planning context and client system. The model is interactive in that decisions made at any step can influence decisions at any other step. The model is derived from prescriptive and descriptive models. It is linear in the sense that it is based on the logic of systematic planning in which certain elements logically precede or logically follow other elements.

The program planning model offered in the current chapter draws heavily upon Caffarella (1988) and Sork (1990), as well as previous research (Mazmanian, 1980; Pennington & Green, 1976) and the experience of the authors. A seventh step of carrying out the program is added to Sork's conceptualization. Also, decisions and activities that tend to cluster around each step of the process are described and enumerated.

Step One: Analyze Planning Context and Client System

The mix of forces at play in the organizational environment of cognitive rehabilitation therapy as well as the forces affecting change and learning in the practices of persons providing cognitive rehabilitation services should be analyzed by those who plan and those who attend continuing education activities. Analysis of the planning context involves developing a detailed understanding of the organizational environment in which planning occurs. The organization in which the planner works has a structure, leadership, policies and procedures, and other characteristics that may have important implications for later steps of planning. Understanding the political, economic, and social climate of the organization is important because the planning process is substantially influenced by this climate and the constraints imposed by the organization.

The planning context extends beyond the organization itself. It includes consideration of the personal, professional, and social forces that influence change and learning for cognitive rehabilitation therapy providers (Cervero, 1988; Fox, Mazmanian, & Putnam, 1989; Nowlen, 1988). Personal forces include the individuals' curiosity, desire for good health, and desire for

financial well-being. Professional forces include the individuals' desire to be a competent health care worker, as well as the diagnostic and therapeutic advances that become available in the clinical environment. Social forces include regulations that might affect behavior, as well as the individuals' relationships with colleagues, supervisors, family, and community. Analyzing the planning context includes continuously scanning the interests of others holding a stake in effective performance (e.g., patients/clients, their families, and insurers). The missions and related activities of scholastic and occupational associations, governmental agencies with regulatory responsibilities, special interest groups, and competing organizations also must be considered.

Decisions

Both the planner and learner should consider the following questions:

1. What are the most current and effective assessment and intervention techniques related to cognitive rehabilitation therapy? Who generated them? Who uses them?
2. What are the most current and effective educational programs associated with cognitive rehabilitation therapy? Who provides them?
3. What would be the major force driving a learner's participation in a selected continuing education or training activity? Desire to interact with peers? Desire to be a competent clinician? Compelled by supervisors to attend?
4. What would prevent the learner from participating in a program? Scheduling of the program? Location? Lack of interest in the topic? Lack of support by the employer?
5. What social, economic, and political factors influence the current status of cognitive rehabilitation and continuing education? Is there pressure to prove the effectiveness of cognitive rehabilitation therapy? Is continuing education mandatory for licensure, practice privileges, or membership in associated occupational or scholastic societies?

Activities

The education and experience of planners and learners weigh heavily in analyzing the planning context and client system. Even though planners and learners need not know every detail associated with every effective clinical technique, social movement, or economic decision, they should be involved enough in their occupations to be sensitive to the major issues that affect the provision of cognitive rehabilitation services and continuing education. Journal reading, participation in selected societies, consultation with colleagues, and careful listening to clients are methods often used to support analysis of context and client systems.

Step Two: Justify and Focus Planning

In most planning models, this step would be called "needs assessment." The typical process of needs assessment involves identifying discrepancies between existing and desired capabilities and determining the relative priority of discrepancies. As such, it is much more than an information-gathering exercise, since identifying desired capabilities and setting priorities both involve making value judgments. In cognitive rehabilitation therapy, the client's needs may be the basis for the potential trainee's needs. Yet, the decision to provide a continuing education activity may depend in large measure upon the provider organization's available and required resources, and its willingness to invest in the provision of a selected continuing education activity.

Program ideas may originate from forces external or internal to the continuing education provider unit. Externally generated ideas include those arising from:

1. Contractual obligations to funding agencies
2. Requests for educational planning services from formal organizations such as rehabilitation facilities, specialty societies, or advocacy groups
3. Requests for topics or educational planning services from informal groups of cognitive rehabilitation therapy providers
4. Requests or suggestions from academic faculty or intervention staff acting independently
5. Requests or suggestions from representatives of higher education acting in association with their academic units

Internally generated program ideas may come from:

1. A history and/or tradition of offering a particular educational activity
2. An organizational mission to provide continuing education or staff training and development
3. A commitment to research in cognitive rehabilitation or education related to cognitive rehabilitation therapy
4. Costs of maintaining the organizational unit charged with providing continuing education or training

In varying degrees and combinations, each of these sources and forces effectively serves to generate program ideas.

Decisions

Planners encounter several decision points in justifying the program idea and planning for implementation of the program. Having generated or been presented with the program idea, planners must decide:

1. Whether or not to continue to develop the idea
2. Whether the idea is appropriate to an educational intervention or some other type of intervention such as medical or administrative
3. Whether the program idea is appropriate for development by the continuing education/ staff training unit, another internal unit such as quality assurance, or an external agency such as the state licensing board or the American Occupational Therapy Association
4. Whether or not the program idea might be of interest to those who provide cognitive rehabilitation services
5. Whether the developed program idea might be of need to those who provide cognitive rehabilitation services

Learners must consider their reasons for participating in the program. Adults often attend continuing education programs to complete educational or occupational requirements. However, they also expect to break the routine of daily practice, test their current knowledge and skills against that of experts in their field, and share information with colleagues. Learners must consider their major reasons for participation and assess the likelihood that those needs will be addressed.

Activities

The needs assessment data-gathering techniques of educational program planners are well documented (Caffarella, 1988; Knowles, 1980; Levine, Cordes, Moore, & Pennington, 1984). Direct mail surveys and postprogram-administered questionnaires provide helpful information. Interviews and informal but purposeful discussions with experts and practitioners have a long history of use and offer planners valuable information in helping to determine what might be needed. Recently, knowledge tests, practice audit, situation analysis, market demand, and peer review have gained increased attention as methods for identifying possible new program ideas.

Planners should be skilled in their ability to utilize all these methods and knowledgeable regarding the strengths and weaknesses of each. The value of the needs assessment is in part dependent upon the planner's best interpretation of data that might help determine what is needed. Resolution of the issue of need is central to needs assessment and objective setting.

Step Three: Develop Objectives

Objectives are more or less detailed descriptions of expected program outcomes. They may describe behaviors expected of the learner following the program or they may be a more general description of what the planner hopes will happen as a result of the program.

> There has been considerable debate about the merits of using "behavioral" versus "non-behavioral" objectives in educational planning. Since the influence of behaviorism has waned, the debate seems to have all but disappeared, but the issue has never been settled. On the one hand, it can be argued that any change in human capability can only be confirmed if the learner's behavior changes in some way. Even quite abstract outcomes such as to raise consciousness, change conceptions, empower people, and transform perspectives can only be understood by the changes in behavior manifested by the learners. On the other hand, it can be argued that people may learn a great many things without ever changing their behavior and that only the most trivial kinds of learning can be described using behavioral objectives. Notwithstanding the merits of the arguments against using behavioral or other forms of objectives and planning, essentially every planning model incorporates the development of objectives as a necessary element. (Sork, 1990, p. 79)

Objectives should be clear and realistic in order to be useful to the planner and the learner.

Planning groups or committees often are formed to help assess needs, determine objectives, and identify an appropriate instructional design. Such groups might include cognitive rehabilitation therapy practitioners, academicians, members of occupational or scholarly associations, educational planners, clients, and others interested in the education and training of those working to provide cognitive rehabilitation therapy. It is not unusual for the continuing education planner to acquire assessments of need from statements of objectives by planning group members. Techniques include (Mazmanian, 1980):

1. Instructing planning group members to determine and write objectives for "important" issues in the practice of cognitive rehabilitation therapy
2. Directing planning group discussions with questions concerning:
   a. what the planners want practitioners to know or be able to do as a result of attending the program
   b. the reasons why practitioners should have the knowledge or be able to perform the task
3. Suggesting ideal outcomes and guiding the planning group toward determining objectives by continually reminding them of their expertise and sensitivity to learning needs of the target group
4. Asking planning groups to consider adopting and/or adapting previously determined objectives

Needs assessment is more often a reformulation and retrospective justification of the program idea than a scientifically identified range of information, skills, or attitudes to be addressed through an educational intervention. Developing objectives usually includes writing, or instructing planning groups to write, a proposal describing the ideal characteristics of a learner who has attended the program.

Decisions

Both the planner and learner should consider the following questions:

1. Who should be involved in program planning? Should the process be committee driven? If so, who should participate?
2. Should objectives be stated in behavioral or other terms? How will objectives be used in relation to evaluation and subsequent program development?

Activities

It is a tenet of adult education that the learner should be involved in all stages of planning. Adults have their own learning agendas, related to their personal, professional, and social roles. It is important, then, to include the viewpoints of individual learners and ideas from the systems in which these individuals function (Caffarella, 1988). For educational activities involving one provider of cognitive rehabilitation therapy or a small group of providers, direct participation in planning often is less difficult than for activities such as conferences designed for many learners. In the case of the latter program design, a compilation of survey and other data reflecting trends is appropriately provided to program planning committees.

The steps involved in developing objectives for the program include:

1. Scheduling the appointment with each participant for the planning group session
2. Securing a facility for the planning session
3. Arranging for the provision of informational materials to planning group members

To the extent that learners openly and constructively participate in developing objectives, they are likely to better inform planners and faculty of their learning needs and expectations of the program to be offered. Many educators (Caffarella, 1988; Houle, 1972; Knowles, 1980) believe that the likelihood of success for learners is tied to their participation in generating concise statements of their learning objectives.

Step Four: Formulate Instructional Plan

All the activities considered necessary to bring about the desired learning constitute the instructional plan.

> This step of planning is where the wealth of research dealing with learning styles, motivation, instructional techniques, conditions of learning, instructional design, media selection, developmental stages, and so on, is applied by the planner to develop the educative structure of the program. This is where "theories" about how adults learn are applied and where characteristics of the client group have the greatest impact on the plan. We know very little about how instructional design decisions are made in practice. It is likely in the health professions that instructional designs for continuing education programs follow the patterns established with professional preparation, whether or not such patterns are the most effective. (Sork, 1990, p. 80)

Decisions

Most professionals are comfortable with lectures and lectures predominate in most continuing education programs, even though behavior modeling might be more appropriate for enabling attainment of some learning objectives. The common assumption among adult educators is that there is no one best way of assisting people to learn (Houle, 1972; Robinson, 1979). Rather, there are seven major factors to be considered when choosing instructional techniques:

1. Instructional Objectives. Is the focus of the objective knowledge acquisition, skill building, or attitude change?
2. Instructor. Is the instructor capable of using the technique and does he or she feel comfortable in doing so?
3. Content. Is the content material abstract or concrete? What is the level of complexity and comprehensiveness of the material?
4. Trainees. How many trainees will there be? What expectations do the trainees have in terms of the techniques to be used and are they capable of learning through those techniques?
5. Time. What time period is available?
6. Cost. Are the costs, if any, associated with the techniques chosen realistic?
7. Space, Equipment, and Material. Is the space, equipment, and/or material necessary to use the techniques readily available? (Caffarella, 1988, p. 168)

Caffarella suggested that of the seven factors, the first two are key: the focus of instructional objectives and the capability of the instructor to use the chosen technique.

To help attain their goals of enhancing the knowledge, skills, and attitudes of cognitive rehabilitation practitioners, educational planners must match appropriate instructional techniques with expected learning outcomes. Certain techniques are better suited than others for enabling predetermined objectives. Each technique has apparent strengths and weaknesses in operationalizing objectives. Caffarella (1988) offered a description of 25 selected instructional techniques matched to categories of learning outcomes. Nine of those instructional techniques appear in Table 4.1, which outlines the types of decisions that educational planners must make in formulating the instructional plan.

Activities

Within the structure of the planning group, resolution of the issue of need is signaled by compilation of the program design. Such a compilation is often found in the form of the planner's notes or minutes of the planning session. Justification of the program idea indicates a settling of the issue of need, a juncture in testing, and reformulation and refinement of the program plan. Activities of the planner include:

1. Estimating a program budget that influences the plan of the continuing education activity
2. Registering in some permanent form the program idea, justification of the program idea, and techniques for presenting the subject matter

The content of the program should build upon the past knowledge and experiences of the participants and be, where appropriate, problem oriented and practical. The potential participant decides whether the program objective, instructional techniques, and other program components fit his or her personal learning preferences and goals.

Step Five: Formulate Administrative Plan

Financial parameters for planning and implementing the program, the promotional strategy for assuring participation of the learner group,

and the administrative tasks required to implement the plan are considered in this step.

> Financial dimensions include estimating the costs of the resources to be used in the program, determining how these costs will be recovered, and setting program fees. Concepts such as threshold pricing; break-even points; fixed, variable, and sunk costs; direct, indirect, and overhead costs; margin, surplus, and deficit; and opportunity costs are used to understand the myriad calculations and considerations involved in program finance. (Sork, 1990, p. 80)

Decisions

Planners must decide or help to decide:

1. Who will serve as instructor(s)? Who will recruit and confirm their participation?
2. Where will the educational activity be conducted?
3. What types of instructional materials are suitable? Worksheets? Content outlines? Programmed texts?
4. What type of audiovisual support is necessary? Flipcharts? Slide projectors? Videotapes? Videodiscs? Transparencies? Projectionist? Production services?
5. How will the program be announced? Direct mail? Telephone marketing? Journal advertisement? Posters?
6. Will instructors be paid? If so, how much will they receive?
7. Will travel and lodging costs be incurred by the program account?
8. What sorts of amenities will be provided? Refreshments? Visits to local sites of interest?

Activities

Planners may assign or be assigned administrative activities associated with gathering information or deciding each of these questions. Such activities may include recruitment of faculty, negotiation of contracts, and selection as well as acquisition of appropriate goods and services. Ordinarily, the planner must acquire or generate a budget that assures adequate resources to implement the program. Some programs are contracted and face little risk of running over budget. Others are developed on speculation, presuming the number of paying participants will enable the program account to break even

Table 4.1.   Selected instructional techniques by category of learning outcomes

Learning outcome	Instructional technique	Description
Knowledge acquisition	Lecture	A one-way, organized, formal talk given by a resource person for the purpose of presenting a series of events, facts, concepts, or principles.
	Debate	A presentation of conflicting views by two people or two teams of people for the purpose of clarifying the argument between them.
	Screened speech	Small groups of participants develop questions they wish resource persons to respond to extemporaneously.
Skill building	Demonstration with return demonstration	A resource person performs an operation or a job, showing others how to do a specified task. The participants then practice the same task.
	Behavior modeling	A model or ideal enhancement of a desired behavior presented via an instructor, a videotape, or film. This is usually followed by a practice session on the behavior.
	Action mazes	A case study that has been programmed, involving a series of decision points with options at each point.
Attitude change	Simulation	A learning environment that simulates a real setting with the focus on attitudes and values related to the situation presented.
	Games	An activity characterized by structured competition to provide insight into the attitudes, values, and interests of the participants.
	Critical incident	Participants are asked to describe an important incident related to their work lives. This is then used as a base for analysis.

Adapted from Caffarella (1988).

financially or to realize revenue beyond total costs of the program.

Assuring participation in programs is usually a challenge. A well-conceived instructional plan can assure intellectual participation in programs, but assuring physical presence in a program depends on communicating the character of the program in such a way that it is attractive and inviting to those who learn about it (Sork, 1990). Continuing educators, for many years, have been applying concepts and principles from marketing research literature, most notably the specialized literature on marketing in nonprofit organizations. Many planners regularly maintain frequency response and financial data on types of mailers (e.g., two-color brochures mailed at bulk rate to a general market segment versus signed personal letters sent with first-class post-

age to a targeted subset of the market segment). In addition, direct mail response data are analyzed often by zip code, occupation, or age of program enrollees. The expenses, revenue, and response rates generated by efforts such as journal advertisements, telephone marketing calls, and other promotional activities enable some planners to be better informed for difficult decisions regarding the promotion of their educational programs.

Step Six: Develop Evaluation Plan

How should evaluation be carried out? Why are some programs successful while others are not? A considerable body of literature exists to help answer each of these questions and to provide techniques and strategies for answering these questions in relation to individual programs.

Since the intent of most continuing professional education is to improve performance, evaluation models that focus on determining changes in practice in the work environment of the practitioner are most relevant. Evaluation designs that allow conclusions to be drawn about relationships between an educational program and changes in practice are expensive and complex so they must be constructed with care. (Sork, 1990, p. 81)

Decisions

To support these activities, educational planners must ask:

1. Who will be involved in planning and overseeing the evaluation?
2. What is the purpose of the evaluation? How will the results be used?
3. What will be judged? Learning? Performance?
4. Which evaluation design will be used?
5. What data collection techniques will be used?
6. How will results be analyzed?

The determination of how evaluative data will be used and by whom tends to guide the evaluation process. Questions of how the evaluation is to be carried out, and criteria for measuring change involve two elements of research. The first is *measurement,* the determination by objective means of the extent to which learners have achieved the criteria of evaluation. The second part is *appraisal,* a subjective judgment of how well the purposes of the program have been achieved (Houle, 1972).

Activities

There are two general approaches used for program evaluation. The *quantitative approach* involves numerical measurement. The *qualitative approach* involves verbal or written descriptions. Evaluation techniques primarily associated with the quantitative approach include: 1) paper-and-pencil tests, 2) performance tests, 3) written questionnaires, 4) review of organizational records and documents, and 5) cost-benefit analysis. Techniques suitable for both quantitative and qualitative approaches include: 1) observation, 2) interviews, and 3) review of products generated by the learner (e.g., a cognitive rehabilitation therapy practitioner's neuropsychological assessment of a client).

There are several standard quantitative designs for evaluation (Cook & Campbell, 1979; Kerlinger, 1986). These designs include the one-group post-test only design, whereby data are gathered from a single group in a postprogram procedure; also included are the one-group pretest/post-test, the time series, and the control group designs. With the one group pretest-post-test design, data are collected before and after the educational program in an effort to measure changes in the individual's or group's performance. The time series design features multiple observations or tests administered over time. The observations or tests may include the same group of learners or a similar group, with the expected outcome that knowledge, skills, or attitudes will change after training. The control group design involves preintervention testing of two similar groups. One group receives education followed by a post-test and the other group receives only the post-test, to determine levels of change attributable to participation in the educational activity.

The qualitative approach to evaluation provides in-depth descriptions (Patton, 1990), usually reported in written form. Data may be gathered through individual or group interviews, observations, videotaping, or reviewing documents and records. The data are usually analyzed for recurring ideas or themes that appear throughout the gathered information. Reports often include quotations from interviewees to illustrate major points. A qualitative approach is well suited for evaluating programs intended to build self-confidence or interpersonal communication skills. Regardless of whether quantitative or qualitative methods are to be used, it is important that the evaluation plan is in place before the educational activity begins.

Step Seven: Carry Out Program

Most personnel who coordinate training programs agree that the actual carrying out of the program can be a very hectic and busy time. All the program arrangements must be checked and thought must be given to how the program should be opened, monitored, and closed. One person may be responsible for all these tasks, including the instructional portion of the program, or a number of people may be involved, depending on the complexity of the training event. (Caffarella, 1988, p. 209)

It is important at the opening of any continuing education or training program to create a positive and comfortable climate for learning.

Decisions

Planners must ask:

1. Are participants welcomed and greeted in a warm way?
2. Is someone available to introduce participants to one another?
3. Are those responsible for on-site registration able to generate name tags, issue instructional materials, provide needed services, and maintain a friendly demeanor?
4. Does the coordinating staff seem to be in control?

These activities tend to orient learners to the learning environment, but it is also important that as a result of the orientation and opening comments, instructors and learners have a clear understanding of: 1) the objectives of the program, 2) the program requirements as they relate to the instructional plan, and 3) the expectations the instructors have for participants and the participants' expectations for instructors (Nadler, 1982).

Activities

To help assure that the program is implemented in an efficient manner, the educational planner must assure the following (Caffarella, 1988):

1. All resource people have arrived and are prepared.
2. Rooms continue to be arranged as requested.
3. Equipment is available and working.
4. Refreshments are delivered on time and are well prepared.
5. Adequate training materials are available.
6. Appropriate evaluation data are being collected as planned.
7. The schedule is being followed by presenters.

Closing the program includes assuring that all data needed for evaluation have been collected and learners and instructors are recognized for their participation in the program. In general, the educational planner has responsibility for assuring that each detail of the program is completed by its end.

DIRECTIONS FOR RESEARCH AND ACTION

Research on the current practice of cognitive rehabilitation therapy may enable the generation of standards of practice to be adapted by all those who provide cognitive rehabilitation services. It may also enable better identification of the differences between ideal and current levels of practice. Having identified those discrepancies, undergraduate, graduate, and continuing education programs may better serve the needs of potential learners. Research into the organizational activities and backgrounds of those who provide cognitive rehabilitation therapy services may guide the continuing education of individual practitioners. It may also shed light on the political paths taken and to be taken by those interested in moving cognitive rehabilitation therapy toward a more prominent professional position.

The complexity of factors affecting cognitive rehabilitation therapy and continuing education ought to stimulate a variety of new investigations and actions. Empirical study is needed to improve the techniques of cognitive rehabilitation therapy and the tools of continuing education. What will be discovered will be worth knowing, since the ability of cognitive rehabilitation therapy providers to learn new and better ways of performing their roles governs the rate of progress in cognitive rehabilitation. The responsibility of the educator is to challenge that ability, encourage learning, and facilitate progress.

REFERENCES

Abreu, B.C., & Toglia, J.P. (1987). Cognitive rehabilitation: A model for occupational therapy. *American Journal of Occupational Therapy, 41,* 439–448.

Alexandre, A., Columbo, F., Nertempi, P., & Bene-detti, A. (1983). Cognitive outcome and early indices of severity of head injury. *Journal of Neurosurgery, 59,* 751–761.

American   Speech-Language-Hearing   Association

(1990). Interdisciplinary approaches to brain damage. *Journal of the American Speech-Language-Hearing Association, 32*(Suppl. 2), 3.

Boake, C. (1989). A history of cognitive rehabilitation of head-injured patients, 1915 to 1980. *Head Trauma Rehabilitation, 4,* 1–8.

Bottcher, S.A. (1989). Cognitive retraining: A nursing approach to rehabilitation of the brain injured. *Nursing Clinics of North America, 24*(1), 193–208.

Bracy, O.L. (1984). Cognitive rehabilitation survey results. *Cognitive Rehabilitation, 2,* 12–13.

Caffarella, R.S. (1988). *Program development and evaluation resource book for trainers.* New York: John Wiley & Sons.

Cervero, R.M. (1988). *Effective continuing education for professionals.* San Francisco: Jossey-Bass.

Commission on Accreditation of Rehabilitation Facilities (CARF). (1990). *Standards manual.* Tucson, AZ: Author.

Cook, T.D., & Campbell, D.T. (1979). *Quasi-experimentation design and analysis issues for field setting.* Chicago: Rand McNally.

Flexner, A. (1915). Is social work a profession? *School and Society, 1,* 901–911.

Fox, R.D., Mazmanian, P.E., & Putnam, R.W. (1989). *Changing and learning in the lives of physicians.* New York: Praeger.

Frangicetto, T. (1989). Northampton Community College: Cognitive retraining program. *Cognitive Rehabilitation, 7,* 10–16.

Goldstein, K. (1942). *Aftereffects of brain injury in war.* New York: Grune & Stratton.

Harley, P. (1989, September). *American Psychological Association Standards of Practice.* Paper presented at 3rd annual conference, Cognitive Rehabilitation and Community Reintegration, Clearwater Beach, FL.

Houle, C.O. (1972). *The design of education.* San Francisco: Jossey-Bass.

Houle, C.O. (1980). *Continuing learning in the professions.* San Francisco: Jossey-Bass.

Kerlinger, F.N. (1986). *Foundations of behavioral research* (3rd ed). New York: Holt, Rinehart & Winston.

Knowles, M.S. (1980). *The modern practice of adult education.* New York: Cambridge.

Knox, A.B. (1985). Adult learning and proficiency. In D. Kleiber & M. Maehr (Eds.), *Advances in motivation and achievement: Vol. 4. Motivation in adulthood* (pp. 251–295). Greenwich, CT: JAI Press.

Kreutzer, J. (Ed.). (1989). Cognitive rehabilitation. [Special issue]. *Journal of Head Trauma Rehabilitation 4*(3).

Kreutzer, J.S., & Boake, C. (1987). Addressing disciplinary issues in cognitive rehabilitation. *Brain Injury, 1,* 199–202.

Levine, H.G., Cordes, D.L., Moore, D.E., & Pennington, F.C. (1984). Identifying and assessing needs to relate continuing education to patient care.

In J.S. Green, S.Y. Grosswald, E. Suter, & D.B. Walthall (Eds.), *Continuing education in the health professions* (pp. 152–173). San Francisco: Jossey-Bass.

Mazmanian, P.E. (1980). A decision-making approach to needs assessment and objective setting in continuing medical education. *Adult Education, 31,* 3–17.

Mazmanian, P.E., Martin, K.O., & Kreutzer, J.S. (1991). Training and practice in cognitive rehabilitation: Organizational analysis. *Cognitive Rehabilitation, 9*(1).

Nadler, L.L. (1982). *Designing training programs: The critical events model.* Reading, MA: Addison-Wesley.

National Head Injury Foundation. (1989). *Proceedings of the Annual Meeting of the National Head Injury Foundation.* Chicago: Author.

Nowlen, P.M. (1988). *A new approach to continuing education for business and the professions.* New York: Macmillan.

Parenté, R. (1989, September). *Training and degree programs for practitioners.* Paper presented at 3rd annual conference, Cognitive Rehabilitation and Community Reintegration, Clearwater Beach, FL.

Parenté, R., & Bennett, T. (1989). Training of cognitive rehabilitation specialists: Reflections by two psychologists. *Cognitive Rehabilitation, 7,* 18–20.

Patton, M.Q. (1990). *Qualitative evaluation and research methods* (2nd ed.). New York: Sage.

Pennington, F., & Green, J. (1976). Comparative analysis of program development processes in six professions. *Adult Education, 27,* 13–23.

Proceedings of the 13th Annual Postgraduate Course on Rehabilitation of the Brain Injured Adult and Child. (1988). Williamsburg: Medical College of Virginia.

Proceedings of the 14th Annual Postgraduate Course on Rehabilitation of the Brain Injured Adult and Child. (1989). Williamsburg: Medical College of Virginia.

Proceedings of the 15th Annual Postgraduate Course on Rehabilitation of the Brain Injured Adult and Child. (1990). Williamsburg: Medical College of Virginia.

Robinson, R.D. (1979). *An introduction to helping adults learn and change.* Milwaukee, WI: Omnibooks.

Rosenthal, M., & Berrol, S. (1989). From the editors. *Journal of Head Trauma Rehabilitation, 4,* vii.

Schudson, M. (1980). A discussion of Magali Sarfatti Larson's *The rise of professionalism:* A sociological analysis. *Theory and Society, 9,* 215–229.

Society for Cognitive Rehabilitation, Inc. (1990). *Bylaws of the Society for Cognitive Rehabilitation, Inc.* Decatur, GA: Author.

Sohlberg, M.M., & Mateer, C.A. (1989). *Introduction to cognitive rehabilitation: Theory and practice.* New York: Guilford Press.

Sork, T.J. (1990). Theoretical foundations of education program planning. *Journal of Continuing Education in the Health Professions, 10,* 73–83.

Tyler, R.W. (1949). *Basic principles of curriculum and instruction.* Chicago: University of Chicago Press.

Uzzell, B.P., & Gross, Y. (Eds.). (1986). *Clinical neuropsychology of intervention.* Boston: Martinus Nijhoff.

Walker, D. (1971). A naturalistic model of curriculum development. *School Review, 80,* 51–65.

Wilensky, H.L. (1964). The professionalization of everyone? *American Journal of Sociology, 70,* 137–158.

PERSONALITY, BEHAVIOR, OUTCOME, AND HOLISTIC INTERVENTION

Often, cognitive rehabilitation is intended to benefit basic skills including memory, attention, hand-eye coordination, and visual perception. These basic skills underlie successful performance of more complex skills required for activities of daily living.

A complexity of interrelated factors underlies clinicians' ability to achieve therapeutic benefits. Furthermore, the tremendous variability among persons with brain injury contributes to difficulties designing appropriate intervention plans.

Awareness of factors that influence postinjury outcome, therapeutic planning, and therapy effectiveness is critical for practitioners. This section of the text includes comprehensive information regarding the sequelae of traumatic brain injury. Varying levels of injury severity, as well as areas of ability including language, cognition, and behavior, are discussed in detail. In addition, a description of assessment strategies critical to therapy planning is presented.

Notably, behavioral problems are common following brain injury. Research and anecdotal evidence suggest that behavioral difficulties may have a greater influence on psychosocial outcome than cognitive factors. Consequently, information is provided about preinjury personality characteristics and their apparent relationship to postinjury behavioral and cognitive sequelae. Practical information is also provided about managing psychosocial and behavioral difficulties within the context of cognitive rehabilitation.

Finally, many persons with traumatic brain injury regularly take prescription drugs. Practitioners must be aware of the potential benefits and side effects of pharmacological measures and how they may influence the outcome of cognitive rehabilitation therapy.

CHAPTER 5

Neurobehavioral Outcome Following Traumatic Brain Injury

Review, Methodology, and Implications for Cognitive Rehabilitation

JEFFREY S. KREUTZER, CATHERINE W. DEVANY, STEFANIE L. MYERS, AND JENNIFER HARRIS MARWITZ

Persons with traumatic brain injury represent a diverse group. To some extent, diversity is a function of preinjury differences in personality, social roles, and intellect (Mayer, Keating, & Rapp, 1986). Additionally, diversity arises from postinjury differences in pathophysiology and associated sequelae (Levin, Benton, & Grossman, 1982). Regarding somatic, cognitive, social, and behavioral outcome, researchers have routinely reported significant individual differences among clients (Dodwell, 1988).

Practitioners in the field of cognitive rehabilitation are faced with the challenge of providing clients with efficacious therapy. Therapy goals are developed through consideration of clients' strengths and limitations as well as medical information and environmental factors (Diller & Gordon, 1981). The task of cognitive rehabilitation is complicated by the need to ascertain which therapeutic interventions are appropriate for the markedly diverse population of persons with brain injury.

A primary purpose of this chapter is to outline the diversity of neurobehavioral outcome following traumatic brain injury as well as the implications for cognitive rehabilitation. Review of the literature is focused on physical, cognitive, behavioral, and communication difficulties. Findings from a large neurobehavioral outcome study including persons with mild, moderate, and severe injury are included. The outcome investigation is intended to illustrate a useful assessment strategy and to provide information regarding the typical consequences of injury. Discussion centers on the role of neurobehavioral assessment in the practice of cognitive rehabilitation.

REVIEW OF NEUROBEHAVIORAL OUTCOME RESEARCH

Many readers are familiar with the Glasgow Coma Scale (GCS) developed by Teasdale and Jennett (1974). The scale comprises three subscales that provide information regarding verbal responsiveness, motor functioning, and the intensity of stimuli required to elicit eye opening. Initially developed as an objective measure of consciousness, the coma scale is now an integral part of the neurological examination completed soon after injury.

The Glasgow Coma Scale (Teasdale & Jennett, 1974) has proven useful as an early prognostic indicator and has been used to classify levels of injury severity (Levin et al., 1982). Severe injury corresponds to a score of 8 or less, moderate injury corresponds to a score of 9–12, and mild injury corresponds to a score of 13–15

This work was partially supported by Grants #G0087C0219 and #H133B80029 from the National Institute on Disability and Rehabilitation Research, United States Department of Education. Partial support was also provided through a grant awarded by International Business Machines Corporation. Appreciation is expressed to Bruce E. Leininger, Ph.D. and Kathleen O'Kane Martin, M.Ed. for comments that were helpful in the preparation of this chapter.

(Rimel, Giordani, Barth, Boll, & Jane, 1981, 1982). Perhaps because of the obvious, adverse long-term consequences, most traumatic brain injury outcome studies have focused on persons with severe injury. Considerably more is known about persons with brain injury admitted for hospitalization with a GCS score of 8 or less. To a lesser extent, researchers have also focused on persons with moderate and mild injury.

Historically, researchers have incorporated two assessment methodologies to describe the neurobehavioral consequences of traumatic brain injury. A group of researchers have used questionnaires and interviews to elicit family members' and clients' perceptions regarding the effects of injury (e.g., Brooks, Campsie, Symington, Beattie, & McKinlay, 1986; Thomsen, 1984). Partly because of concerns related to diminished self-awareness arising from injury, most investigators have relied primarily on family members' rather than clients' reports. Neuropsychological assessment procedures have also been used extensively to describe the diverse cognitive, intellectual, sensory, motor, linguistic, and perceptual skills of persons with traumatic brain injury (e.g., Lezak, 1983; Reitan & Davison, 1974).

Each assessment methodology is subject to bias and uncertain validity. Psychological denial may cause relatives and clients to minimize difficulties. Client perceptions of disability may be affected by memory deficits and impairment of self-awareness arising from pathophysiological changes. Psychological distress may contribute to exaggerated reports by relatives. Neuropsychological tests are clearly more objective than self-report measures and avoid the issue of biased reporting. Unfortunately, several factors contribute to uncertainties regarding the value of neuropsychological assessment. A clear relationship between neuropsychological test scores, ability to perform daily living activities, and clients' and relatives' perceptions of sequelae has not been demonstrated (e.g., Acker, 1986; Hart & Hayden, 1986). Furthermore, neuropsychological assessment procedures represent an unusual and highly structured situation. As such, test results may not provide a good representa-

tion of characteristic behavior evident in daily living activities.

Efforts to enhance the validity of conclusions regarding neurobehavioral outcome and the complexity of interrelationships among outcome variables have contributed to an increased reliance upon a combination of assessment methodologies. Following is a review of research derived from the two commonly used methodologies.

Family and Client Perceptions of Neurobehavioral Outcome

Most research pertaining to perceptions of outcome following brain injury has been carried out in Europe. Both cross-sectional and longitudinal investigations from England, Denmark, and Scotland have focused on persons with severe brain injury. More recently, investigators have studied persons with mild injury, and to a lesser extent, moderate injury.

Mild and Moderate Brain Injury

Although the incidence of mild brain injury is relatively high, there is continuing debate regarding the long-term effects of such insults on cognitive processes. Several investigators have argued that there is little evidence of long-term impairment in abilities required for work, academic functioning, and avocational activity (e.g., Dikmen, Temkin, & Armsden, 1989). These researchers have cited the fact that nearly all persons with mild brain injury return to preinjury vocational and prevocational activities within 1 year postinjury. Other investigators have proposed that cognitive impairment can persist following mild brain injury and are beginning to accept the validity of clients' claims regarding disability (e.g., Leininger, Gramling, Farrell, Kreutzer, & Peck, 1990; Rimel et al., 1981).

In a recent review of the literature, Rutherford (1989) reported on patterns of "postconcussion" symptoms evident in the acute and late stages of mild brain injury. Headache, visual impairment, fatigue, and dizziness were commonly reported during both the late and early stages of injury. Nausea and vomiting were uniquely associated with the early stages of injury. Irritability, anxiety, depression, and memory impairment were commonly reported in studies of late outcome. Notably, these symptoms have also been reported as common sequelae of severe brain injury (e.g., Brooks, Campsie, Symington, Beattie, & McKinlay, 1987; Oddy, Coughlan, Tyerman, & Jenkins, 1985). Rutherford also reported that poor hearing and insomnia were commonly observed late postconcussion symptoms.

Investigations of sequelae following moderate brain injury (admission GCS: 9–12) are few. Rimel and colleagues (1982) provided limited data on neurobehavioral sequelae following moderate injury. At 3 months postinjury, 93% of 197 clients suffered from a persistent headache. Problems with memory (90%), activities of daily living (87%), transportation (62%), and finances were also reported. Forty-two percent reported difficulties in two or more areas, and the overall unemployment rate was 69%.

Severe Brain Injury

Thomsen (1974, 1984) completed a series of outcome studies delineating brain-injured persons' difficulties at 2–5 years and 10–15 years postinjury. At the 10–15 year follow-up, relatives of 28 males and 12 females with severe brain injury completed a series of interviews and questionnaires. Reportedly, 10% were aphasic and 38% were dysarthric. Additionally, a majority were described as demonstrating personality and

emotional changes (65%), diminished concentration (53%), social isolation (68%), slowness (53%), fatigue (50%), disinterest (55%), and low stress tolerance (55%). Comparisons with early follow-up data obtained at 2–5 years postinjury yielded no evidence of substantial improvement. A summary of research describing problems most frequently reported by relatives is presented in Table 5.1.

In Scotland, Neil Brooks and his colleagues (Brooks et al., 1987) reported on a group of 134 persons with severe traumatic brain injury. Using structured interviews and questionnaires, follow-up data pertaining to neurobehavioral sequelae were obtained from clients and relatives between 2 and 7 years postinjury. Approximately 75% of relatives reported that clients had difficulties related to slowness, personality, memory, and irritability. Between 54% and 65% indicated that clients had problems with depression, anxiety, coordination, restlessness, and mood changes. Head injury–related problems most often reported by clients included memory (66%), irritability (62%), fatigue (43%), concentration (41%), and anxiety (35%). For every area, a greater proportion of relatives reported problems, with differences ranging from 10% (memory) to 36% (coordination).

Oddy and his colleagues (1985) reported on neurobehavioral outcome 7 years following se-

Table 5.1. Head injury–related problem areas reported by a majority of relatives in a series of late outcome follow-up studies

Thomsen (1984)	Oddy, Coughlan, Tyerman, and Jenkins (1985)	Brooks, Campsie, Symington, Beattie, and McKinlay (1987)
Memory	Memory	Slowness
Sociability	Concentration	Personality
Personality	Speech	Memory
Stress tolerance		Irritability
Disinterest		Fatigue
Concentration		Anxiety
Slowness		Concentration
Fatigue		Depression
		Coordination
		Restlessness

Note: Within each study, problem areas are ranked hierarchically from most to least frequently reported.

vere traumatic brain injury. Interviews and checklists were used to obtain information from family members and persons with traumatic brain injury. Relative to all other areas, memory problems (79%) were most frequently reported by family members. Fifty-percent of family members also reported sequelae affecting concentration and speech. Relatives also reported that clients had problems with fatigue (43%), disinterest (43%), impatience (43%), childishness (40%), and denial (40%). As in the Brooks et al. study (1987), clients reported many fewer problems in every area than did relatives. Difficulties with memory (53%), concentration (46%), coordination (31%), temper (31%), and conversation following (28%) were most frequently reported by persons with head injury.

In summary, problems arising from severe brain injury apparently persist for at least 7–15 years postinjury. Most frequently reported problems are related to memory, concentration, fatigue, coordination, slowness, personality, and disinterest. Furthermore, family members routinely report a greater frequency of head injury–related problems than do the clients themselves.

Neuropsychological Tests and Outcome Research

Neuropsychological tests are often used to provide quantitative and descriptive information regarding client outcome. As such, they represent a subset of neurobehavioral assessment strategies. Many neuropsychological tests have normative data available. Often, descriptive information is available for healthy populations as well as for persons with a variety of neurological disorders. Initially, clinicians used neuropsychological tests to aid in the diagnosis of neurological conditions. Test interpretations also provided information regarding lesion localization and rate of disease progression (Lezak, 1983; Mapou, 1988). With advances in medical technology, the role of neuropsychological testing has begun to veer away from diagnosis and toward assessing the efficacy of various therapies, including cognitive rehabilitation (e.g., Gordon, 1987; Ruff et al., 1989).

Given the availability of several excellent resources, the present discussion of neuropsychological outcome following brain injury is limited. For a more comprehensive review, the reader is referred to recent works written and edited by Levin and his colleagues (e.g., Levin et al., 1982; Levin, Eisenberg, & Benton, 1989; Levin, Grafman, & Eisenberg, 1987).

Mild Brain Injury

Intensified interest in mild traumatic brain injury during the last decade was stimulated by a group of researchers at the University of Virginia (Barth et al., 1983; Rimel et al., 1981). Extensive neuropsychological evaluations were performed on a group of 71 clients at 3 months post– mild brain injury. The Halstead-Impairment Index derived from the Halstead-Reitan Neuropsychological Test Battery was used to designate severity of brain dysfunction (Reitan & Wolfson, 1985). Reportedly, 31% of the persons with mild head injury sustained moderate or severe impairment, and 31% sustained mild impairment. Among clients who were employed preinjury, approximately one third returned to work postinjury. Furthermore, probability of returning to work was related to Halstead-Impairment Indices. The authors concluded that "minor head injuries may not be minor after all" (Barth et al., 1983, p. 529).

Following a review of research regarding symptoms after mild head injury, Binder (1986) concluded there was considerable uncertainty regarding the persistence of cognitive dysfunction beyond the acute stages of injury. He argued that elderly persons as well as those with lower socioeconomic status or previous head injuries may have a worse prognosis.

Binder (1986) and Levin et al. (1987) provided evidence of neuropsychological deficits in the subacute period following mild brain injury. Levin and his colleagues (1987) conducted a multicenter study to compare neuropsychological outcome of persons with mild head injury and a matched control group. Evaluation of verbal learning, attention, verbal memory, immediate digit recall, and information processing was conducted at baseline (resolution of posttraumatic amnesia), and at 1 and 3 months postinjury. Relative to controls, persons with mild brain injury demonstrated neuropsychological impairment on all measures at baseline. Significant improvement was evident at 1 month postinjury, and there were no neurobehavioral differences evident between clients and controls at 3 months postinjury.

Recently, Leininger and his colleagues (1990) revealed evidence of significant neuropsychological dysfunction among persons with symptomatic mild brain injury who ranged from 1 to 20 months postinjury. Comparison of neuropsychological test results with a matched group of controls revealed impairments on measures of information processing, visuomotor construction, complex problem solving, verbal learning, and memory for designs. From their investigation, the authors concluded that "neuropsychological evaluation of patients with postconcussive symptoms will often provide justification for many complaints which might erroneously be attributed to neuroticism or greed" (Leininger et al., 1990, p. 296).

In summary, researchers generally agree that neuropsychological impairment is most often observed within the first several weeks following mild injury. Long-term effects have been observed and are documented most frequently among the elderly as well as those with a history of brain injury or psychiatric illness.

Moderate and Severe Brain Injury

Investigation of the neuropsychological consequences of brain injury has focused predominantly on persons with severe injury (Rimel et al., 1982). Few investigations have focused solely on persons with moderate brain injury and most studies either compare persons with moderate and severe injury or combine them into a single group.

Among the existing research on moderate brain injury is the work of Rimel et al. (1982). Rimel and her colleagues reported Halstead-Reitan Neuropsychological Test Battery (Reitan & Wolfson, 1985) findings for a group of 32 persons with moderate brain injury at 3 months postinjury. Of the eight scores derived from the test battery, a majority of clients scored in the

impaired range on seven. Impairment indices derived by combining the eight test scores revealed that 45% showed overall evidence of brain dysfunction.

Tabbador, Mattis, and Zazula (1984) investigated neuropsychological outcome in a comparative study of persons with moderate ($n = 29$) and severe ($n = 39$) brain injury. Measures of intelligence (Wechsler Adult Intelligence Scale–Revised [WAIS-R], Wechsler, 1981), visual naming, language comprehension, fine motor coordination, and memory were performed. Initial examination at an average of 21 days postinjury revealed substantial impairment in every functional area while between-group differences were notably minimal. Among functional areas, impairment was most prominent on tests of fine motor skills and memory and relatively less pronounced on language and intellectual skills. Furthermore, while there was evidence of intellectual and linguistic recovery at reevaluation 1 year postinjury, there was little evidence of improvement in memory or fine motor abilities.

Dikmen, Machamer, Temkin, and McLean (1990) conducted a prospective outcome study of moderate and severe brain injury at 1, 12, and 24 months postinjury. Neuropsychological tests were administered to 31 consecutive adults admitted for traumatic brain injury and a group of matched controls. Testing consisted of the Halstead-Reitan Neuropsychological Test Battery (Reitan & Wolfson, 1985), selected subtests of the Wechsler Memory Scale (Wechsler, 1945), the Selective Reminding Test (National Institutes of Health, 1982), and the WAIS-R (Wechsler, 1981). The investigators observed that substantial improvement occurred during the first year. However, improvement slowed thereafter and pervasive deficits were observed at a 2-year follow-up. Relative to controls, poor performance was observed on nearly every measure at 2 years postinjury. Conclusions regarding injury reported by Dikmen and colleagues (1990) are similar to those reported in the exhaustive review of the literature by Levin et al. (1982).

Considered as a whole, neuropsychological investigations of outcome following brain injury yield a number of conclusions. First, moderate and severe brain injury causes diverse impairments of cognitive abilities. Although improvement may be substantial in the first 12 months following injury, serious impairments often remain at 2 years postinjury. Second, impairments observed among persons with moderate brain injury are nearly equal in severity to those observed following severe brain injury. Finally, there is evidence of impairment following mild brain injury, but a majority of persons recover to preinjury levels of functioning within 3–6 months.

PROTOCOL FOR NEUROBEHAVIORAL ASSESSMENT: INVESTIGATION, METHODOLOGY, AND OUTCOME

Researchers have provided information regarding various aspects of neurobehavioral outcome following traumatic brain injury. Investigators relied on neuropsychological assessment, structured interviews, and/or questionnaires to describe outcome. Most studies have focused on severe injury. A few have provided information on mild injury, and fewer still have provided information on moderate injury.

Undoubtedly, clinicians practicing cognitive rehabilitation will be required to address the diverse needs of persons with varying levels of disability. Disability levels are dependent on acuity as well as the initial pathophysiology of injury. Each clinician will necessarily develop a method for evaluating a heterogeneous group of clients. The process of developing appropriate evaluation methods is often formidable.

Within this section, the reader is presented with a description for a neurobehavioral evaluation methodology. The evaluation procedure involves neuropsychological assessment as well as questionnaires administered to persons with brain injury and primary caregivers. Experience has demonstrated the efficacy of this methodology for persons with mild, moderate, or severe injury and varying acuity levels. To better illustrate this assessment procedure, outcome data are presented for a relatively large and heterogeneous sample of persons with head injury who were evaluated at a major trauma center. Exam-

ination of the data yields important descriptive information regarding brain injury outcome. Additionally, readers who choose to adopt all or a portion of the methodology can use the descriptive data for comparison with their own clients.

Participants

Participants were 135 persons referred for neuropsychological evaluation through the Medical College of Virginia's Department of Rehabilitation Medicine. The sample was predominately male (71.1%) and white (82.2%). Ages ranged from 16 to 64 years ($M = 32.4$; $SD = 10.6$) and years of education from 7 to 20 years ($M = 12.6$; $SD = 2.3$). More than two thirds of the participants were single, divorced, or separated. The majority of the sample (54.8%) were unemployed.

To qualify for inclusion in the study, clients were required to meet the following criteria: 1) no prior incident of brain injury predating the injury for which the client was receiving evaluation and/or therapy, 2) no history of neurological or major psychiatric disorder, and 3) no premorbid history of substance abuse treatment.

Participants were categorized according to severity of injury as defined by the Glasgow Coma Scale (Teasdale & Jennett, 1974). Severe injury was denoted by a score of 8 or less ($N = 72$) on hospital admission. Persons with admission coma scores ranging from 9 to 12 ($N = 28$) were labeled as having a moderate injury, and those with scores of 13 and above ($N = 33$) were labeled as having a mild injury. In cases where a GCS score was not available, an estimate was made by reviewing medical records.

Referral sources included professionals in the community (56.3%) as well as a university-based supportive employment program (43.7%). A majority of the individuals were evaluated within 36 months postinjury (71.4%), while 20% were 6 or more years postinjury. The mean length of time since injury for the entire sample was 42.5 months ($SD = 57.7$).

Neurobehavioral Evaluation Instruments

A battery of 23 neuropsychological tests was administered to each participant. The neuropsychological battery consisted of tests that provide information relevant to a broad range of cognitive skill areas including attention, concentration, memory, information processing, learning, and visuoperceptual skills. Academic skills were evaluated as well. A brief listing of each test along with corresponding primary skill areas and dependent measures derived from each is presented in Table 5.2.

Many readers are aware that a wide variety of neuropsychological tests are available (e.g., Hartlage, Asken, & Hornsby, 1987; Lezak, 1983). Selection criteria for tests included: 1) availability of normative data especially for persons with brain injury, 2) feasibility of administration to persons with widely varying levels of disability; and 3) demonstrated sensitivity to pathophysiological and functional changes.

Neurobehavioral outcome was also assessed using the General Health and History Questionnaire (GHHQ) (Kreutzer, Leininger, Doherty, & Waaland, 1987; Kreutzer & Wehman, 1990). A primary caregiver, typically a relative or close friend, completed the questionnaire, which provided information regarding a variety of brain injury sequelae. Informants ($N = 135$) were predominantly parents (40%) and spouses (29.6%). The remaining questionnaires were completed by other relatives (13.4%), friends (12.6%), and rehabilitation personnel (4.4%). Complete descriptions of neuropsychological tests and the GHHQ are presented in the appendix at the end of this chapter.

Procedure

Demographic and injury-related information was gathered from medical charts and interviews with the participants. Neuropsychological tests were administered by one of four experienced neuropsychological technicians with master's degrees in psychology. Standard administration and scoring protocols were followed for all tests. GHHQ (Kreutzer et al., 1987; Kreutzer & Wehman, 1990) data were obtained from significant others within a limited amount of time following administration of the test battery to the client. Responses to questionnaires were reviewed by investigators who, in turn, attempted to obtain any missing information via interview.

Results

General Health and History Questionnaire

Informants provided information about clients in the following problem areas: 1) somatic, 2) cognitive, 3) behavioral, and 4) communication and social. Items in each category were ranked according to frequency of occurrence. An item was considered a problem if endorsed as occurring "sometimes," "often," or "always." Table 5.3 lists the top 10 problem items in each area, ranked according to percentage of endorsement.

The somatic problem reported most often (85%) for persons with traumatic brain injury was "tired." "Moves slowly" ranked second highest (74%), followed by "loses balance" and "headaches" (71%). Several items were apparently not problematic for the majority of clients. For example, a significant proportion of family members reported that the clients never experienced blackout spells (89%) or seizures (86%), or picked their nose or skin (85%).

Items related to cognitive functioning were seen as more problematic overall than were somatic, behavioral, or communication problems. The vast majority of all clients (94%) were reportedly suffering from some degree of confusion. "Misplaces things" and "loses train of thought" were also commonly reported problems (78%). Difficulties related to cognitive functioning that were endorsed as "never" occurring in most cases were "trouble following instructions" (87%) and "forgets to eat" (75%).

Reportedly, behavioral difficulties that were most frequent for clients included being "frustrated" (87%), "bored" (85%), and "restless" (77%). Violent acting-out behaviors were among those items endorsed least frequently, including "hits or pushes others" (13%), "threatens to hurt self" (14%), and "threatens to hurt others" (16%). In the area of communication and social functioning, most clients experienced some difficulty with retrieval of words (81%). Nearly two thirds of the sample (65%) argued on a regular basis. The communication problem endorsed least often for the entire sample, yet still occurring in nearly one fourth of the cases, was nonsensical speech.

Table 5.2. Neuropsychological tests, primary skill areas measured, and dependent measures

Test (Abbreviation)	Dependent measure
Attention	
Trail Making: Part A (Trail Making A)	Completion time (seconds)
Trail Making: Part B (Trail Making B)	Completion time (seconds)
Symbol Digit Modalities—Written (Symbol digit written)	Number correct
Symbol Digit Modalities—Oral (Symbol digit oral)	Number correct
Digit Span Forward (Digits forward)	Maximum digits
Digit Span Backward (Digits backward)	Maximum digits
Paced Auditory Serial Addition—Revised (Serial addition)	Number correct (sum of 4 trials)
Word fluency	
Controlled Oral Word Association (Word association)	Corrected score
Verbal memory	
Kreutzer Memory Paragraph—Immediate Recall (Paragraph immediate recall)	Number correct
Kreutzer Memory Paragraph—10-Minute Recall (Paragraph delayed recall)	Number correct
Verbal learning	
Auditory Verbal Learning (Verbal learning)	Number correct (sum of 5 trials)
Visual construction	
Complex Figure—Copy (Complex figure copy)	Number correct
Block Design	Age-scaled score
Visual memory	
Complex Figure—3-minute Recall (Complex figure recall)	Number correct
Nonverbal reasoning	
Category	Total errors
Academic abilities	
Arithmetic	Age-scaled score
Spelling	Age-scaled score
Reading Accuracy	Age-scaled score
Reading Comprehension	Age-scaled score
Motor speed	
Grooved Pegboard—Dominant (Pegboard dominant)	Completion time (seconds)
Grooved Pegboard—Nondominant (Pegboard nondominant)	Completion time (seconds)

(continued)

Table 5.2   *(continued)*

Hand strength (unilateral)	
Grip Strength–Dominant	Kilograms
Grip Strength–Nondominant	Kilograms

Sources of tests: Arithmetic and Spelling (Wide Range Achievement Test–Revised [WRAT-R]; Jastak & Wilkinson, 1984); Auditory Verbal Learning Test (Rey, 1964; Taylor, 1959); Block Design (Wechsler Adult Intelligence Scale–Revised [WAIS-R]; Wechsler, 1981); Category Test (Halstead, 1947); Complex Figure Test: Copy and 3-Minute Recall (Osterrieth, 1944; Rey, 1941; Taylor, 1959); Controlled Word Association Test (Benton & Hamsher, 1976); Digit Span: Forward and Backward (WAIS-R; Wechsler, 1981); Grip Strength: Dominant and Nondominant (Halstead, 1947); Grooved Pegboard: Dominant and Nondominant (Mathews & Klove, 1964); Kreutzer Memory Paragraph: Immediate Recall and 10-Minute Recall (Kreutzer, 1986); Paced Auditory Serial Addition Test–Revised (Levin, 1983); Reading Accuracy and Reading Comprehension (Gray Oral Reading Test–Revised [GORT-R]; Wiederholt, 1986); Symbol Digit Modalities Test: Written and Oral (Smith, 1968, 1973); Trail Making Test: Parts A and B (Reitan, 1958).

Neuropsychological Test Outcome

Neuropsychological tests and dependent variables included in the present analyses are summarized in the appendix at the end of this chapter. While these tests are known to measure a variety of interrelated skills (Lezak, 1983), they are listed according to primary skill areas. Assignment to primary skill areas is done for organizational purposes, and the possibility that some debate may exist regarding grouping is acknowledged.

Table 5.4 lists descriptive statistics for the sample, including means, standard deviations, and ranges. Also included in this table are the percentage of participants scoring in the impaired range for each test. Impairment is defined as scoring less than one standard deviation below the normal population (i.e., at or below the 15th percentile). Normative data were gathered from test manuals and other well-established references (Bigler, 1984; Fromm-Auch & Yeudall, 1983; Jastak & Wilkinson, 1984; Leininger et al., 1990; Lezak, 1983; Wechsler, 1981; Weins, McMinn, & Crossen, 1988; Wiederholt, 1986). The cutoff scores used as the criteria for impairment are also presented in Table 5.4.

Neuropsychological tests were also grouped according to the percentage of participants scoring within the impaired range. On only one of the 23 tests administered, WAIS-R Block Design (Wechsler, 1981), did fewer than one fourth of all clients demonstrate impaired performance. Those tests on which 25%–49% of participants were

impaired are listed in Table 5.5. Within this group, most persons (48%) showed notably deficient nonverbal reasoning skills, as measured by the Category Test (Halstead, 1947). Table 5.5 also lists tests on which 50%–74% of the sample were impaired. Nearly three quarters of the participants scored within the substandard range on both the written and oral versions of the Symbol Digit Modalities Test (Smith, 1968, 1973). There were no tests on which greater than 75% of the individuals obtained a significantly impaired score.

Univariate analysis of variance was used to compare clients with mild, moderate, and severe injury on the basis of neuropsychological test performance. In order to correct for familywise error rate and an artificial alpha inflation as a result of running multiple analyses, a Scheffé correction was computed (Keppel, 1982). The procedure involves calculating a stringent critical F value to be used when evaluating the significance of the obtained F. The critical F value is determined based on degrees of freedom within and between groups as well as the number of subjects ($N = 133$) and groups ($N = 3$) (Keppel, 1982). The Scheffé correction adjusted the F value from the standard critical values of $F = 3.07$ ($p < .05$) and $F = 4.79$ ($p < .01$) to $F = 6.14$ and $F = 9.58$ ($p < .05$ and $p < .01$, respectively), thus providing a conservative standard for testing significance.

Means for persons with head injury on each of the neuropsychological tests are reported in Table 5.6 along with F values comparing the

Table 5.3. Most frequently reported problems of persons with traumatic brain injury

Item	Percentage reporting
Somatic problems	
Tired	85%
Moves slowly	74%
Loses balance	71%
Headaches	71%
Muscles ache	59%
Drops things	55%
Weak	55%
Trouble falling asleep	51%
Dizziness	50%
Muscles tingle or twitch	49%
Cognitive problems	
Confused	94%
Misplaces things	78%
Loses train of thought	78%
Thinks slowly	77%
Trouble making decisions	77%
Poor concentration	75%
Forgets if he or she has done things	75%
Forgets what he or she reads	74%
Forgets people's names	72%
Easily distracted	72%
Behavioral problems	
Frustrated	87%
Bored	85%
Restless	77%
Impatient	75%
Sad, blue	74%
Lonely	73%
Complains	72%
Difficulty getting things started	71%
Misunderstood by others	70%
Jumpy, irritable	64%
Communication and social problems	
Difficulty thinking of the right word	81%
Argues	65%
Makes spelling mistakes	61%
Difficulty pronouncing words	53%
Uncomfortable around others	52%
Writes slowly	51%
Trouble understanding conversation	46%
Difficulty making conversation	45%
Writing is hard to read	45%
Does not participate in sports	42%

three groups. Significant differences were found between groups of persons with mild, moderate, and severe head injury on 13 of the 23 administered tests. Among those tests that differentiated head-injured groups most substantially were Symbol Digit Modalities Test–Written ($F = 26.71, p < .01$) and Symbol Digit Modalities Test–Oral (Smith, 1968, 1973) ($F = 17.92, p < .01$) as well as the Auditory Verbal Learning Test (Rey, 1964) ($F = 15.41, p < .01$). Tests that did not discriminate between the three groups included WAIS-R Digit Span Forward (Wechsler, 1981) ($F = 0.10$), the Category Test (Halstead, 1947) ($F = 0.11$), and Grip Strength–Dominant ($F = 0.25$) and Grip Strength–Nondominant (Halstead, 1947) ($F = 0.89$). In considering the primary skill areas measured by each test, those measures of learning and memory distinguished severity groups more consistently than did tests of other areas of ability.

Additional comparisons were made between severity groups by computing the total number of 23 possible tests on which each individual performed in the impaired range. This calculation provided an index of proportional impairment, that is, a ratio of impairment scores to the full battery. For example, a client who scored in the impaired range on 7 of the 23 possible tests would obtain a 30% impairment index, suggesting that performance was defective on nearly one third of the battery. Using this calculation, performance between severity groups was compared across the full battery of tests. The percentage of clients in each group who scored in the impaired range on greater than 50% of the battery (i.e., 12 or more tests) was computed. Only 27% of persons with mild injury and 33% of those with moderate injury met this criteria. However, 59% of persons with severe injury performed in the defective range on more than half of the administered tests.

Persons with mild, moderate, and severe injury were further contrasted using analysis of variance to compare mean number of defective test scores for each group. The ANOVA revealed significant differences between mild ($M = 7.9$), moderate ($M = 8.8$), and severe ($M = 11.7$) groups ($F = 7.57, p < .05$) on total number of impaired tests.

Table 5.4. Descriptives for neuropsychological tests and percentage of individuals with impaired performance

Test	Mean	SD	Range	% Impaired	Criterion score
Attention					
Trail Making A	47.63	32.06	10–180	43%	>39
Trail Making B	109.83	69.82	30–300	61%	>73
Symbol digit written	36.83	14.63	0–69	73%	<46
Symbol digit oral	43.40	16.40	10–95	74%	<53
Digits forward	6.03	1.29	4–9	40%	<6
Digits backward	4.25	1.19	2–8	28%	<4
Serial addition	60.99	24.54	0–100	65%	<74
Word fluency					
Word association	34.62	11.52	12–71	30%	<28
Verbal memory					
Paragraph immediate recall	6.67	2.98	1–15	28%	<5
Paragraph delayed recall	6.90	3.98	0–15	30%	<5
Verbal learning					
Verbal learning	42.05	12.83	9–68	53%	<44
Visual construction					
Complex figure copy	16.32	7.89	0–31	43%	<30
Block design	9.39	3.38	1–19	21%	<7
Visual memory					
Complex figure recall	28.67	5.73	0–36	50%	<17
Nonverbal reasoning					
Category	45.91	34.98	10–150	48%	>35
Academic abilities					
Arithmetic	7.10	3.09	1–15	42%	<7
Spelling	8.16	3.60	1–15	36%	<7
Reading accuracy	7.54	4.60	1–18	50%	<8
Reading comprehension	8.92	4.39	1–18	36%	<8
Motor speed					
Pegboard dominant	104.55	59.36	47–300	54%	>80
Pegboard nondominant	116.33	71.06	45–300	64%	>78
Hand strength (unilateral)					
Grip strength dominant	37.20	16.23	0–69	51%	<44
Grip strength nondominant	33.82	13.86	0–61	58%	<45

Note: Abbreviations of text names are used in this table. See Table 5.2 for complete names of tests and authors of tests.

Impairment is defined as scoring less than 1 standard deviation below the mean of the normative sample (criterion score).

SD = Standard deviation.

SUMMARY, CONCLUSIONS, AND IMPLICATIONS

Neurobehavioral outcome research has demonstrated that persons with brain injury manifest a wide variety of problems, which are particularly apparent in the acute stages of injury. Research has also demonstrated that the adverse neurobehavioral consequences of injury can preclude successful performance of important daily living activities (Ben-Yishay, Silver, Piasetsky, & Rattok, 1987; Lezak, 1987).

Table 5.5. Neuropsychological tests on which 25%–49% and 50%–74% of persons with head injury were impaired

Test	Percentage
25%–49%	
Attention	
Trail Making A	43%
Digits forward	40%
Digits backward	28%
Word fluency	
Word association	30%
Verbal memory	
Paragraph immediate recall	28%
Paragraph delayed recall	30%
Visual construction	
Complex figure copy	43%
Nonverbal reasoning	
Category	48%
Academic abilities	
Arithmetic	42%
Spelling	36%
Reading comprehension	36%
50%–74%	
Attention	
Trail Making B	61%
Symbol digit written	73%
Symbol digit oral	74%
Serial addition	65%
Verbal learning	
Verbal learning	53%
Visual memory	
Complex figure recall	50%
Academic abilities	
Reading accuracy	50%
Motor speed	
Pegboard dominant	54%
Pegboard nondominant	64%
Hand strength (unilateral)	
Grip strength dominant	51%
Grip strength nondominant	58%

Note: Abbreviations of test names are used in this table. See Table 5.2 for complete names of tests and authors of tests.

The value of neurobehavioral assessment in conjunction with cognitive rehabilitation therapy is significant for a variety of reasons. Comprehensive neurobehavioral assessment helps provide the therapist with a broad perspective of the client's strengths and limitations. Neuropsychological evaluation yields information about behavior in structured settings. Client and family reports complement these test data by revealing the ability to carry out activities of daily living, in addition to interpersonal skills. Taken together, this information provides a comprehensive profile of the client and establishes an agenda for therapy as well as a basis for its evaluation.

Establishing Goals and Priorities for Therapy

The investigation reported in this chapter included persons with all levels of injury severity and revealed that 25%–75% of clients performed in the impaired range on every test, with the exception of the WAIS-R Block Design (Wechsler, 1981). These data are indicative of the diversity of impairment associated with diffuse brain injury. Given the considerable variability among these clients, neurobehavioral assessment may help to establish the unique characteristics of each individual. Additionally, many clients have a number of well-preserved areas of functioning despite their difficulties. Certainly, clients' strengths are important, apparent in the evaluation process, and should be considered in therapy planning.

Providers of cognitive rehabilitation therapy can use assessment data to decide which problems should receive immediate attention. Therapists may choose to focus on a single set of cognitive difficulties as a priority. For example, improvement of attentional skills may be viewed as a prerequisite to improvement of memory problems.

Parenté and Anderson (1984) suggested that assessment data are also useful in predicting the likely success of cognitive rehabilitation. Parenté and Anderson proposed that memory and learning abilities are especially important. For example, a skills training approach dependent on extensive practice may not be appropriate for persons with especially severe memory loss. In such cases, maintenance of therapy gains over time or generalization is likely to be minimal. Alternatively, development and use of compen-

Table 5.6. Comparisons of neuropsychological tests among head injury groups

Test	Means			F	p
	Mild	Moderate	Severe		
Attention					
Trail Making A	34.6	42.2	61.0	7.44	<.05
Trail Making B	82.2	99.4	137.5	6.73	<.05
Symbol digit written	47.8	43.3	29.8	26.71	<.01
Symbol digit oral	52.1	52.5	36.6	17.92	<.01
Digits forward	6.0	6.1	6.0	0.10	ns*
Digits backward	4.4	4.7	4.1	2.17	ns
Serial addition	66.2	69.4	50.6	5.37	ns
Word fluency					
Word association	36.7	37.6	32.6	2.63	ns
Verbal memory					
Paragraph immediate recall	7.9	7.5	5.8	7.71	<.05
Paragraph delayed recall	9.0	7.5	5.7	9.52	<.01
Verbal learning					
Verbal learning	49.1	46.8	37.0	15.41	<.01
Visual construction					
Complex figure copy	31.0	29.0	27.4	4.77	ns
Block design	11.2	10.6	8.3	10.65	<.01
Visual memory					
Complex figure recall	19.7	18.1	13.9	7.61	<.05
Nonverbal reasoning					
Category	43.9	46.5	47.3	0.11	ns
Academic abilities					
Arithmetic	8.7	7.5	6.2	7.71	<.05
Spelling	9.4	7.9	7.6	2.95	ns
Reading accuracy	10.6	8.4	6.0	12.09	<.01
Reading comprehension	11.8	9.4	7.6	10.14	<.01
Motor speed					
Pegboard dominant	86.3	94.0	117.9	3.93	ns
Pegboard nondominant	82.7	95.6	137.8	9.58	<.01
Hand strength (unilateral)					
Grip strength dominant	35.6	37.0	38.2	0.25	ns
Grip strength nondominant	32.8	31.6	35.8	0.89	ns

Note: Abbreviations of test names are used in this table. See Table 5.2 for complete names of tests and authors of tests.

ns = nonsignificant.

satory strategies for clients with severe memory dysfunction may prove most useful.

Often clients have a variety of behavioral and social problems. Personality and emotional changes, including depression, have been identified as problems—especially for persons with severe brain injury. Low frustration tolerance, restlessness, and irritability are also commonly identified problems. Within holistic cognitive rehabilitation programs, behavioral difficulties are often addressed. Therapists work to improve personality and behavioral difficulties within the context of individual therapy sessions. For example, frustration tolerance and aggressive difficulties can interfere with progress in therapy. Behavioral management techniques can be applied in the context of cognitive rehabilitation to address such interferences and benefit overall performance. Additionally, social skills training in group contexts using role playing and videotape feedback has proven to be useful.

If behavioral problems are especially severe, psychopharmacological treatment may be necessary. However, medications often have side effects that impair cognitive functioning (see Chapter 7, this volume). A close working relationship with the prescribing physician is necessary to help in the selection of medications with greatest overall benefits. For less severe problems, interdisciplinary rehabilitation may occur concurrently. Chronic fatigue, post-traumatic seizures, poor balance, insomnia, and dizziness are relatively common sequelae of traumatic brain injury. Generalized muscular pain and headache are also common. Cognitive remediation therapists are encouraged to be aware of potentially valuable medical and rehabilitation services including physical therapy, occupational therapy, and vocational rehabilitation. Communication among treating professionals is essential for coordinated service delivery.

Measurement of Therapy Progress

Neurobehavioral assessment provides potentially valuable information regarding the benefits of therapy. For example, neuropsychological evaluations are often used as indicators of therapy generalization (Gordon, 1987). Extensive research has indicated that neuropsychological tests including the Trail Making (Reitan, 1958), Symbol Digit Modalities (Smith, 1968, 1973), Kreutzer Memory Paragraph (Kreutzer, 1986), WAIS-R Block Design (Wechsler, 1981), and Arithmetic (Jastak & Wilkinson, 1984) tests are most sensitive to level of injury severity. As such, these tests may prove most sensitive to functional improvements in the context of cognitive rehabilitation. Greater evidence of therapeutic effectiveness exists if clients show improvement on neuropsychological measures in addition to improved performance on related therapy training tasks.

Neurobehavioral measures can be used to plot the natural history of improvement following brain injury and serve as a baseline for determination of therapy efficacy. Improvement normally occurs following injury, especially in the acute stages. Therapists must be cautious in their attempts to discriminate accurately between spontaneous recovery and improvement attributable to therapy. To address this issue, Ruff and his colleagues (1989) described a neuropsychological methodology that helps delineate actual therapy benefits.

In the final analysis, neurobehavioral assessment provides standardized criteria for evaluating therapy. By measuring client change according to these criteria, therapists may find either justification for their therapy regime or cause for its alteration or termination.

Conclusions

Neurobehavioral assessment is most often utilized as a means of describing outcome following brain injury. To a lesser extent, assessment data have demonstrated value in the measurement of therapy efficacy. Ideally, therapy gains should be most apparent on measures that reflect abilities that are the focus of therapy. Least improvement is anticipated on measures that are unrelated to therapy tasks. For example, a therapist working to improve memory skills should anticipate significant improvement on measures of memory function. Less improvement or no improvement should be anticipated on measures of hand-eye coordination and visuoperceptual abilities.

Uncertainties remain about the relationships between reported performance in activities of daily living and quantitative information derived from neuropsychological testing. Within the investigation reported in this chapter, neuropsychological testing revealed greatest difficulty for clients on measures of sustained attention, information processing, and motor speed. These findings are consistent with other investigations of neurobehavioral outcome and, furthermore, correspond with client and family perceptions.

In some instances, clinicians may see improvement in test scores following intervention, while the client or family report fails to corroborate these impressions. In other cases, clients and family members may report improvement that is not revealed by testing. The most valid deductions can be drawn when similar information regarding improvement is derived from all sources. Nevertheless, additional data are needed to help establish the value of diverse outcome assessment methodologies in establishing the benefits of cognitive rehabilitation.

REFERENCES

Acker, M.B. (1986). Relationships between test scores and everyday life functioning. In B.P. Uzzell & Y. Gross (Eds.), *Clinical neuropsychology of intervention* (pp. 85–118). Boston: Martinus Nijhoff.

Barth, J.T., Macciocchi, S.N., Giordani, B., Rimel, R., Jane, J.A., & Boll, T.J. (1983). Neuropsychological sequelae of minor head injury. *Neurosurgery, 13,* 529–533.

Benton, A.L., & Hamsher, K. des. (1976). *Multilingual Aphasia Examination.* Iowa City: University of Iowa.

Ben-Yishay, Y., Silver, S., Piasetsky, E., & Rattok, J. (1987). Relationship between employability and vocational outcome after intensive holistic cognitive rehabilitation. *Journal of Head Trauma Rehabilitation, 2*(1), 35–48.

Bigler, E. (1984). *Diagnostic clinical neuropsychology.* Austin: University of Texas Press.

Binder, L.M. (1986). Persisting symptoms after mild head injury: A review of the postconcussive syndrome. *Journal of Clinical and Experimental Neuropsychology, 8,* 323–346.

Brooks, N., Campsie, L., Symington, C., Beattie, A., & McKinlay, W. (1986). The five year outcome of severe blunt head injury: A relative's view. *Journal of Neurology, Neurosurgery, and Psychiatry, 49,* 764–770.

Brooks, N., Campsie, L., Symington, C., Beattie, A., & McKinlay, W. (1987). The effects of head injury on patient and relative within seven years of injury. *Journal of Head Trauma Rehabilitation, 2*(3), 1–13.

Dikmen, S., Machamer, J., Temkin, N., & McLean, A. (1990). Neuropsychological recovery in patients with moderate to severe head injury: 2 year follow-up. *Journal of Clinical and Experimental Neuropsychology, 12,* 507–519.

Dikmen, S., Temkin, N., & Armsden, G. (1989). Neuropsychological recovery: Relationship to psychosocial functioning and postconcussional complaints. In H.S. Levin, H.M. Eisenberg, & A.L. Benton (Eds.), *Mild head injury* (pp. 229–244). New York: Oxford University Press.

Diller, L., & Gordon, W.A. (1981). Interventions for cognitive deficits in brain-injured adults. *Journal of Consulting and Clinical Psychology, 49,* 822–834.

Dodwell, D. (1988). The heterogeneity of social outcome following head injury. *Journal of Neurology, Neurosurgery, and Psychiatry, 51,* 833–838.

Fromm-Auch, D., & Yeudall, L.T. (1983). Normative data for the Halstead-Reitan neuropsychological tests. *Journal of Clinical Neuropsychology, 5,* 221–238.

Gordon, W.A. (1987). Methodological considerations in cognitive remediation. In M. Meier, A. Benton, & L. Diller (Eds.), *Neuropsychological rehabilitation* (pp. 111–131). New York: Guilford Press.

Gregory, R.J., Paul, J.J., & Morrison, M.W. (1979). A short form of the Category Test for adults. *Journal of Clinical Psychology, 35,* 795–798.

Halstead, W.C. (1947). *Brain and intelligence.* Chicago: University of Chicago Press.

Hart, T., & Hayden, M.E. (1986). The ecological validity of neuropsychological assessment and remediation. In B.P. Uzzell & Y. Gross (Eds.), *Clinical neuropsychology of intervention* (pp. 21–50). Boston: Martinus Nijhoff.

Hartlage, L.C., Asken, M.J., & Hornsby, J.L. (Eds.). (1987). *Essentials of neuropsychological assessment.* New York: Springer.

Jastak, S., & Wilkinson, G.S. (1984). *Wide Range Achievement Test–Revised: Administration manual.* Wilmington, DE: Jastak Associates.

Keppel, G. (1982). *Design and analysis: A researcher's handbook* (2nd ed.). Englewood Cliffs, NJ: Prentice-Hall.

Kreutzer, J.S. (1986). *The Story Recall Test.* Unpublished manuscript, Virginia Commonwealth University, Medical College of Virginia, Richmond.

Kreutzer, J.S., Leininger, B.E., Doherty, K., & Waaland, P.K. (1987). *General Health and History Questionnaire.* Richmond: Medical College of Virginia, Rehabilitation Research and Training Center on Severe Brain Injury.

Kreutzer, J.S., & Wehman, P. (Eds.). (1990). *Community integration following traumatic brain injury.* Baltimore: Paul H. Brookes Publishing Co.

Leininger, B.E., Gramling, S.E., Farrell, A.D., Kreutzer, J.S., & Peck, E.A. (1990). Neuropsychological deficits in symptomatic head injury patients after concussion and mild concussion. *Journal of Neurology, Neurosurgery, and Psychiatry, 53,* 293–296.

Levin, H.S. (1983). *The Paced Auditory Serial Addition Task–Revised.* Unpublished test, University of Texas at Galveston.

Levin, H.H., Benton, A.L., & Grossman, R.G. (1982). *Neurobehavioral consequences of closed head injury.* New York: Oxford University Press.

Levin, H.S., Eisenberg, H.M., & Benton, A.L.

(Eds.). (1989). *Mild head injury.* New York: Oxford University Press.

Levin, H.S., Grafman, J., & Eisenberg, H.M. (Eds.). (1987). *Neurobehavioral recovery from head injury.* New York: Oxford University Press.

Levin, H.S., Mattis, S., Ruff, R., Eisenberg, H.M., Marshall, L.F., Tabaddor, K., High, W.M., & Frankowski, R.F. (1987). Neurobehavioral outcome following minor head injury: A three center study. *Journal of Neurosurgery, 66,* 234–243.

Lezak, M.D. (1983). *Neuropsychological assessment* (2nd ed.). New York: Oxford University Press.

Lezak, M.D. (1987). Relationships between personality disorders, social disturbances, and physical disability following traumatic brain injury. *Journal of Head Trauma Rehabilitation, 2*(1), 57–69.

Livingston, M.G., Brooks, D.N., & Bond, M.R. (1985). Three months after severe head injury: Psychiatric and social impact on relatives. *Journal of Neurology, Neurosurgery, and Psychiatry, 48,* 870–875.

Mapou, R.L. (1988). Testing to detect brain damage: An alternative to what may no longer be useful. *Journal of Clinical and Experimental Neuropsychology, 10,* 271–278.

Mathews, C.G., & Klove, H. (1964). *Instruction manual for the Adult Neuropsychological Test Battery.* Madison: University of Wisconsin Medical School.

Mayer, N.H., Keating, D.J., & Rapp, D. (1986). Skills, routines, and activity patterns of daily living: A functional nested approach. In B.P. Uzzell & Y. Gross (Eds.), *Clinical neuropsychology of intervention* (pp. 205–222). Boston: Martinus Nijhoff.

National Institutes of Health. (1982). Selective Reminding Test. (Unpublished test). In *National Trauma Coma Data Bank test administration manual.* Bethesda, MD: Author.

Oddy, M., Coughlan, T., Tyerman, A., & Jenkins, D. (1985). Social adjustment after closed head injury: A further follow-up seven years after injury. *Journal of Neurology, Neurosurgery, and Psychiatry, 48,* 564–568.

Oddy, M., Humphrey, M., & Uttley, D. (1978). Subjective impairment and social recovery after head injury. *Journal of Neurology, Neurosurgery, and Psychiatry, 41,* 611–616.

Osterrieth, P.A. (1944). Le Test de Copie d'une Figure Complexe [The Complex Figure Copying Test]. *Archives de Psychologie, 30,* 206–356.

Parenté, F.J., & Anderson, J.K. (1984). Use of the Wechsler Memory Scale in predicting success in cognitive rehabilitation. *Cognitive Rehabilitation, 2,* 12–15.

Reitan, R.M. (1958). Validity of the Trail Making Test as an indication of organic brain damage. *Perceptual and Motor Skills, 8,* 271–276.

Reitan, R.M., & Davison, L.A. (1974). *Clinical neuropsychology: Current status and applications.* New York: Hemisphere.

Reitan, R.M., & Wolfson, D. (1985). *The Halstead-Reitan Neuropsychological Test Battery: Theory and clinical interpretation.* Tucson, AZ: Neuropsychological Press.

Rey, A. (1941). L'examen psychologique dans les cas d'encephalopathie traumatique [The psychological examination for head injury]. *Archives de Psychologie, 28,* 286–340.

Rey, A. (1964). *L'examen clinique en psychologie* [The clinical examination in psychology]. Paris: Presses Universitaries de France.

Rimel, R.W., Giordani, B., Barth, J.T., Boll, T.J., & Jane, J.A. (1981). Disability caused by minor head injury. *Neurosurgery, 9,* 221–228.

Rimel, R.W., Giordani, B., Barth, J.T., Boll, T.J., & Jane, J.A. (1982). Moderate head injury: Completing the clinical spectrum of brain trauma. *Neurosurgery, 11,* 344–351.

Ruff, R.M., Baser, C.A., Johnston, J.W., Marshall, L.F., Klauber, S.K., Klauber, M.R., & Minteer, M. (1989). Neuropsychological rehabilitation: An experimental study with head injured patients. *Journal of Head Trauma Rehabilitation, 4*(3), 20–36.

Rutherford, W.H. (1989). Postconcussion symptoms: Relationship to acute neurological indices, individual differences, and circumstances of injury. In H.S. Levin, H.M. Eisenberg, & A.L. Benton (Eds.), *Mild head injury* (pp. 217–222). New York: Oxford University Press.

Smith, A. (1968). The Symbol Digit Modalities Test: A neuropsychologic test for screening of learning and other cerebral disorders. *Learning Disorders, 3,* 83–91.

Smith, A. (1973). *Symbol Digit Modalities Test manual.* Los Angeles: Western Psychological Services.

Tabbador, K., Mattis, S., & Zazula, T. (1984). Cognitive sequelae and recovery course after moderate and severe head injury. *Neurosurgery, 14,* 701–708.

Taylor, E.M. (1959). *The appraisal of children with cerebral deficits.* Cambridge, MA: Harvard University Press.

Teasdale, G., & Jennett, B. (1974). The Glasgow Coma Scale. *Lancet, 2,* 81–84.

Thomsen, I.V. (1974). The patient with severe head injury and his family. *Scandinavian Journal of Rehabilitation Medicine, 6,* 180–183.

Thomsen, I.V. (1984). Late outcome of very severe blunt head trauma: A 10–15 year second follow-up. *Journal of Neurology, Neurosurgery, and Psychiatry, 47,* 260–268.

Wechsler, D. (1945). A standardized memory scale for clinical use. *Journal of Psychology, 19,* 87–95.

Wechsler, D. (1981). *Wechsler Adult Intelligence Scale–Revised manual.* New York: Psychological Corporation.

Weins, A.N., McMinn, M.R., & Crossen, J.R. (1988). Rey Auditory-Verbal Learning Test: Developmental norms for healthy young adults. *Clinical Neuropsychologist, 2,* 67–87.

Wiederholt, J.L. (1986). *Gray Oral Reading Test– Revised manual.* Austin, TX: PRO-ED.

APPENDIX

Descriptions of Neurobehavioral Outcome Measures

Arithmetic and Spelling (Jastak & Wilkinson, 1984) Taken from the Wide Range Achievement Test–Revised (WRAT-R) (Jastak & Wilkinson, 1984), these subtests yield an index of academic abilities in the areas of arithmetic and spelling. For the Arithmetic subtest, individuals are asked to solve increasingly difficult mathematical problems with paper and pencil within a 10-minute time period. The Spelling subtest requires individuals to spell words that have been presented orally. Raw scores, based on number of correct responses, are converted to standard scores. Standard scores are, in turn, transformed to scaled scores using a procedure similar to that of the Wechsler Adult Intelligence Scale–Revised WAIS-R (Wechsler, 1981) (maximum score = 19).

Auditory Verbal Learning Test (AVLT) (Rey, 1964; Taylor, 1959) This test measures verbal learning and memory by asking individuals to recall a list of 15 common nouns presented in identical order across five trials. The score is the sum of correctly recalled words for all trials (maximum score = 75). Scores for individual trials can also be considered in evaluating learning and memory.

Block Design (Wechsler, 1981) This WAIS-R subtest measures visual construction as well as reasoning abilities. Individuals are timed as they arrange four or nine blocks to resemble various geometric designs presented on cards. Speed and accuracy determine scores, which are based on age (maximum score = 19).

Category Test (Halstead, 1947) Originally developed as part of the Halstead-Reitan Neuropsychological Battery (Reitan & Wolfson, 1985), the Category Test provides information relevant to nonverbal reasoning, hypothesis testing, and decision making. Stimuli, organized according to different principles and grouped into five subtests, are presented. Individuals, in turn, must decide which of four possible responses correctly reflects the appropriate principle. The examiner notes when each new subtest has begun in order to alert the individual that the principle may have changed. Individuals are given feedback throughout the test as to the correctness of each response. No additional cuing is provided. A short form consisting of 120 items (Gregory, Paul, & Morrison, 1979) was used in the study presented in this chapter. Scores, based on total number of errors, were adjusted using a conversion table (Gregory et al., 1979) in order to estimate performance on the original, unabridged test (maximum score = 208).

Complex Figure Test: Copy and 3-Minute Recall (Osterrieth, 1944; Rey, 1941; Taylor, 1959) In the first phase of the test, individuals are asked to copy a complex geometric design that provides information regarding visual construction abilities. Three minutes after the drawing is completed, individuals are told to draw the figure from memory, having received no prior warning that they would be asked to do so. Scores are based on detail presence, location, and accuracy for each drawing (maximum score = 36). The memory component reflects incidental (versus intentional) memory.

Controlled Oral Word Association Test (COWA) (Benton & Hamsher, 1976) This test of verbal fluency requires individuals to generate words beginning with a consonant provided by the examiner. A total of three trials are administered, each lasting for 60 seconds. Scores are based on total words generated across the three trials, with a correction added for age and education (no maximum score).

Digit Span: Forward and Backward (DSF, DSB) (Wechsler, 1981) Subtests from the WAIS-R, the DSF and DSB measure ability to recall series of digits in correct sequence. Each series is presented orally with the length increasing by one digit every two trials. For the DSF, individuals recall the digits in the same order in which they were presented. For the DSB, individuals must reverse the order of presentation. The final score is based on the maximum number of digits correctly recalled (DSF maximum score = 9; DSB maximum score = 8).

General Health and History Questionnaire (GHHQ) (Kreutzer, Leininger, Doherty, & Waaland, 1987; Kreutzer & Wehman, 1990) The GHHQ was developed to provide information regarding a broad spectrum of somatic, cognitive, social, and behavioral difficulties arising from brain injury. The self-report instrument was developed following a thorough examination of the outcome literature (e.g., Livingston, Brooks, & Bond, 1985; Oddy, Humphrey, & Uttley, 1978), and extensive interviews with brain-injured persons and their families.

The 105-item questionnaire is available in both client and family versions. In cases where family members are unavailable, information can be obtained from friends or others who know the client well. Individual items provide descriptions of problems within the following areas of functioning: 1) somatic, 2) cognitive, 3) behavioral, and 4) communication and social. Respondents use a 4-point scale ranging from "not at all" to "always" to indicate the frequency of experienced difficulties (e.g., "confusion" or "headaches").

Grip Strength: Dominant and Nondominant (Halstead, 1947) Taken from the Halstead-Reitan Neuropsychological Test Battery (Reitan & Wolfson, 1985), this test evaluates unilateral strength of grip for both the dominant and nondominant hand. Individuals are given a hand dynamometer and asked to hold the instrument at their side and squeeze the handle as hard as possible. Scores are assigned for each hand based on kilograms of pressure (maximum score = 100).

Grooved Pegboard: Dominant and Nondominant (Mathews & Klove, 1964)   This test of motor speed and manual dexterity requires individuals to place 25 metal pegs, one at a time, into a pegboard. Each hole in the pegboard has a groove and the pegs must be rotated in order to fit the hold properly. A trial is conducted for each hand, dominant and nondominant, and scores reflect completion time in seconds. A maximum of 300 seconds is permitted for completion with each hand and the maximum score is assigned for those who exceed the limit.

Kreutzer Memory Paragraph—Immediate Recall and 10-Minute Recall (Kreutzer, 1986)   This short paragraph provides a context for evaluation of contextual memory. Individuals are asked to recall a set of instructions similar to those that might be given to patients at a doctor's office. Individuals are asked to repeat instructions related to scheduling a hypothetical appointment immediately following presentation. After the immediate recall trial, the paragraph is read a second time. Ten minutes later, individuals are again asked to repeat the instructions. Both administrations allow assessment of intentional memory, because individuals are told to try and remember as much as possible prior to administration. Scores reflect the number of information points correctly recalled for each trial (maximum score = 15).

Paced Auditory Serial Addition Test–Revised (PASAT-R) (Levin, 1983)   Individuals are required to add serially 26 consecutive digits presented on a cassette tape for each of four trials. In each trial, speed of stimulus presentation increases (i.e., 2.8 seconds, 2.4 seconds, 2.0 seconds, and 1.6 seconds). The final score is based on the total number of correct responses across the four trials (maximum score = 100).

Reading Accuracy and Reading Comprehension (Wiederholt, 1986)   Originating from the Gray Oral Reading Test–Revised (GORT-R) (Wiederholt, 1986), these subtests tap different aspects of academically based reading ability. Individuals are instructed to read aloud a maximum of 13 short stories. Reading Accuracy is scored for mispronunciations, omissions, repetitions, and completion time. Reading Comprehension scores are based on ability to answer questions regarding story content correctly. Independent scores are assigned for each subtest and scaled according to age (maximum score = 19).

Symbol Digit Modalities Test: Written and Oral (SDMT) (Smith, 1968, 1973)   A test of attention, visuomotor tracking, and speed of information processing, the SDMT requires individuals to rapidly match numbers corresponding to symbols using a key. Both a written (individuals write the matching number underneath the appropriate symbol) and oral (individuals state the corresponding number aloud) version of the test are administered. Individuals work for 90 seconds and scores reflect the number of symbols matched correctly for each trial (maximum score = 110).

Trail Making Test: Parts A and B (Reitan, 1958)   Considered to be highly sensitive to brain dysfunction (Lezak, 1983), both portions of the Trail Making Test require sustained attention, motor speed, and visuomotor tracking. Individuals are required to draw a line connecting circles on a 8½″ × 11″ piece of paper. Part A involves connecting the circles in ascending numerical order. For Part B, individuals must alternate between numbers and letters (i.e., "1—A—2—B...13"). Each trial is scored according to completion time in seconds and instructions are given to work as quickly as possible. Testing is discontinued if time exceeds 300 seconds for either part, and the maximum score is assigned.

CHAPTER 6

Cognition, Language, Attention, and Information Processing Following Closed Head Injury

BRENDA L.B. ADAMOVICH

The ability to communicate or to exchange information between individuals requires intrinsic relationships between cognition, language, attention, and information processing. Skills in these areas may be impaired as a result of traumatic brain injury.

Cognitive skills include the ability to discriminate two or more stimuli (e.g., those pertaining to a situation or conversation), the ability to meaningfully organize information presented or received from others, the ability to generate appropriate responses, and the ability to problem solve in logical steps. *Language skills* include the use of symbols specific to a particular group to communicate thoughts and feelings. *Attention skills* range from the ability to initiate attention to the ability to attend to salient features in order to convey or comprehend information. *Information processing skills* range from the recognition of information or stimuli to the use of internal and external feedback in order to generate responses. Stimulus recognition depends on the ability to make comparisons with past experiences. Accurate stimulus recognition is essential for meaningful conversations and interactions. Internal feedback results through a speaker's evaluation of the response of others, either through questions asked or through the reading of gestural/behavioral responses (e.g., disinterested or confused looks and head nods). External feedback includes direct suggestions by individuals or groups of individuals regarding specific content, methods of conveying content, or specific pragmatic behaviors. Information processing skills also include the rate of responding and the amount of information an individual is capable of holding in short-term storage.

In the sections that follow, the processes of cognition, language, attention, and information processing are discussed in greater detail.

COGNITION

Cognition is always inferred from behavior (Mann & Sabatino, 1985). Cognition includes the use of processes and the knowledge base to: 1) make decisions as to the most appropriate and functional way of interacting with the environment, 2) execute these decisions, 3) monitor responses to determine the appropriateness and accuracy of these decisions, and 4) adjust behavior if it is determined to be inappropriate and/or inaccurate ("Cognitive Rehabilitation Guidelines," 1986).

Cognitive processes that are often impaired after closed head injury include: arousal/alerting, perception/low-level selective attention, discrimination, organization, memory, and high-level thought processing (Adamovich, Henderson, & Auerbach, 1985). This hierarchy was designed based on research with head-injured persons (Adamovich, 1978; Adamovich & Henderson, 1982, 1983, 1984) in an attempt to establish an organized approach to the rehabilitation of attention, information processing, and cognition. A division between the levels is somewhat artificial in that the clinician may be working on the most difficult tasks at one level and the easiest activities at the next level. Although attention is the focus of early intervention, it is essential that attention skills continue to improve as the client moves through the therapy continuum. Memory skills must also continually improve as more complex processing places a greater load on memory.

Cognitive breakdowns of normal children and children with learning disabilities, as well as research regarding successful methods of rehabilitating these breakdowns, may serve as a starting point for work with closed head injury clients. However, hierarchies of cognitive complexity for subjects with brain injury may not always correspond to hierarchies of complexity for children. For example, with regard to antonyms and synonyms, Muma (1978) found that children selected objects that were the same when asked to choose one that was the same, yet they also selected a similar object when asked to choose one that was different. It was suggested that the ability to identify synonyms develops before the ability to identify antonyms. Adamovich and Henderson (1982, 1983) found that individuals with closed head injury also showed this pattern of task difficulty. However, Adamovich and Brooks (1981) found that the reverse was true with subjects who sustained right hemisphere damage secondary to cerebrovascular accidents. These subjects experienced more success providing antonyms than synonyms.

Specific information regarding the cognitive processes typically impaired following closed head injury is provided next.

Arousal/Alerting

Arousal refers to a continuum extending from sleep to wakefulness. Factors to be considered include arousal, attentiveness, and vigilance. The reader is referred to the section titled "Attention" for specific intervention suggestions.

Perception

Perception refers to the integration and interpretation of information received at the sense organs based on an internal or stored representation of the stimulus. People perceive according to how they classify or represent experiences based on prior knowledge (Kirby, 1980; Shaw & Cutting, 1980). Specific perceptual abilities include visual and auditory tracking, sound recognition, shape recognition, and word perception. Brooks (1974) suggested that individuals with closed head injury were unable to identify previously displayed items as familiar, possibly due to poor initial learning or to their adopting strict criteria, whereby items were identified only if they exactly met the criteria.

Specific perceptual therapy activities include visual and auditory tasks such as:

1. Tracking an auditory stimulus or scanning a visual stimulus such as a line
2. Perceiving and recognizing environmental sounds and words and pointing to corresponding pictures
3. Tracing or copying a figure followed by a word
4. Drawing within boundaries (e.g., drawing two parallel lines with a dotted line between it)
5. Bisecting lines by drawing a line through the midpoint of the horizontal lines
6. Following simple commands (e.g., "Open your eyes," "Close your mouth")
7. Naming objects or familiar items, beginning with meaningful visual stimuli (e.g., pictures of a person's home, animals, family, friends, school, neighborhood) as well as familiar sounds (e.g., the person's dog barking, voices of familiar people)

Discrimination

Discrimination refers to the ability to differentiate two or more stimuli. Wetzel and Squire (1982) indicated that discriminations are differentiations between an individual and a world of experience. Cognitive distancing (i.e., freeing an individual from direct experience to rely more on representations of experience) is based on a continuum that progresses from the discrimination of concrete to abstract items (e.g., objects to pictures to words). Discrimination skills include the visual discrimination of color, shape, and/or size followed by the discrimination of pictures, words, sentences, and situations.

Intervention should focus on gradually increasing the number and degree of similarity of stimuli. First, items that differed only in one salient feature (color, shape, or size) would be presented. The number of items would gradually be increased. Next, three items would be presented with two discriminating variables, such as color plus shape, and the number of items would gradually be increased. This process would be continued, gradually increasing the number of discriminating variables as well as the number of stimuli in the response set.

Organization

Organization refers to the ability to deal with discrete actions or components that must be grouped or sequenced according to the priority of each component, using a learned strategy. General organizational skills include *categorization, closure,* and *sequencing.* Categorization refers to the sorting of information into groups. Categorization tasks are those in which the individual is required first to identify optimal categories, then to recognize subtle differences, and finally to switch sets. Objects and pictures may be sorted according to physical attributes, meaningful units, function, and likenesses and differences. Closure refers to the completion of incomplete visual information (e.g., filling in missing parts of pictures, missing letters of words, missing words of a sentence, missing sentences of a paragraph) and the completion of incomplete aural information such as that in which sounds are presented one at a time and an individual must mentally put the sounds together to form a word. Sequencing refers to the ability to order information temporally or spatially. The process begins with sequencing according to size (e.g., smallest to largest) and color (e.g., lightest to darkest), and progresses to the sequencing of letters, words, sentences, and steps to functional activities.

Memory

Memory deficits occur due to ineffective encoding of information, inadequate storage of information, difficulty retrieving information using recognition, cued recall or free recall, and/or a lack of strategies to deal with interferences. Various types of memory play important roles in an individual's ability to function and to communicate successfully. The various types of memory include semantic memory, episodic memory, immediate recall, delayed recall, recall with interference, and long-term memory (Bellugi & Studdert-Kennedy, 1980; Marshall & Newcombe, 1980; Neisser, 1976).

Adamovich and Henderson (1982, 1984) compared 32 persons with closed head injury to persons who had sustained left and right cerebrovascular accidents and to non-brain-injured control groups. The individuals with closed head injury used fewer strategies to generate words and tended to change strategies during the task more often than all of the other experimental and control groups, possibly due to an inability to maintain attention over time.

Memory therapy should focus on the provision of compensatory strategies to cope with lasting memory difficulties. These strategies should include techniques to facilitate initial encoding of information to ensure adequate initial storage of material as well as techniques that facilitate retrieval of stored information (Geschwind, 1982; Norman, 1979; Patten, 1982). Specific internal retrieval strategies consist of the following:

1. Verbal description
2. Visual imagery
3. Chunking activities, in which information is visually or aurally organized into segments that coincide with the individual's memory span
4. Categorization or appropriate grouping of information to be recalled
5. Rehearsal, in which information to be recalled is drilled or practiced
6. Use of associations based on semantic relationships (e.g., cane-crutches and day-night), acoustic relationships (e.g., dew-shoe), or visual relationships (e.g., desk-drawer)
7. Temporal or spatial ordering, in which events in episodic and semantic memory are recalled by remembering certain landmark events associated with the event to be recalled or those that occurred at a similar point in time
8. Primacy and recency benefits, in which the first and last items have a greater chance of being recalled when compared to information presented in the middle of an information string
9. Preview-question-read-state-test (PQRST) approach

Mnemonic devices consisting of specific memory tricks used to increase associative learning through paired association may also be utilized. During encoding, new words or bits of information are chained or paired to a preestablished set of key words and phrases or a familiar sequence of known locations. This can be referred to as a peg system in which new items are "pegged" to existing items (e.g., rhyming peg: one equals bun; phonetic peg: two equals n because it has two down strokes; loci peg: items are linked to familiar locations). The substitute word system is based on linking a visual image with a word (e.g., to remember the name Cameron, visualize a *camera on* his balding head [outstanding facial feature]). The Link System (Lorayne & Lucas, 1974) links lists of items together in a funny way to facilitate retrieval (e.g., to remember bologna and milk, picture a cow eating bologna as the farmer milks it).

Generally, persons with closed head injury must learn to rely on external compensatory aids to assist memory. These include: calendars, appointment books, note pads, daily logs/diaries, memo books, lists, structure/routines, alarms to remind a person to refer to an appointment book, tape recorders that deliver sequences of instructions to be followed, and microcomputers. (The reader is referred to Chapters 12 and 19, this volume, for further discussion of memory intervention strategies.)

High-Level Thought Processing

Reasoning and problem solving require the generation of responses based on relevant information to formulate a solution to a problem that must then be checked or tested as to the appropriateness of the solution. Such high-level thought processing includes the following:

1. *Convergent thinking* This refers to the recognition and analysis of relevant and missing information in visually or aurally presented sentences, paragraphs, conversations, and stories to identify the central theme or main point. For example, if presented with the statements "Jack opened the door to his home and was greeted by a houseful of people. The room was decorated with crepe paper and balloons and on the table sat a cake with candles," the individ-

ual should identify the central theme as being a surprise birthday party for Jack.

2. *Deductive reasoning* This refers to the drawing of conclusions regarding a given situation based on premises or general principles, in a step-by-step manner. For example, given the following facts, "It does not open things, it is made of metal, it becomes hot, and it is not used in the preparation of food," the individual should be able to select the correct item: can opener, iron, toaster, blender, or coffee maker.

3. *Inductive reasoning* This involves the formulation of a solution based on details that lead to, but do not necessarily support, a standard conclusion. Inductive reasoning tasks include the formulation of antonyms and synonyms; analogous thinking; the recognition of cause-and-effect relationships; and open-ended problem solving, including story completion tasks.

4. *Divergent thinking* This involves the generation of unique abstract concepts or hypotheses that deviate from standard concepts or ideas. Divergent thinking tasks include the recognition and interpretation of homographs, idioms, absurdities, proverbs, similes and metaphors, poetry, fables, puns, jokes, and riddles.

Cognitive Characteristics of High-Level Clients with Closed Head Injury

High-level clients with closed head injury often forget appointments as well as activities completed during the previous day. Activities or tasks often are not initiated, partly due to an inability to decide what needs to be done first, second, and so forth, and partly due to an inability to get going. All or portions of conversations tend to be repeated, often several times, with no real acknowledgement that this is occurring. Generally, immediate memory is only mildly impaired, if at all, at this level. Recall after a short period of interfering activity is usually impaired. Pre-traumatic and post-traumatic amnesia (i.e., recall of events immediately prior to and following the accident) are only mildly impaired. Remote memory or recall of old information from before the injury is remarkably good. Subtle cognitive deficits of high-level clients often become apparent during group interactions. Unfamiliar situations are particularly stressful. Specific behaviors that emerge include:

1. Inability to understand the point of view of others
2. Rigidity in modifying an opinion
3. Difficulty recognizing the main point of a conversation
4. Inability to question or clarify in an attempt to gain additional information necessary to form an appropriate conclusion
5. Difficulty taking turns
6. Difficulty giving and receiving feedback
7. Concern for self-goals, causing difficulty accepting group decisions
8. Presentation of too little or excessive information
9. Difficulty switching from one topic to another
10. Lack of self-esteem and self-appraisal
11. Inability to connect short-term goals and long-term goals, such that the individuals fail to see the relevancy of therapy tasks or group activities to their life in general
12. Establishment of unrealistic individual goals and aspirations due to a denial of deficits

Group Remediation Techniques

Group therapy sessions may be useful for all levels of head-injured individuals—to provide peer support, peer review, and practice of conpensatory techniques in more natural settings. However, high-level clients, in particular, tend to benefit from group therapy that focuses on interpersonal interaction, including pragmatic skills such as situationally appropriate behavior, eye contact, and turn taking. Group therapy should also focus on social skills, empathic abilities, personal social adjustment, and life skills (e.g., shopping, utilizing public transportation, emergency skills). The impact of cognitive processes on pragmatic/functional/social behaviors and metalinguistic skills (e.g., humor, figurative language) becomes most apparent when higher functioning individuals attempt to reintegrate into their home, community, peer group, and workplace. Ongoing observations should be made in each appropriate area if behaviors interfering with integration are to be discovered and

dealt with appropriately. Therapeutic community outings are particularly valuable in preparation for real-life situations. (For further discussion of group intervention, the reader is referred to Chapter 15, this volume.)

Use of Computers

Computers can be helpful in therapy for attention, concentration/persistence, visual localization, visual scanning, visual tracking, reaction time, memory, hand-eye coordination, discrimination, and organization, and for various problem-solving tasks. Although many of these activities can be presented via workbooks, younger clients with head injury tend to enjoy using the computer and are, therefore, motivated to complete therapy activities. (For further discussion of computer-assisted intervention, the reader is referred to Chapter 13, this volume.)

LANGUAGE VERSUS COGNITION

Language disturbances secondary to diffuse brain damage following closed head injury usually stem from underlying disturbances in attention, cognition, and information processing. These disturbances differ from the linguistic deficits due to focal brain lesions typically resulting due to left cerebrovascular accidents. Language and cognition both require adequate attending skills and the ability to process information effectively. An impairment of language may impair other cognitive processes; likewise, an impairment of other cognitive processes such as the ability to discriminate, organize, and remember may impair communication (e.g., a person will not be able to convey or comprehend information if unable to remember the first part of a conversation by the time the conversation has been completed). Several theories regarding the relationship between cognition and language are described next.

Theories of Cognition and Language

Cognition Precedes Language

Some investigators feel that cognitive development is a significant determiner in the development of language (Bates, 1976; Piaget, 1962).

An example in support of this theory was provided by Clarke (1973), who suggested that the comprehension of physical space terms such as "a *long* stick" is cognitively less complex and must be acquired prior to the comprehension of temporal space terms such as "it took a *long* time."

Language Determines Thoughts and Cognition

Proponents of a second theory regard language as an important determiner of one's thoughts and cognitions. The Sapir-Whorf hypothesis (Bruner, 1975) suggests that the language an individual speaks directly determines major aspects of thought such as time. For example, a language such as English that codes verbs into tenses objectifies time as if it were a ribbon with various spaces marked off. In contrast, verbs are not coded into tenses in the Hopi language, and so, Hopi Indians have a very different concept of time. Time is important as it pertains to the pragmatic aspects of life, such as planting season, harvesting season, and so forth: Verbs simply describe these seasons or significant events.

Parallel Development of Language and Cognition

A final theory of language and cognitive development is that language and thought develop in parallel, and then merge in early childhood. Language and verbal behavior are regarded as cognitive processes (Muma, 1978). Justification of this theory includes the following examples. The developmental sequence for both concept development and naming skills are essentially the same. An object would first be identified, followed by the identification of important relationships and the identification of new concepts by noting similar, stable, and salient characteristics. Finally, a name or word would be attached to the concept. Muma (1978) suggested a similar hierarchy in the development of naming skills: 1) anticipation/reference on previous experiences, 2) object permanence/figure-ground, 3) knowledge, 4) mental imaging, 5) reversibility or lack of reliance on action of objects, 6) concept knowledge, and 7) word knowledge. Similar techniques are utilized in cognition as well as language intervention.

Additionally, both concept acquisition and linguistic acquisition require the ability to generalize information based on the presentation of meaningful and explicit feedback, the provision of direct instructions regarding strategies, and the provision of general strategies to supplement specific strategies (Meichenbaum, 1980). Both cognition and language require the reinforcing and strengthening of previously learned patterns of decision making, problem solving, and responding, or the establishment of compensatory mechanisms when functional return is not possible. The interrelation between language and other cognitive processes serves as a basis for effective communication.

Cognitive-Communicative Impairments

Cognitive-communicative impairments, or those communicative disorders that result from deficits in linguistic and nonlinguistic cognitive processes, best describe the communication problems experienced by persons with closed head injury. Head-injured persons usually fail to communicate due to generalized cognitive, information processing, and attentional factors rather than purely linguistic factors. For example, Hagen (1981, 1983) suggested that head-injured persons fail to convey meaning due to irrelevancy, confabulation, circumlocution, tangential thoughts, no logiosequential order, and general disorganization.

Sarno (1980) studied 56 persons with closed head injury postinjury for the presence and nature of verbal deficits. Subjects ranged from 3 weeks to 8 weeks postinjury, with the length of coma ranging from 10 minutes to 5 months. Three subtests of the Neurosensory Center Comprehensive Examination for Aphasia (NCCEA) (Spreen & Benton, 1969) were administered: Visual Naming, Word Fluency, and Sentence Repetition. Results suggested that all persons within the study evidenced some degree of verbal impairment. Eighteen (32%) presented with extensive lesions, the lowest word fluency scores, and classical symptoms of aphasia. Twenty-one (38%) has dysarthria, and 17 (30%) had no discernible aphasic deficits in spontaneous speech but showed clear evidence of verbal deficits on testing. Among the aphasic individuals, 39% were fluent, 38% were nonfluent, 11% were anomic, and 11% were globally impaired. Almost half of the group had focal lesions of the left hemisphere, as evidenced by right-handed subjects with right hemiplegia. There was little relationship between severe aphasia and lesion sites.

Levin, Grossman, Sarwar, and Meyers (1981) conducted a longitudinal study of persons with closed head trauma with acute aphasia. Of 12 individuals with residual language deficits, 6 showed specific language deficits and 6 had language deficits secondary to more general cognitive disturbances. The individuals who fully recovered from aphasia or who exhibited a specific language deficit were within average ranges on the Weschler Adult Intelligence Scale (WAIS) (Weschsler, 1955). Individuals with generalized language deficits had intellectual deficits on the Verbal and Performance subtests of the WAIS.

Many of the behaviors described in the literature as language deficits following closed head injury may actually be secondary to more generalized cognitive, attentional, and/or information processing problems. The distinction of linguistic versus cognitive disturbances is difficult following both generalized brain damage secondary to closed head injury and focal brain damage secondary to left cerebrovascular accidents. Resulting behaviors may be due to either linguistic or cognitive deficits. For example, confabulation, tangential speech, and perseveration are commonly reported language disturbances experienced by aphasic individuals following left cerebrovascular accidents. Yet these same behaviors occur following closed head injury, due to a cognitive disturbance such as attention deficits. Linguistic deficits may result in word-finding problems or difficulty in sequencing and/or comprehending information. However, sequencing errors may also be due to cognitive deficits, such as organizational or memory difficulties. Word-finding problems and comprehension deficits may be due to a linguistic disturbance or to memory disturbances.

In summary, head-injured individuals have predominant cognitive disturbances, which are responsible for the majority of resulting behaviors. Yet, it is possible that the extensive cognitive disturbances may mask less obvious linguistic disturbances. The reverse tends to be true for aphasic individuals with focal left hemisphere brain lesions. These individuals evidence predominant linguistic disturbances, which may mask less obvious cognitive disturbances.

ATTENTION

Attention Disturbances After Closed Head Injury

Attentional systems include arousal, activation, and effort to control attention (Pribram, 1975). After closed head injury, the manipulation of the focus of attention tends to be impaired in three basic ways: 1) initiating and sustaining attention, 2) shifting the focus of attention when appropriate, and 3) inhibiting the inappropriate shifting of the focus of attention (S.H. Auerbach, personal communication, March 14, 1984). Effort accompanies only those attentional processes that change the representational organization of the information processing mechanism or the patterned memory trace representative of an experienced stimulus. Initially, cognitive effort is due to the origin and activation/manifestation of peripheral muscular mechanisms. As problem solving progresses and problem-solving skills develop, the effort becomes more and more a concomitant of the brain processes involved apart from the peripheral manifestation, and thus becomes truly cognitive.

Geschwind (1982) referred to these attentional disturbances experienced by individuals following closed head injury as "global" disorders of attention or "confusional states." Confusional states were defined as disorders in which there is a loss of the normal coherence of thought or action. Emphasis was placed on the differentiation of these disorders from unilateral disorders of attention, which are confined to one side of space, resulting primarily in neglect of the left side of space and of the body (Geschwind, 1982). Geschwind also differentiated global disorders of attention from disorders of attention that occur due to lesions primarily within the reticular formation of the brain stem, which result in a lack of arousal or unresponsiveness to stimuli. Striking clinical features of global disorders of attention, according to Geschwind, include:

1. Loss of coherence or the disruption of the overall pattern of action or topic of discus-

sion despite the correct performance of individual fragments

2. Paramnesia or the distortion of memory resulting in incorrect answers with elements of the correct answer present (e.g., reduplicative paramnesia in which certain items are duplicated such that the hospital is regarded as a school and the therapists as teachers)
3. Propagation of errors in which items in the environment are brought into apparent coherence with an error
4. Occupational jargon such that if the hospital is identified as the place of work, people and things are given occupational labels and functions
5. Inattention to environmental stimuli or failure to use environmental information, which could result in impulsivity, inappropriate social judgment, lack of insight, literal interpretations, and impaired memory
6. Isolated or predominant disturbance of writing characterized by spatially abnormal, incorrect words; misspellings; and letters that contain multiple, perseverative loops
7. Unconcern with or denial of illness
8. Playful behavior, characterized by unintentional humor restulting from incoherent speech that appears amusing

Geschwind (1982) further stated that the striking clinical features of global attentional disorders are due to breakdowns in the following attentional systems:

1. Selectivity, or the limited handling of stimuli
2. Coherence, or the maintenance of stimuli over time
3. Distractibility, or the appropriate and inappropriate shifting of focus
4. Universality, or the registering of as many unattended stimuli (external and internal) as possible
5. Sensitivity, which depends on a person's state at a given time

Although supportive data are lacking, S.H. Auerbach (personal communication, March 14, 1984) suggested a linear relationship between the improvement of mental control or attention deficits and the improvement of cognitive or thought-processing deficits over time post–closed head injury. He used this as a basis to propose that closed head injury causes specific attentional disruptions rather than cognitive deficits. He further suggested that it is the attentional disruptions that interfere with cognitive abilities. Mental control deficits, as defined by S.H. Auerbach, clearly exist in head-injured persons. It is suggested, however, that these deficits, as well as "global" attention deficits, as defined by Geschwind (1982), exist independent of cognitive deficits. All three areas of difficulty interfere with information processing. Attentional disorders are often the focus of therapy with low-level clients (i.e., with severe impairment). The attention deficits may mask impairments in other areas such as information processing and cognition. Many different attentional skills are impaired at this low level of mental functioning, including basic arousal, ranging from sleep to wakefulness; vigilance or maintenance of attention; and selective attention to enable the integration and interpretation of information. As attentional disorders recover, many information processing and cognition deficits become apparent, and thus become the focus of therapy.

Remediation of Low-Level Attention Deficits

Initial remediation of attention deficits should focus on multimodality stimulation (e.g., tactile, visual, gustatory, oral-verbal, auditory, vestibular) to achieve reflexive responding, which is gradually brought under voluntary control. Auditory and verbal stimulation progress from the presentation of gross nonspeech sounds (e.g., bells, buzzers) to more finely discriminated speech sounds. Oral-verbal stimulation includes passive stretching and the use of facilitative exercises for increasing the range of the articulators (e.g., licking a lollipop). Tactile stimulation includes the use of hot and cold temperatures and a variety of textures. Visual stimulation begins with the use of bright lights, colors, and familiar items. Gustatory stimulation requires foods that include bitter, sour, sweet, salty, and bland flavors. Olfactory stimulation begins with strong noxious and familiar smells. Vestibular stimulation is provided during positioning and balancing activities.

Remediation of High-Level Attention Deficits

Ben-Yishay (1978) suggested that individuals must have maximum attention, concentration, and persistence to participate in verbal logical reasoning. Problem solving is impaired if adequate attention is not devoted to analyzing the stimulus, problem, or situation completely. An individual's ability or inability to direct attention is an essential determinant of the success or failure of any practical operation. As attention improves or expands, individuals become capable of reconstructing their perception and, therefore, become free from the auditory or visual field.

Higher level attention deficits tend to result in more pragmatic and interactive or interpersonal disruptions. Attentional disturbances experienced by persons with closed head injury functioning at a higher cognitive level may result in behavior that appears to be egocentric, rude, impulsive, disinhibited, denying, and lacking in coherence (i.e., information conveyed both verbally and graphically is out of sequence). Conversations tend to turn on and off, with frequent, off-the-track interjections. The off-the-track interjections often become new topics, leaving the previous topic abandoned and incomplete. Distractibility also interferes with task completion. The performance of high-level head-injured persons deteriorates when distractions occur or if they are given too much information or stimulation, causing them to become overwhelmed and unable to proceed effectively.

Tasks to test for difficulties in this area include observations of clients while performing real or simulated jobs (e.g., serving as a secretary/receptionist in the clinic or performing other jobs that require the completion of several tasks simultaneously). It should be noted that, initially, clients may tend to become flustered by distractions, which results in inaccurate telephone messages, concrete responses to questions, and what appears to be rudeness.

INFORMATION PROCESSING

Quite often, persons with closed head injury lack the skills necessary to process and give order to information. This results in difficulty interacting with the environment and learning from it (Parrill-Burnstein, 1981). Additional difficulty occurs because of an inability to assimilate and accommodate new information. Assimilation refers to the interpretation of objects and events according to a person's current way of thinking or past experiences. Accommodation refers to the revision of concepts and opinions based on new experiences.

Theories

Information processing theory most appropriate to persons with head injury refers to the analysis and synthesis of information in sequential steps. Guilford and Hoepfner (1971) suggested that there are four kinds of information that must be processed: 1) figural or concrete information, 2) symbolic or abstract information, 3) semantic or meaningful information, and 4) behavioral or pragmatic information. Information processing theorists have suggested that no matter what kind of information is being processed, various stages or steps of information processing are necessary if the information is to be learned or to become meaningful (Bates & Rankins, 1976; Greenfield, 1978; Mayer, 1981; Parrill-Burnstein, 1981; Pea, 1979). Initially, verbal information is processed in an analytical manner and visual information is processed in a holistic manner. Next, information is processed based on an internal or stored representation of the stimuli according to past experiences and prior knowledge. A stimulus is then integrated with stored information, a response is generated, the response is executed, and, based on feedback, the response is revised when necessary (Parrill-Burnstein, 1981). Mayer suggested that a stimulus progresses to the short-term sensory store, then to short-term memory/working memory, and then to long-term memory, or a response.

Parrill-Burnstein (1981) suggested that information processing during problem solving involves several stages—including reception, perception, discrimination, organization, and memory—before an individual can generate a solution to a problem, evaluate that solution using feedback or results, and generate a new solution if indicated. This model in information processing is appropriate to persons with head injury. Breakdown at any stage, due to attention and cognitive deficits, results in an inability to solve problems adequately (Adamovich et al., 1985; Bates & Rankins, 1976; Greenfield, 1978; Pea, 1979).

Intervention team members should be aware of the way in which each individual best processes information. Consideration should be given to the fact that the right hemisphere processes information in a more holistic, gestalt, or simultaneous fashion; and the left hemisphere is responsible for more analytical, linear, or sequential processing (Bever, 1975; Galin, 1974; Gazzaniga, 1979). Kirby (1980) suggested that: 1) simultaneous processing takes place in both cerebral hemispheres, with involvement of the parieto-occipital areas in verbal and nonverbal tasks; 2) successive processing takes place in the frontotemporal areas of both hemispheres; and 3) the prefrontal lobes of both hemispheres are considered to be responsible for the planning and programming of behavior after incoming information is analyzed.

Remediation Techniques

On the one hand, teaching a transfer to a person who processes best from a right hemisphere perspective should first include the presentation of the overall task (e.g., "We are now going to move from this chair to the bed") before all of the individual steps are presented. On the other hand, if left hemisphere information processing is more intact, each individual step might be given, after which the overall purpose of the activity would be stressed. Consideration of each individual's best method of processing information by all treating clinicians will provide for greater success in therapy programs. Kirby (1980) pointed out that both types of processing, perhaps in different proportions, are required in both verbal and nonverbal tasks. Individuals seem to vary in their abilities to use simultaneous or successive processing; however, the effectiveness of performance is often dependent on the ability to utilize both types and to select the appropriate mode given a particular situation.

Specific information processing intervention considerations appropriate to persons with head injury include: stimuli selected to accomplish each task, the mode of presentation of the stimuli (e.g., simultaneous versus sequential), the stimulus presentation rate, response time, and the utilization of feedback to modify responses.

SUMMARY

Cognitive processes include perception, discrimination, organization, recall, and problem solving. The affect of cognitive processing on day-to-day real-life activities can be illustrated by the task of taking a shower. The individual must recognize the task at hand, the goal of the activity, and the items to be used in the activity such as a washcloth, soap, and a towel, based on past experience. Next, the individual must be able to discriminate between these items based on physical attributes and function. Placing white soap, a white washcloth, and a white towel on a white sheet makes it difficult for the client to differentiate individual items. Using soap with unusual shapes or oversized washcloths with undersized towels would also make it difficult for clients to recognize individual items and to discriminate between the items.

Organization skills come into play with the categorization or grouping of items that go together for an activity such as showering, and the sequencing of individual steps in the correct order to complete the activity successfully. Persons with head injuries frequently have sequencing difficulties.

It is not uncommon for a client to get into a shower with his or her clothes on or to put shoes on before socks. Clients who sit all day and think about performing an activity such as taking a shower are often diagnosed as having initiation problems; frequently, however, they have sequencing deficits in which they are unable to determine what needs to be done first, second, and so on. A task such as taking a shower is overwhelming for persons who are unable to sequence multiple steps.

The cognitive processes necessary to take a shower apply in all functional activities such as brushing teeth, dressing, toileting, eating, meal preparation, and shopping. If a client is only capable of discriminating between two items, a tray of food containing seven items would be too complex and could result in frustration and agitation. Obtaining a few items from a grocery store can take hours if a client is unable to organize. A client lacking organization skills will begin at one end of the store and will search each aisle, looking at every single product until the first item on the list is located. Once an item is located, the client will go back to the first aisle and repeat the process to obtain the next item. There is frequently no recognition of organization within the store (e.g., dairy section, a produce section, a soup section).

Memory and problem-solving skills are necessary if the client is to manage a home, raise children, function in the community, and/or return to work. These skills are important determiners of the client's overall level of independence. Likewise, adequate attention is essential for the successful completion of all tasks and activities. A client's ability to progress to more demanding cognitive tasks depends on a corresponding improvement in attention.

The most effective method of information processing for each client should be determined by all clinicians. For example, some clients will learn best by experiencing an activity and others will benefit by understanding the theory. Some people process information in a step-by-step sequential fashion, which others process in an overall gestalt fashion. A client's ability to process information might be impaired if information is presented too quickly or if an adequate response time is not given. If information is not adequately processed initially, the storage of the information for later use is likely to be impaired. Also important is the use of feedback regarding the effectiveness of a response, with a corresponding modification of responses as necessary. Persons with head injury frequently experience difficulty recognizing and using feedback.

In conclusion, cognitive rehabilitation professionals should assist each client in reaching the greatest level of independence in functional activities in the home, community, and workplace. Levels of cognition, language, attention, and information processing must be a primary focus of intervention, as they will determine each client's overall level of independence in all activities.

REFERENCES

Adamovich, B.B. (1978). A comparison of the processes of memory and perception between aphasic and non-brain injured adults. In R.H. Brookshire (Ed.), *Clinical Aphasiology Conference proceedings* (pp. 327–337). Minneapolis, MN: BRK Publishers.

Adamovich, B.B., & Brooks, R. (1981). A diagnostic protocol to assess the communication deficits of patients with right hemisphere damage. In R.H. Brookshire (Ed.), *Clinical Aphasiology Conference proceedings* (pp. 244–253). Minneapolis, MN: BRK Publishers.

Adamovich, B.B., & Henderson, J.A. (1982, November). *An investigation of the cognitive changes of head trauma patients following a treatment period.* Paper presented at the American Speech-Language-Hearing Association Annual Convention, Toronto, Canada.

Adamovich, B.B., & Henderson, J. (1983, November). *Cognitive deficits post traumatic head injury: Diagnostic and treatment implications.* Paper presented at the American Speech-Language-Hearing Association Annual Convention, Cincinnati, OH.

Adamovich, B.B., & Henderson, J.A. (1984). Can we learn more from word fluency measures with aphasic, right brain injured, and closed head trauma patients? in R.H. Brookshire (Ed.), *Clinical Aphasiology Conference proceedings* (pp. 124–131). Minneapolis, MN: BRK Publishers.

Adamovich, B.B., Henderson, J.A., & Auerbach, S. (1985). *Cognitive rehabilitation of closed head injured patients.* San Diego: College-Hill Press.

Bates, E. (1976). Pragmatics and sociolinguistics in child language. In D.M. Morehead & A.E. Morehead (Eds.), *Normal and deficient child language* (pp. 79–102) Baltimore: University Park Press.

Bates, E., & Rankins, J. (1976). Morphological development in Italian: Connotation and denotation. *Journal of Child Language, 6,* 29–52.

Bellugi, U., & Studdert-Kennedy, M. (Eds.). (1980, March). *Signed and spoken language: Biological constraints on linguistic form.* Report of the Dahlem Workshop, Berlin, Germany.

Ben-Yishay, Y. (1978, June). *Working approaches to remediation of cognitive deficits in brain damaged patients* (Monograph 59). New York: New York University Medical Center, Institute of Rehabilitation Medicine, Department of Behavioral Sciences.

Bever, T.G. (1975). Cerebral asymmetrics in humans are due to the differentiation of two incompatible processes: Holistic and analytic. *Annals of the New York Academy of Sciences, 265,* 252–262.

Brooks, D. (1974). Recognition memory and head trauma. *Journal of Neurology, Neurosurgery and Psychiatry, 37,* 794–801.

Bruner, J.S. (1975). From communication to language. A psychological perspective. *Cognition, 3,* 255–287.

Clarke, H.H. (1973). Space, time semantics, and the child. In T. Moore (Ed.), *Cognitive development and acquisition of language* (pp. 27–63). New York: Academic Press.

Cognitive Rehabilitation Guidelines of Acute Hospitals, Outpatient Rehabilitation Departments, Rehabilitation Agencies, and C.O.R.F.'s (1986). *Medicare Provider Bulletin, #217.*

Galin, D. (1974). Implications for psychiatry of left and right cerebral specialization. *Archives of General Psychology, 1,* 572–583.

Gazzaniga, M. (1979). *Handbook of behavioral neurobiology: Vol. 2. Neuropsychology.* New York: Plenum.

Geschwind, H. (1982). Disorders of attention: A frontier in neuropsychology. *Philosphical Transactions of the Royal Society of London, 298,* 173–185.

Greenfield, P.M. (1978). Informativeness, presupposition, and semantic choice in single-word utterances. In N. Waterson & C. Snow (Eds.), *Development of communication: Social and pragmatic factors in language acquisition* (pp. 71–92). New York: John Wiley & Sons.

Guilford, J.P., & Hoepfner, R. (1971). *The analysis of intelligence.* New York: McGraw-Hill.

Hagen, C. (1981, January). *Diagnosis and treatment of language disorders secondary to closed head injury.* Paper presented at the Conference on Models and Techniques of Cognitive Rehabilitation, Indianapolis, IN.

Hagen, C. (1983). Language disorders secondary to closed head injury: Diagnosis and treatment. In A.L. Holland (Ed.), *Language disabilities in adults* (pp. 78–96). Boston: College-Hill Press.

Kirby, J.R. (1980). Individual differences and cognitive processes: Instructional application and methodological difficulties. In J.R. Kirby & J.B. Biggs (Eds.), *Cognition, development, and instruction* (pp. 119–139). New York: Academic Press.

Levin, H.S., Grossman, R.G., Sarwar, M., & Meyers, C.A. (1981). Linguistic recovery after closed head injury. *Brain and Language, 12,* 360–374.

Lorayne, H., & Lucas, J. (1974). *The memory book.* New York: Ballantine Books.

Mann, L., & Sabatino, D.A. (1985). *Foundations of cognitive process in remedial and special education.* Rockville, MD: Aspen.

Marshall, J.C., & Newcombe, F. (1980, March). The structuring of language by biological and neurological processes. Group report. In U. Bellugi & M. Studdert-Kennedy (Eds.), *Signed and spoken language: Biological constraints on linquistic form* (pp. 345–358). Report of the Dahlem Workshop, Berlin, Germany.

Mayer, R.E. (1981). *The promise of cognitive psychology.* San Francisco: W.H. Freeman.

Meichenbaum, D. (1980). Cognitive behavior modification with exceptional children: A promise yet unfulfilled. *Exceptional Education Quarterly, 1.*

Muma, J.R. (1978). *Language handbook: Concepts assessment and intervention.* Englewood Cliffs, NJ: Prentice-Hall.

Neisser, V. (1976). *Cognition and reality: Principles and implications of cognitive psychology.* San Francisco: W.H. Freeman.

Norman, D.A. (1979). Descriptions: An intermediate state in memory retrieval. *Cognitive Psychology, 11,* 107–123.

Parrill-Bernstein, M. (1981). *Problem solving and learning disabilities: An information processing approach.* New York: Grune & Stratton.

Patten, B.M. (1982). *Modality specific memory disorders.* New York: Neurological Institute.

Pea, R.D. (1979). Can information theory explain early word choice? *Journal of American Language, 6,* 397–410.

Piaget, J. (1962). *Play, dreams and imitation in childhood.* New York: W.W. Norton.

Pribram, K.H. (1975). Effort and the control of attention. *Psychological Review, 82*(2), 116–149.

Sarno, M.T. (1980). The nature of verbal impairment after closed head injury. *Journal of Nervous and Mental Disease, 168,* 685–692.

Shaw, R.E., & Cutting, J.E. (1980, March). Clues from an ecological theory of event perception. In U. Bellugi & M. Studdert-Kennedy (Eds.), *Signed and spoken language: Biological constraints on linguistic form* (pp. 57–83). Report of the Dahlem Workshop, Berlin, Germany.

Spreen, O., & Benton, A.L. (1969). *Neurosensory Center Comprehensive Examination of Aphasia (NCCEA): Manual of directions.* Victoria, British Columbia: University of Victoria, Neuropsychology Laboratory.

Wechsler, D. (1955). *Manual for Wechsler Adult Intelligence Scale (WAIS).* New York: Psychological Corporation.

Wetzel, C.D., & Squire, L.R. (1982). Cued recall in anterograde amnesia. *Brain and Language, 15,* 70–81.

CHAPTER 7

Pharmacological Aspects of Cognitive Function Following Traumatic Brain Injury

NATHAN D. ZASLER

Cognition is a complex phenomenon encompassing many different aspects of brain function. Whether transient or permanent, cognitive dysfunction following traumatic brain injury is generally the rule rather than the exception. Cognitive function deficits in memory and learning commonly have the greatest impact on day-to-day activities.

Much of our knowledge regarding cognitive deficits following brain injury has been derived from animal research. There is still much that is unknown. Strides are being made daily in gaining a better understanding of the neurophysiology, neuroanatomy, and neurochemistry of cognitive processes in the normal (noninjured) brain. We have just begun to gain a very preliminary understanding of aberrations in memory and learning processes after traumatic brain injury.

From a functional standpoint, the cognitive problems seen as a consequence of traumatic brain injury tend to produce problems in all aspects of daily life, potentially making even routine activities major life obstacles. As rehabilitation physicians (physiatrists) and neural scientists gain a better understanding of how to integrate their respective knowledge bases, better insight will be gained into both the potential benefits and the adverse effects of pharmacological agents on cognitive function. This chapter briefly reviews some of the advances being made in the understanding of the basic neural science aspects of cognitive functions and the potential role of pharmacotherapy in remediation of cognitive dysfunction.

NEURAL MECHANISMS OF COGNITION

Different parts of the brain make specific contributions to memory and learning. The neuroanatomical corrrelates for these cognitive processes are quite plastic, allowing for rapidly adaptable alterations in behavior in response to short-term internal and external environmental changes. Some of the phenomena that have been proposed to account for the witnessed cognitive neural plasticity include: collateral sprouting, long-term potentiation, dendritic spines formation, increased receptor density, and formation of new synapses. Brain neurons seemingly translate environmental stimuli into relatively long-lasting neurochemical changes. The collection of neural changes representing memory is commonly known as the engram. It is presently hypothesized that memory (or for that matter the engram itself) is stored in the same neural systems that participate in the perception, analysis, and processing of any learned information. The idea that information storage is localized in specific cortical areas is in contradistinction to older views that promulgated a more integrated memory storage process.

It must be remembered that learning and memory fall along a continuum, and since learning depends on information storage, all types of learning are based on memory. One must there-

This work was partly supported by Grant #H133B80029 from the National Institute on Disability and Rehabilitation Research, United States Department of Education.

fore recognize that there are multiple processes occurring concomitantly that involve integration of acquisition of information, ultra-short-term retention, short-term memory, long-term memory, and retrieval (Cowan, 1988; Rusted & Warburton, 1989). Ultimately, regardless of the exact specifics of the processes in question, the final common denominator is theorized to be biochemically medicated.

NEUROANATOMICAL CORRELATES OF COGNITION

Most of what is now known regarding memory function has been acquired secondary to knowledge garnered through the recent development of animal models of human amnesia in primates and other animals, as well as the neuroanatomical information presently available about these relevant brain regions in primates (Squire, 1986). Theory holds that the critical structures involved in memory function are the hippocampus, amygdala, and their diencephalic targets, as well as the anterior nucleus of the thalamus and the mediodorsal thalamic nucleus. Other related structures hypothesized to be involved include the mammillary nuclei, ventromedial frontal cortex, and basal forebrain. The locus ceruleus, which gives rise to a significant number of ascending activating noradrenergic fibers (which form part of the reticular activating system), and the amygdala may be important in selective attention as well.

The hippocampus, which receives input from both the amygdala and locus ceruleus, is the only subcortical structure that exhibits long-term potentiation and is additionally felt to play an integral role in human memory function. Some researchers have hypothesized that the role of the hippocampus may be to transfer short-term information into a more permanently coded long-term storage. The hippocampus has also been theorized to play a role in spatial and temporal cognitive mapping of environmental stimuli. Diencephalic damage, particularly to the inner portions of the dorsomedial, anteroventral, and pulvinar nuclei of the thalamus, as well as the mamillary bodies, have all been associated with memory impairment. The cerebral

cortex is not 100% essential for all types of learning, as different types of associative learning (e.g., operant and classical conditioning) can still occur in the absence of intact cortical function (Graff-Radford, Tranel, Van Hoesen, & Brandt, 1990; Markowitsch, 1988).

Ultimately, an accurate and detailed understanding of the integral neural mechanisms involved in the mediation of cognitive processes will be gained. For now, satisfaction must be had with the fact that our knowledge regarding these processes continues to grow at an extremely rapid rate. This explosion of knowledge should have an impact on our ability to "manipulate" aberrations in the function when they occur.

THEORETICAL NEUROCHEMICAL MEDIATORS OF COGNITIVE PROCESSES

Although single neurochemical mechanisms for cognition have been proposed, in reality, cognition is most likely a set of processes mediated via the interaction of a variety of neurochemical systems. Some of the neurochemical substrates that have been proposed to be involved in the mediation of cognitive processes (both facilitory and inhibitory) include: cholinergic, catecholaminergic, neuropeptidergic (vasopressin, thyrotropin releasing hormone [TRH], endogenous opioids, neuropeptide Y, and adrenocorticotropic hormone [ACTH], gabaminergic, and hormonal systems (Black et al., 1987; Erickson, 1990; McGaugh, 1983). Other substances (i.e., vitamin co-factors and trace metals) have also been theorized to play important roles in allowing normal neurophysiological reactions to proceed unabated (O'Shanick, 1986).

DIFFERENTIAL DIAGNOSIS OF COGNITIVE IMPAIRMENT FOLLOWING TRAUMATIC BRAIN INJURY

Before any pharmacological agent is administered in an attempt to improve cognitive function, one must first establish whether or not the individual's internal and external environments have been "maximized" and "stabilized" (O'Shanick, 1991).

The examination of the internal environment should be composed of assessing the individual's present neuromedical condition. Neuromedical issues that could present with alterations in cognitive function include: basic metabolic abberations, nutritional depletion, occult infection, neuroendocrine dysfunction, suboptimal cerebral blood flow and/or oxygenation, post-traumatic hydrocephalus, late extra-axial collections, and unrecognized post-traumatic seizure disorders. Other critical internal factors include the neuroanatomic correlates of injury elucidated via either static or dynamic imaging technologies; postinjury medical history (i.e., significant hypoxic-ischemic injury, elevated intracranial pressures); and preinjury factors such as prior brain injury, substance abuse, learning disability, or psychiatric illness.

The examination of the external environment must take into consideration the extent of "stimulation" and the cognitive-behavioral status of the individual at that particular time. It must be recognized that whether structured or not, the extent and complexity of environmental stimulation must be gauged by the individual's cognitive-behavioral profile. An individual who is highly destructible, easily irritated, or hyperaroused will do better with less stimulation than with more. An individual who tends to be at the lower end of the functional scale, or who becomes more confused in unfamiliar surroundings will perform better, cognitively speaking, when provided with more structured stimulation in a familiar environment. Many times, individuals with brain injury who are severely disabled from a physical standpoint are also assumed to be severely disabled from a cognitive standpoint; this is not always the case. In these types of individuals, cognitive performance may actually suffer secondary to inadequate environmental stimulation, sometimes close to the point of environmental sensory deprivation.

It is also critical to consider issues of aging with respect not only to the potential response of an individual to medication (Gordon & Preiksaitis, 1988) following traumatic brain injury but also to the inherent decline in learning ability and retenion of new information that is known to occur with aging. Additionally, certain situational variables appear to influence the performance of geriatric clients; specifically, older persons perform more poorly when task difficulty is high, or when complex encoding strategies or mnemonics are required.

MODIFICATION OF COGNITIVE FUNCTION VIA PHARMACOLOGICAL AGENTS

Facilitation

Many drugs have been advocated to improve memory, learning, and cognitive function in general. Disappointingly, there is as yet no "magic bullet." In all probability, this is more a reflection of the nature of the basic neurophysiological and neurochemical processes in question rather than a representation of a lack of adequate understanding on the part of researchers regarding cognitive processes. Of the agents that have been studied, the response rates have seemingly been quite variable, or the sample populations and/or experimental methodologies have been suboptimal. Ultimately, a "cognitive enhancement cocktail" combining various agents in an attempt to normalize and even maximize the neurochemical environment deemed to be most conducive to enhancement of cognitive processes may be found. At present, however, there does not appear to be one single cognitive enhancing drug (CED) that works *all* the time for *every* individual with postinjury cognitive deficits.

Neuropeptides

In recent years, there has been a fairly extensive body of literature examining the potential influence of hypothalamic and pituitary neuropeptides on learning and memory (Greidanus, van Wimersma, Jolles, & DeWied, 1985). ACTH and vasopressin analogs have been reported to improve memory and learning in numerous testing situations in several species of animals and humans. One hypothesis is that ACTH and melanocyte stimulating hormone (MSH) affect attentional and motivational processes, whereas vasopressin is more directly involved in memory processes per se. Opioids, specifically beta-endorphin and met-enkephalin, seem to have amnestic qualities that can be reversed via administration of opioid antagonists such as naloxone or naltrexone (Serby et al., 1986; Zager & Black, 1985).

The only published double-blinded, placebo-controlled study that specifically examined the utility of vasopressin in persons with traumatic brain injury found no benefit with regard to shortening the length or magnitude of post-traumatic amnesia (Reichert & Blass, 1982). Regardless of ultimate efficacy, the electrolytic effects of vasopressin on sodium homeostasis may be the limiting factor in clinical application of this cognitive enhancing drug. More recent research on the utility of TRH and vasopressin has been conducted at the University of Washington in the Department of Rehabilitation Medicine as part of the Rehabilitation Research and Training Center in Traumatic Brain Injury (Zasler, 1991b). Preliminary data seem encouraging regarding a potential role of these agents in memory enhancement, possibly mediated via cholinergic systems.

Cholinergic Agonists

Of all neurotransmitter systems proposed to play a role in memory function, the cholinergic system has without question received the most attention. Most of the work in this area emanates from research in senile dementia, Alzheimer's type (SDAT). Although the scientific literature is mixed regarding the role of cholinergic pathways in memory function, there are an increasing number of drug studies in humans and animals that suggest that pretreatment with anti-cholinergic drugs disrupts memory storage, whereas cholinergic agonists may actually produce dose-dependent facilitation or disruption. There has also been some research suggesting that a neurochemical dissociation of cholinergic memory systems exists, such that cholinergic neurotransmission is required for declarative but not procedural memory (Nissen, Knopman, & Schacter, 1987). Interestingly, there may actually be a "therapeutic window" for cholinergic agents in which beneficial effects are present at middle-range doses and are absent at low-range doses, and high doses lead to impaired cognitive function (Davis et al., 1978).

The approach to treatment of cognitive deficits referable to cholinergic system augmentation may take one of three main routes: precursor

agents such as choline or lecithin, anticholinesterases such as physostigmine or tetrahydro-aminoacridine (THA), or direct cholinergic agonists such as bethanecol or oxotremorine (Hock, 1987). There have only been a few scattered studies with rather mixed results specifically addressing the utility of cholinergic agents in persons with traumatic brain injury (Goldberg et al., 1982; Levin et al., 1986; Weinberg, Auerbach, & Moore, 1987). Tetrahydro-9-aminoacridine, a potent anticholinesterase, may be a cholinergic "drug of the future" secondary to the fact that it can be administered orally, has a relatively long half-life, and has a reasonable side-effect profile (Summers, Majovsky, Marsh, Packiki, & Kling, 1986). Although the utility of this class of agents is yet to be clarified, the pharmacological side effects and suboptimal modes of administration of many of these agents may ultimately limit their clinical usefulness (Zasler, 1991a).

Catecholaminergic Agonists

A large body of evidence indicates that catecholamines may be involved in the modulation of learning and memory. According to a number of drug studies, drugs that disrupt catecholamine systems disrupt memory storage, while catecholamine agonists produce dose-dependent facilitation or disruption. As an example, amphetamine has been shown to have no effect at low doses, improvement at restricted dosages ranges, and impairment at higher doses (Zornetzer, 1978). The major catecholaminergic neurotransmitters are norepinephrine and dopamine.

It is possible to change the net balance of neurotransmitter effects as well as turnover through the administration of agents that ultimately affect the net activity at the postsynaptic receptor site. Drugs may exert their effect by increasing release from presynaptic stores (methylphenidate), increasing production and release from the prepresynaptic vesicles (L-dopa/carbidopa), decreasing reuptake into presynaptic vesicles (nortriptyline, desipramine), or acting directly at the postsynaptic receptor site (bromocriptine) (Zasler, 1991b). Some agents, such as amantadine, may act at both the pre- and postsynaptic receptor via a variety of mechanisms to bring about their ultimate agonistic effect (Gualtieri,

Chandler, Coons, & Brown, 1989). The use of psychostimulants such as amphetamine or ritalin typically results in improved concentration and performance, a suppression of fatigue, and elevated mood. These noradrenergic drugs may also produce adverse side effects in terms of anorexia, hyptertension, tachycardia, and aberrant behavioral changes (i.e., euphoria or dysphoria).

Although there are multiple studies that have utilized catecholaminergic agonists after brain injury, very few have specifically assessed their utility for remediation of cognitive dysfunction (Gualtieri & Evans, 1988; Lal, Merbitz & Grip, 1988). One case study involving the assessment of clonidine (a central alpha-2 noradrenergic agonist) did not find any benefit to this particular pharmacological intervention (McIntyre & Gasquoine, 1989).

Nootropics and Vasoactive Agents

Nootropics are a relatively new class of central nervous system–active drugs whose functional direct impact is on the higher integrative mechanism of the brain. A few of the nootropic-like drugs that have been advocated to improve cognitive function include piracetam, etiracetam, aniracetam, pramiracetam, vincamine, dihydroergotamine, and centrophenoxine. Their chemical structures are quite different and their specific mechanisms of action are still unknown. Some of the proposed mechanisms of nootropic action include: facilitation of dopamine release, increasing acetylcholine turnover, and inhibition of alpha-adrenoreceptors (Coper & Herrmann, 1988). One study in traumatic brain injury demonstrated some beneficial effects of pramiracetam (McLean, Stanton, Cardenas, & Bergerud, 1987). Unfortunately, most of the more promising nootropic agents are still not clinically available for general use in the United States.

The beneficial effects of Hydergine, a dihydrogenated ergot alkaloid, were reviewed by McDonald (1980), who concluded that it produced some global improvement in memory tests. Interestingly, however, a recent well-controlled study using ergoloid mesylates for Alzheimer's disease failed to show any significant memory benefit (Jenike, Albert, Heller, Lo-Castro, & Gunther, 1986). There are no studies

that have specifically assessed the utility of this drug for treatment of cognitive dysfunction in persons after traumatic brain injury.

Numerous drugs aside from Hydergine have been utilized to improve cognitive function secondary to their presumptive beneficial effects on cerebrovascular blood flow. These drugs include papaverine hydrochloride, cyclanedelate, naftidrofuryl, and pentoxifylline. Although literature exists suggesting a beneficial effect of these agents in geriatric populations with concomitant "dementia" (Hock, 1987), there has been no substantial exploration of the benefits of these agents in persons with cognitive dysfunction following traumatic brain injury.

Inhibition

Given the neurochemical complexity of cognitive processes, it should not be surprising that pharmacological agents may have the potential to impair cognitive processes in both noninjured and injured brains. It is critical to remain aware of the relative risks of certain pharmacological agents in terms of their potential to impede cognitive processing.

There are basically three main classes of drugs that are felt to have the potential to interfere with cognitive functioning via their basic neurochemical mechanisms of action: Catecholaminergic antagonists, gabaminergic agonists, and cholinergic antagonists. Agents that block catecholaminergic receptor sites have been linked with deficits in attention, concentration, and memory. The main drug categories in this group are neuroleptics and antihypertensives. Neuroleptics such as haloperidol, thiothixene, and thorazine are used primarily for treatment of behavioral disturbances and act via dopaminergic blockade. Ideally, they should only be used for treatment of acute agitation and are rarely needed for long-term behavioral management. Antihypertensives such as methyldopa, propranolol, and prazosin act via noradrenergic blockade and therefore may impair cognitive function in the individual with brain injury. If at all possible, attempts should be made to avoid these agents given the availability of multiple other antihypertensives that act peripherally and are just as clinically effective (e.g., angiotensin converting enzyme [ACE] inhibitors, calcium channel blockers) (O'Shanick & Zasler, 1990).

Gabaminergic agonists have multiple potential clinical uses including: seizure management, spasticity treatment, control of aggression, and as adjuvants for procedural sedation or hypnotics. The adverse cognitive effects that have been reported with this class of drugs include: state-dependent learning, paradoxical agitation, and transient global amnesia (TGA) (Barron & Sandman, 1985; Healey, Pickens, Meisch, & McKenna, 1983). One must therefore realize that medications such as Valium, baclofen, clonazepam, lorazepam, and temazepam are not necessarily innocuous agents with regard to their potential cognitive side effects.

The association of anticholineric use and cognitive impairment is by no means foreign to most practicing physicians. The fact that antidepressants are so commonly prescribed following traumatic brain injury indicates a need for judicial use of this class of medications as well as an awareness of the relative anticholinergic potencies of specific agents (O'Shanick & Zasler, 1990). Given the fact that newer, and less anticholinergic agents, are now available (i.e., fluoxetine and trazodone), it would seem reasonable to assess the efficacy of these agents in persons with traumatic brain injury to assess their true efficacy in the treatment of organic affective disorders (Glenn & Wroblewski, 1989).

CONCLUSIONS

It should be evident from review of the information presented in this chapter that the exact mechanisms of cognitive function have yet to be clarified. Obviously, less is known about the mechanisms of cognitive dysfunction associated with brain injury regardless of the specific etiology. We do, however, have a working knowledge of some of the more basic mechanisms of cognitive function, allowing us to gain better insight into the potential benefits as well as adverse effects of particular pharmacological interventions. The future of pharmacological intervention of cognitive deficits following traumatic brain injury looks promising indeed. We must therefore continue to strive to clarify the basic neural science aspects of cognitive function, and secondarily address the aberrations that occur concomitant with traumatic brain injury.

Rehabilitationists must approach the therapy of persons with brain injury as well as the individuals themselves from a holistic perspective. One cannot attempt to address all issues regarding cognitive dysfunction after brain injury if there is not an appreciation of the potential utility of pharmacological rehabilitation with cognitive enhancing drugs.

REFERENCES

Barron J., & Sandman, C.A. (1985). Paradoxical excitement to sedative-hypnotics in mentally retarded clients. *American Journal of Mental Deficiency, 90,* 124–129.

Black, I.B., Adler, J.E., Dreyfus, C.F., Friedman, W.F., LaGamma, E.F., & Roach, A.H. (1987). Biochemistry of information storage in the nervous system. *Science, 236,* 1263–1268.

Coper, H., & Herrmann, W.M. (1988). Psychostimulants, analeptics, nootropics: An attempt to differentiate and assess drugs designed for the treatment of impaired brain functions. *Pharmacopsychiatry, 21,* 211–217.

Cowan, N. (1988). Evolving conceptions of memory storage, selective attention, and their mutual constraints within the human information-processing system. *Psychological Bulletin, 104,* 163–191.

Davis, K.L., Mohs, R.C., Tinklenberg, J.R., Pfeffer-

baum, A., Hollister, L.E., & Kopell, B.S. (1978). Physostigmine: Improvement of long-term memory processes in normal humans. *Science, 201,* 272–274.

Erickson, K.R. (1990, February). Amnestic disorders; Pathophysiology and patterns of memory dysfunction. *Western Journal of Medicine,* pp. 159–166.

Glenn, M.B., & Wroblewski, B.W. (1989). Update on pharmacology: The choice of antidepressants in depressed survivors of traumatic brain injury. *Journal of Head Trauma Rehabilitation, 4*(3), 85–88.

Goldberg, E., Gerstman, J.L., Mattis, S., Hughes, J.E., Bilder, T.M., & Sirio, C.A. (1982). Effects of cholinergic treatment on post-traumatic anterograde amnesia. *Neurology, 39,* 581.

Gordon, M., & Preiksaitis, H.G. (1988). Drugs and the aging brain, *Geriatrics, 43,* 69–78.

Graff-Radford, N.R., Tranel, D., Van Hoesen, G.W., & Brandt, J.P. (1990). Diencephalic amnesia. *Brain, 113*, 1–25.

Greidanus, Tj., van Wimersma, B., Jolles, J., & De Wied, D. (1985). Hypothalamic neuropeptides and memory. *Acta Neurochirurgica, 75*, 99–105.

Gualtieri, T., Chandler, M., Coons, T.B., & Brown, L.T. (1989) Amantadine: A new clinical profile for traumatic brain injury. *Clinical Neuropharmacology, 12*, 258–270.

Gualtieri, C.T., & Evans, R. (1988). Pharmacotherapy and the neurobehavioral sequelae of traumatic brain injury. *Brain Injury, 2*(2), 101–129.

Healey, M., Pickens, R., Meisch, R., & McKenna, T. (1983). Effects of clorazepate, diazepam, lorazepam, and placebo on human memory. *Journal of Clinical Psychiatry, 44*, 436–439.

Hock, F.J. (1987). Drug influences on learning and memory in aged animals and humans. *Neuropsychobiology, 17*, 145–160.

Jenike, M.A., Albert, M.S., Heller, H., LoCastro, S., & Gunther, J. (1986). Combination therapy with lecithin and ergoloid mesylates for Alzheimer's disease. *Journal of Clinical Psychiatry, 47*, 249–251.

Lal, S. Merbitz, C., & Grip, J. (1988). Modification of function in head-injured patients with Sinemet. *Brain Injury, 2*(3), 225–234.

Levin, H.S., Peters, B.H., Kalisky, Z., High, W.M., Laufen, A.V., Eisenberg, H.M., Morrison, D.P., & Gary, H.E. (1986). Effects of oral physostigmine and lecithin on memory and attention in closed head-injured patients. *Central Nervous System Trauma, 3*(4), 333–342.

Markowitsch, H.J. (1988). Diencephalic amnesia: A reorientation towards tracts? *Brain Research Reviews, 13*, 351–370.

McDonald, R.J. (1980). Hydergine. A review of 26 clinical studies. In J. Guski (Ed.), *Determining the effects of aging on the central nervous system* (pp. 121–138). Berlin: Schering.

McGaugh, J.L. (1983). Hormonal influences on memory, *Annual Review of Psychology, 34*, 297–323.

McIntyre, F.L., & Gasquoine, P. (1989). Effects of clonidine on post-traumatic memory deficits. *Brain Injury, 4*(2), 209–211.

McLean, A., Stanton, K., Cardenas, D., & Bergerud, D. (1987). Memory training combined with the use of oral physostigmine. *Brain Injury, 1*, 145–159.

Nissen, M.J., Knopman, D.S., & Schacter, D.L. (1987). Neurochemical dissociation of memory systems. *Neurology, 37*, 789–794.

O'Shanick, G.J. (1986). Neuropsychiatric complications in head injury. *Advanced Psychosomatic Medicine, 16*, 173–193.

O'Shanick, G.J. (1991). Cognitive function following brain injury: Pharmacologic interference and facilitation. *NeuroRehabilitation: An Interdisciplinary Journal, 1*(1), 44–49.

O'Shanick, G.J., & Zasler, N.D. (1990). Neuropsychopharmacological approaches to traumatic brain injury. In J.S. Kreutzer & P. Wehman (Eds.), *Community integration following traumatic brain injury* (pp. 15–27). Baltimore: Paul H. Brookes Publishing Co.

Reichert, W.H. & Blass, J.P. (1982). A placebo-controlled trial shows no effect of vasopressin on recovery from closed head injury. *Annals of Neurology, 12*, 390–392.

Rusted, J.M. & Warburton, D.M. (1989). Cognitive models and cholinergic drugs. *Neuropsychobiology, 21*, 31–36.

Serby, M., Resnick, R., Jordan, B., Adler, J., Corwin, J., & Rotrosen, J.P. (1986). Naltrexone and Alzheimer's disease. *Progress in Neuropsychology and Biological Psychiatry, 10*, 587–590.

Squire, L.R. (1986). Mechanisms of memory. *Science, 232*, 1612–1619.

Summers, W.K., Majovsky, L.V., Marsh, G.M., Packiki, K., & Kling, A. (1986). Oral tetrahydroaminoacridine in long-term treatment of senile dementia, Alzheimer type. *New England Journal of Medicine, 315*(20), 1241–1287.

Weinberg, R.M., Auerbach, S.H., & Moore, S. (1987). Pharmacologic treatment of cognitive deficits: A case study. *Brain Injury, 1*(1), 57–59.

Zager, E.L., & Black, P.M. (1985). Neuropeptides in human memory and learning processes. *Neurosurgery, 17*(2).

Zasler, N.D. (1991a). Advances in neuropharmacologic rehabilitation of brain dysfunction. *Brain Injury.*

Zasler, N.D. (1991b). *Medical and physical restoration research workshop, brain injury subgroup.* Presented at the National Institute on Disability and Rehabilitation Research, Washington, DC.

Zornetzer, S.R. (1978). Neurotransmitter modulation and memory: A new neuropharmacological phrenology? In M.A. Lipton, A. DiMascio, & K.F. Kilian (Eds.), *Psychopharmacology—A generation of progress* (pp. 637–649). New York: Raven Press.

CHAPTER 8

Premorbid Psychosocial Factors that Influence Cognitive Rehabilitation Following Traumatic Brain Injury

MICHAEL S. ALBERTS AND LAURENCE M. BINDER

The difficult task of cognitive rehabilitation following traumatic brain injury is further complicated in persons with a history of maladaptive psychosocial functioning. Such maladaptive functioning is characterized by a history of psychopathology, substance abuse, and attention deficit hyperactivity disorder (ADHD) or learning disabilities. The incidence of these factors in traumatically brain-injured individuals is of sufficient size to warrant attention and concern from practitioners involved in rehabilitation care. An accurate understanding of an individual's premorbid functioning serves not only as a valuable prognistic indicator for both the speed and potential of progress made in cognitive recovery from head trauma, but also as a warning of factors that might complicate rehabilitation.

DEMOGRAPHICS OF PERSONS WITH TRAUMATIC BRAIN INJURY

It is well known that certain age groups are over-represented among persons with head injury. Kraus and Nourjah (1989) pointed out that the incidence of mild head injury peaks in the 15–24-year-old age group for males, with a rate in their sample of over 300/100,000 in the population. The same age peak applies for females; however, the incidence of mild head injury for females is only one third that of males for the 15–24-year-old group. The age group of 15–29 years accounts for 62% of central nervous system trauma

due to head injury, with males in that age group heavily over-represented (e.g., Rimel, Jane, & Bonds, 1990). The young head-injured group includes a predominance of unmarried, unemployed individuals of low socioeconomic status (Barber & Webster, 1974). Automobile accidents account for the majority of severe injuries (Jennett & MacMillan, 1981).

PRE-EXISTING PSYCHOPATHOLOGY

Until recently, little valid information regarding the epidemiology of psychopathology among adolescents and young adults was available. However, Lewinsohn, Hops, Roberts, and Seeley (1988) collected data on approximately 1,000 adolescents between the ages of 14 and 18. They found that 36.5% of the sample had experienced at least one psychological disorder, at some time in their lives, that met the diagnostic criteria of the *Diagnostic and Statistical Manual of Mental Disorders (DSM-III-R)* (American Psychiatric Association, 1987). The highest rates were in the category of affective disorder (20.5%), followed by childhood/adolescent disorders (14.1%) and substance use disorders (8.6%). At the time of data collection, 9.8% of the sample were experiencing diagnosable psychopathology. Clearly, the incidence of psychopathology among this late adolescent group is of sufficient size to imply that a segment of traumatically brain-injured individuals presenting for cognitive rehabilitation will either have a history of psychopathology or will have been experiencing a psychological disorder at the time of the injury. The data from Lewinsohn's group indicated that certain factors seem to correlate with adolescent depression, in particular. These include involvement in oppositional and antisocial behaviors, suicidal ideation, and a lack of coping skills. Not only might these factors increase the probability of sustaining a head injury, they are likely to be present following an accident, in the cognitive rehabilitation therapy setting.

Other studies have confirmed that psychopathology is common prior to head injury. Malt, Myhrer, Blikra, and Hoivik (1987) studied a group of patients (predominantly young adults) recently admitted to a surgical ward following head injury and found that 37% had a diagnosable psychiatric disorder on admission and 21% had a personality disorder. In adults living in the community, the prevalence of chronic depression is 12%–15% (Scott, 1988). Epidemiological data underscore the importance of investigating premorbid psychological functioning, but such data are insufficient to determine the premorbid functioning of a specific individual. Unfortunately, it is difficult to determine the etiology of personality disturbances based on the post-trauma presentation alone. Clinicians may want to attribute all erratic or dysfunctional behavior seen in rehabilitation clients to the outcome of the injury. However, given the incidence of psychopathology in the demographically injury-prone group, caution is urged in attempting to attribute personality features to the injury alone.

A comprehensive evaluation of premorbid functioning is only possible with the cooperation of family and friends, as well as the gathering of as much objective data (e.g., results of previous psychological or intellectual testing; medical, psychiatric, or school records) as possible. The great variability of emotional changes secondary to both the physiological effects of the injury and the psychological reaction to the limitations imposed by the injury can be extremely difficult to delineate. Neuropsychological deficits can be present in persons presenting with central nervous system pathology, with depression (Roy-

Byrne, Weingartner, Bierer, Thompson, & Post, 1986), or with both.

An in-depth understanding of the client's premorbid psychological functioning can serve several purposes. First, therapy decisions can be influenced by the cause of psychological symptomatology. For example, depressive symptoms known to have originated prior to the head trauma, rather than stemming from a post-trauma syndrome, might be addressed in a way more consistent with the therapy of a physiologically non-impaired individual. Second, expectation of the duration of symptoms might also be different depending on the etiology of the symptoms. As the time course of recovery varies widely for different psychological and neuropsychological functions (Newcombe & Artiola i Fortuny, 1979), emotional changes secondary to the loss of specific neuropsychological functions could also be expected to vary considerably. As Bond (1984) eloquently stated, "It is clear that in all but the very severest injuries pre-traumatic personality traits are evident during recovery and influence the cause of post-traumatic disability" (pp. 170–171).

Lishman (1978) presented a number of case examples demonstrating the relationship of premorbid personality to post-traumatic psychological problems and the difficulty in differential diagnosis. He argued that: 1) the severity of the injury is invaluable in determining the likelihood of behavioral difficulties after trauma, 2) the injury can actualize and exaggerate premorbid traits, 3) certain post-trauma symptoms can be related to specific premorbid personality traits, and 4) current psychosocial stressors must be evaluated as an additional contributor to personality changes.

SUBSTANCE ABUSE

The epidemic of substance abuse in American society has been reflected in the incidence of drug use among young adults with head injury. A sampling of case reviews revealed the incidence of elevated blood alcohol levels to be 63% for a group of persons with mild head injury (Kraus & Nourjah, 1989) and 61% for drivers involved in motor vehicle accidents who were admitted to a hospital trauma unit (Huth, Maier, Simnowitz, & Herman, 1983). Marzuk et al. (1990) reported that 45.1% of traffic fatalities in a group of 16–30-year-olds had alcohol metabolites detected. Of this same group, 11.6% had both alcohol and cocaine metabolites detected.

An elevated blood alcohol level at the time of admission to a trauma center is not proof of alcohol abuse, but clearly there must be a high incidence of alcohol abuse in this population. Persons presenting to rehabilitation units are more likely than the general population to have either a history of substance abuse or a family history of substance abuse.

Some of the regular alcohol-abusing individuals who arrive at the rehabilitation unit could be expected to show characteristic neuropsychological deficits due to the drinking alone, particularly if they are middle-age or elderly (for a discussion of this, see Ryan & Butters, 1986). Among the commonly described deficits are problems with attention, cognitive flexibility, memory, and reasoning (Hillbom & Holm, 1986). These preexisting problems, combined with continued post-trauma alcohol use and a reduced tolerance for alcohol, create a scenario for rehabilitation failure and behavioral problems in the therapy setting. Recent reports, however, have suggested that only about half of physicians representing physical medicine and rehabilitation training programs in the United States who responded to a survey supported routine alcohol and drug screening (Rohe & DePompolo, 1985). Only 65% had a prohibition policy and only 55% routinely provided access to drug counselors. This alcohol-use tolerance by physicians is particularly striking, because the lethal combination of continued alcohol use coupled with brain trauma will reduce the chances of successful rehabilitation of cognitive deficits.

Examination of drinking patterns following the injury has revealed some interesting data. Kreutzer, Doherty, Harris, and Zasler (1989) studied a group of 87 persons with traumatic brain injury. Of this sample, 25.3% were labeled as nondrinkers prior to the injury, compared with 72.3% following the injury. The authors concluded that the number of persons who continue to drink postinjury is sizable. Other factors compound the problem of post-traumatic alcohol abuse. Not only is the issue of substance abuse rarely confronted, but more than 50% of the rehabilitation physicians responding to a survey stated that there were appropriate reasons for ordering alcohol for an inpatient, including vasodilation, appetite stimulation, and increased socialization (Rohe & DePompolo, 1985).

Therefore, drinking behavior among cognitive rehabilitation clients must be addressed as an issue of considerable importance. This necessitates encouraging and allowing access to substance abuse intervention as soon as the individual is cognitively able to participate in a therapy program. This is critical because, as Kreutzer and Harris (1990) noted, when the drinking rehabilitation clients improve, they may find themselves relatively unsupervised, with available transportation and a sizable cash source.

Decreased alcohol consumption following traumatic brain injury and cognitive rehabilitation is likely a significant intermediate step toward reducing the repetition of behaviors that lead to additional injury. The great increase in abstinence from alcohol following brain injury is encouraging (Kreutzer et al., 1989).

LEARNING DISABILITIES AND ATTENTION DEFICIT HYPERACTIVITY DISORDER

The goal of cognitive rehabilitation is to help the client regain the most substantial level of functioning possible. Many intervening variables come into play that may limit the return to function. Among these variables are the severity of the injury, social and emotional support, and the motivation of the client. Ideally, fully recovered functioning in the cognitive, social, and psychological domains is the goal of the cognitive rehabilitation therapy team.

Additionally, it must be recognized that a significant number of individuals with brain trauma were functioning below the median level of intellectual functioning for the population, prior to their injury. Only recently has it been recognized that a history of learning disability is associated with increased risk for traumatic brain injury. Haas, Cope, and Hall (1987) studied 80 persons admitted to an acute care rehabilitation unit following blunt traumatic head injury. Over 44% of those born after 1952 (the date at which learning disability became widely recognized within the educational system), for whom records were available, had poor premorbid academic performance.

Factors hypothesized as explaining the link between premorbid learning disabilities and increased incidence of head injury include the continued presence of the primary symptoms of learning disabilities (distractibility, short attention span), poor frustration tolerance, and generalized neuropsychological dysfunction impairing the ability to process information in a manner that would aid in avoiding accidents (Haas et al., 1987). Some evidence suggests that individuals with learning disabilities are thought to be at greater risk for other lifelong difficulties such as delinquency and emotional disorders, and to end up in lower socioeconomic occupations. An analysis of 18 studies of long-term outcome of learning disabilities reported that 12 of 18 studies showed such unfavorable outcomes (Schonhaut & Satz, 1983). Each of these outcomes alone can be highly problematic, even in the absence of traumatic brain injury.

A generalized deficit in a broad range of neuropsychological functioning (using the Halstead-Reitan Neuropsychological Test Battery [Reitan & Wolfson, 1985] and the Wide Range Achievement Test–Revised [WRAT-R] [Jastak & Wilkinson, 1984]) in individuals with learning disabilities as compared to normals has been supported by controlled research (O'Donnell, Kurtz, & Ramanaiah, 1983). Generally, individuals with learning disabilities do better on neuropsychological tests than individuals with brain injury, but worse than normals (Orsini, Van Gorp, & Boone, 1988).

Because both the rate of progress and upper limit of functioning during rehabilitation will be influenced by premorbid intellectual ability in addition to injury factors, it is imperative that knowledge of premorbid functioning be available to the therapy team. This is best gained by careful gathering of documented information

such as school transcripts and results of previously administered standardized tests. Clinical lore has suggested that such methods as using the highest subtest score from the Wechsler Adult Intelligence Scale–Revised (WAIS-R) (Wechsler, 1981) as an indicator of premorbid ability is adequate. However, follow-up analysis of the WAIS-R standardization sample (made up of persons with no known history of brain injury) indicated that the mean intersubtest scatter was 6.7 (Matarazzo & Prifitera, 1989). This datum, showing a mean range from highest to lowest subtest score of more than two standard deviations, proved that the assumption that the highest subtest score is a reliable measure of premorbid intelligence is erroneous. Other methods of premorbid intellectual functioning estimation have been devised. Such methods include the use of regression equations that take advantage of a variety of demographic characteristics to predict premorbid intelligence (Barona & Chastain, 1986). Clearly, these will not identify individuals with learning disabilities who are of average intelligence.

An additional difficulty in assessing premorbid learning disability is the frequent comorbidity of attention deficit hyperactivity disorder. The cardinal symptoms of this disorder in children are persistent attentional difficulties (being unable to sustain attention to information during classroom activities) and impulsivity. Epidemiological information supports an incidence rate for ADHD of 3%–4% of school-age children (Wender, 1987), with a sex ratio of 5:1, males to females. Higher estimates of prevalence have been made depending on the diagnostic criteria used. Some researchers have considered ADHD a symptom rather than a diagnosis, seeing ADHD as a cluster of behaviors representing a variety of organic and environmental etiologies (Frances & Jensen, 1985). Although no conclusive etiological theory has been accepted, various studies have supported a genetic component to ADHD (Safer, 1973). Morrison and Stewart (1973) compared adoptive and biological parents of hyperactive children, and found that the biological parents had a higher incidence of alcoholism, antisocial personalities, and hysteria.

The most compelling factor to warrant concern about ADHD in traumatically brain-injured individuals is the persistence of the syndrome into adolescence and adulthood. Various studies have reported continued poor academic performance. For example, Weiss, Hechtman, Perlman, Hopkins, and Wener (1979) found continued difficulty with restlessness, impulsivity, and academic performance more prevalent in a group of adults formerly diagnosed with hyperactivity as children, than in controls. Gittelman, Mannuzza, Shenker, and Bonagura (1985) conducted a longitudinal study of 101 males in late adolescence or early adulthood who had been diagnosed with hyperactivity as children, and reviewed 15 follow-up studies of children diagnosed with hyperactivity. Gittelman's group (1985) found ADHD, conduct disorder (including antisocial disorder), and substance abuse disorder significantly more prevalent in the former client group than in the control group. Of the therapy group, 28% had admitted to being dysfunctional at some time because of alcohol or drug use and 45% had a history of conduct disorder (as compared to 16% of the controls). A significant comorbidity of conduct disorder and substance abuse disorder was noted. Formerly hyperactive children were twice as likely to be arrested and nine times as likely to be incarcerated as controls (Manuzza, Klein, Konig, & Giampino, 1989).

Because of the comorbidity of substance abuse disorders, conduct disorders, learning disabilities, and ADHD, adults with a history of diagnosed ADHD probably have a greater risk of traumatic brain injury than the general population. Furthermore, the residual symptoms of adult ADHD (inability to sustain attention, persistent hyperkinetic motor activity, affective liability, short temper, and impulsivity) are easily confused with the symptom cluster following traumatic brain injury. There is little or no evidence suggesting that cognitive rehabilitation is an effective means of reducing symptom manifestation in individuals with ADHD, but methylphenidate may be effective (Wender, Reimherr, Wood, & Ward, 1985).

For this reason, it is imperative that the clinician understand the nature of the syndrome with which he or she is dealing. For ADHD, the information required to establish a premorbid diagnosis is more difficult to obtain than other syndromes. School records, particularly elementary school records, are helpful. However, the clinician must look beyond the grade reports to the observations and subjective comments of teachers. Documentation of frequent reprimands or remedial instructions for behavior problems within the classroom is often found in children with ADHD. Retrospective diagnosis through structured interviews with a parent might also aid in documentation (Wender et al., 1985).

CASE REPORTS

The data in Table 8.1 are from two individuals with a history of a severe head trauma and one individual with no history of trauma or other neurological disease. Case 1, a 47-year-old male with no adverse neurological history and 12 years of education, performed poorly on the Wide Range Achievement Test–Revised (Jastak & Wilkinson, 1984), particularly in the areas of reading and spelling. Such a profile is typical of an individual with a developmental learning disability. This client was referred for neuropsychological evaluation because of chronic problems performing job tasks that required written work. Other testing showed poor verbal memory, difficulty with copying a complex drawing, and mildly perseverative thinking.

Case 2, a 39-year-old woman with 14 years of education, was referred for evaluation of possible sequelae 1 year after traumatic brain injury that resulted in a large intracerebral hemorrhage that resolved spontaneously with time. The data in Table 8.1 and other testing data showed very close to normal neuropsychological abilities. Neither she nor her husband reported any residual problems in daily functioning. She was working full time in her preinjury capacity. She did have subtle neuropsychological deficits, shown by testing data not listed in Table 8.1.

Case 3, an 18-year-old woman with 9 years of education, was also referred because of a previous intracerebral hemorrhage. However, her traumatic brain injury was less severe than Case 2 as judged by the size of the abnormali-

Table 8.1.   Selected neuropsychological data from three cases

Test	Scores		
	Case 1	Case 2	Case 3
Wechsler Adult Intelligence Scale–Revised			
Information	7	12	3
Digit Span	8	14	9
Vocabulary	5	13	5
Arithmetic	7	10	6
Comprehension	7	14	5
Similarities	6	14	5
Picture Completion	6	12	9
Picture Arrangement	12	13	7
Block Design	6	12	10
Object Assembly	11	11	9
Digit Symbol	8	12	9
Verbal IQ	84	117	77
Performance IQ	101	118	82
Full Scale IQ	89	118	82
Wisconsin Card Sort Test			
Perseverative responses	30	N/A	34
Categories	4		5
Trail Making Test: Parts A and B	27/94″	23/77″	34/68″
Complex Figure Test			
Copy	25	34	34
Auditory Verbal Learning Test	6,6,7,6,8,(5),4		5,8,11,10,10,(5),7
Recognition	9, 10 errors	N/A	11, 3 errors
Wide Range Achievement Test–Revised[a]			
Reading	1	N/A	3
Spelling	1		3
Arithmetic	10		1

[a]Percentiles are listed.

Sources of tests: Auditory Verbal Learning Test (AVLT) (Rey, 1964; Taylor, 1959); Complex Figure Test (Osterrieth, 1944; Rey, 1941; Taylor, 1959); Trail Making Test: Parts A and B (Reitan, 1958); Wechsler Adult Intelligence Scale–Revised (WISC-R) (Wechsler, 1981); Wide Range Achievement Test–Revised (WRAT-R) (Jastak & Wilkinson, 1984); Wisconsin Card Sort Test (Heaton, 1981).

ties shown on computerized axial tomography acutely, and the duration of severe confusion (post-traumatic amnesia) following the trauma. The test score deficits of Case 3 are worse than Case 2 because of preexisting educational deficiencies suggested by the limited duration of her educational experience and her current academic achievement. She was unemployed and not attending school, just as she was before her injury. Reading recognition, in particular, should be relatively unaffected by a traumatic brain in-

jury producing neither visual impairment nor language disturbance. The low reading score of Case 3 provided a strong psychometric clue to lifelong learning problems.

These three cases clearly illustrate that the examination of testing data alone is insufficient to assess premorbid functioning. A baseline level of neuropsychological abilities must be derived from all available information, including reports of academic achievement, psychopathology, substance abuse, and learning disabilities in order to provide a context for understanding postinjury abilities.

CONCLUSIONS

The prevalence of the premorbid syndromes of psychopathology, substance abuse, learning disabilities, and ADHD among head-injured individuals, and their possible influence on behavioral manifestations following head injury, warrant a thorough investigation of each individual's premorbid status prior to decision making regarding cognitive rehabilitation therapy. Although this task may be time-consuming, the information derived can have a marked impact on the focus of therapy and the expected results. Based on their experience, the authors of this chapter recommend that the following procedures be carried out with all clients at the onset of cognitive rehabilitation:

1. *Academic transcripts and records of standardized tests should be obtained.* These "hard data" provide valuable insights into the client's lifelong level of academic functioning. Such data are also frequently a measure of potential for recovery that clearly outlines deficits in particular areas of school performance. Results from standardized academic tests are often translated into IQ scores that are moderately correlated with the psychologist's commonly used instruments. Transcripts are the most reliable baseline information available.

2. *Extensive information about the client's premorbid functioning should be gathered from family or other available collaterals.* Particularly valuable information includes the client's drinking/drug use. Evidence cited earlier in this chapter supports the hypothesis that persons with substance abuse problems will not succeed in cognitive rehabilitation unless their substance abuse problems are dealt with first. For that reason, all persons presenting to the emergency room following traumatic head injury should have a blood alcohol level drawn and a urine drug screen. Those individuals with positive results are particularly suspect for drug and alcohol problems, and should be further evaluated.

Drug and alcohol therapy resources should be available to patients in the rehabilitation unit. Close cooperation between these two hospital services can expedite the process of helping the rehabilitation patients deal with their drug/alcohol use, thereby reducing the risk of subsequent accidents and head trauma.

Other important information obtained from the family includes the head-injured individual's daily functioning, with a particular interest in indicators of psychopathology. A history of legal problems, conduct disorder, or depression can provide a helpful perspective in understanding the client's behavior following head trauma. It may also signal the need for a mental health clinician to become involved in therapy.

3. *The nature of the accident should be well documented.* Was the individual engaging in characteristic behaviors (an assault associated with alcohol use, reckless driving, or driving with excessive speed)? Was the accident a suicide attempt (either subtle or overt)? This information can provide valuable hypotheses regarding the premorbid functioning of the individual. If the hypotheses are confirmed through other data, the clinical insights will aid in developing accurate expectancies of behavior during rehabilitation and beyond.

The difficult work of rehabilitation and the process of recovery from traumatic brain injury can be assisted immeasurably by an accurate picture of the individual's premorbid functioning.

REFERENCES

American Psychiatric Association. (1987). *Diagnostic and statistical manual of mental disorders* (3rd ed., rev.). Washington, DC: Author.

Barber, J.B., & Webster, J.C. (1974). Head injuries: A review of 150 cases. *Journal of the National Medical Association, 66*(3), 201–204.

Barona, A., & Chastain, R.L. (1986). An improved estimate of premorbid IQ for blacks and whites on the WAIS-R. *International Journal of Clinical Neuropsychology, 8,* 169–173.

Bond, M.R. (1984). The psychiatry of closed head injury. In N. Brooks (Ed.), *Closed head injury* (pp. 148–177). New York: Oxford University Press.

Frances, A., & Jensen, P.S. (1985). Separating psychological factors from brain trauma in treating a hyperactive child. *Hospital and Community Psychiatry, 36*(7), 711–713.

Gittelman, R., Mannuzza, S., Shenker, R., & Bonagura, N. (1985). Hyperactive boys almost grown up. *Archives of General Psychiatry, 42,* 937–947.

Haas, J.F., Cope, D.N., & Hall, K. (1987). Premorbid prevalence of poor academic performance in severe head injury. *Journal of Neurology, Neurosurgery, and Psychiatry, 50,* 52–56.

Heaton, R.K. (1981). *Wisconsin Card Sort Test manual.* Odessa, CA: Psychological Assessment Resources.

Hillbom, M., & Holm, L. (1986). Contribution of traumatic head injury to neuropsychological deficits in alcoholics. *Journal of Neurology, Neurosurgery, and Psychiatry, 49,* 1348–1353.

Huth, J., Maier, R., Simnowitz, D., & Herman, C. (1983). Effect of acute ethanolism on the hospital course and outcome of injured automobile drivers. *Journal of Trauma, 23,* 494–498.

Jastak, S., & Wilkinson, G.S. (1984). *Wide Range Achievement Test.* Wilmington, DE: Jastak Associates.

Jennett, B., & MacMillan, R. (1981). Epidemiology of head injury. *British Medical Journal, 282,* 101–104.

Kraus, J.F., & Nourjah, P. (1989). The epidemiology of mild head injury. In H.S. Levin, H.M. Eisenberg, & A.L. Benton (Eds.), *Mild head injury* (pp. 8–22). New York: Oxford University Press.

Kreutzer, J.S., Doherty, K.R., Harris, J.A., & Zasler, N.D. (1989). *Alcohol use among persons with traumatic brain injury.* Manuscript submitted for publication.

Kreutzer, J.S., & Harris, J.A. (1990). *Model systems of treatment for alcohol abuse following traumatic brain injury.* Manuscript submitted for publication.

Lewinsohn, P.M., Hops, H., Roberts, R., & Seeley, J.R. (1988, November). *Adolescent depression: Prevalence and psychosocial aspects.* Paper presented at the annual meeting of the American Public Health Association, Boston.

Lishman, W.A. (1978). Psychiatric sequelae of head injuries: Problems in diagnosis. *Journal of the Irish Medical Association, 71,* 306–314.

Malt, U., Myhrer, T., Blikra, G., & Hoivik, B. (1987). Psychopathology and accidental injuries. *Acta Psychiatrica Scandanavia, 76,* 261–271.

Manuzza, S., Klein, R.G., Konig, P.H., & Giampino, T.L. (1989). Hyperactive boys almost grown up: IV. Criminality and its relationship to psychiatric status. *Archives of General Psychiatry, 46,* 1073–1079.

Marzuk, P.M., Tardiff, K., Leon, A.C., Stajic, M., Morgan, E.B., & Mann, J.J. (1990). Prevalence of recent cocaine use among motor vehicle fatalities in New York City. *Journal of the American Medical Association, 263*(2), 250–256.

Matarazzo, J.D., & Prifitera, A. (1989). Subtest scatter and premorbid intelligence: Lessons from the WAIS-R standardization sample. *Psychological Assessment: A Journal of Consulting and Clinical Psychology, 1,* 186–191.

Morrision, J.R., & Stewart, M.A. (1973). The psychiatric status of the legal families of adopted hyperactive children. *Archives of General Psychiatry, 28,* 888–891.

Newcombe, F., & Artiola i Fortuny, A. (1979). Problems and perspectives in the evaluation of psychological deficits after cerebral lesions. *International Journal of Rehabilitation Medicine, 1,* 182–192.

O'Donnell, J.P., Kurtz, J., & Ramanaiah, N.V. (1983). Neuropsychological test findings for normal, learning-disabled, and brain-damaged young adults. *Journal of Consulting and Clinical Psychology, 51,* 726–729.

Orsini, D.L., Van Gorp, W.G., & Boone, K.B. (1988). *The neuropsychology casebook.* New York: Springer-Verlag.

Osterrieth, P.A. (1944). Le Test de Copie d'une Figure Complexe [The Complex Figure Copy Test]. *Archives de Psychologie, 30,* 206–356.

Reitan, R.M. (1958). Validity of the Trail Making Test as an indication of organic brain damage. *Perceptual and Motor Skills, 8,* 271–276.

Reitan, R.M., & Wolfson, D. (1985). *The Halstead-Reitan Neuropsychological Test Battery.* Tucson, AZ: Neuropsychology Press.

Rey, A. (1941). L'examen psychologique dans les cas d'encephalopathie traumatique [The psychological examination for head injury]. *Archives de Psychologie, 28,* 286–340.

Rey, A. (1964). *L'examen clinique en psychologie* [The clinical examination in psychology]. Paris: Presses Universitaries de France.

Rimel, R.W., Jane, J.A., & Bond, M.R. (1990). Characteristics of the head injured patient. In M. Rosenthal, E.R. Griffith, M.R. Bond, & J.D. Miller (Eds.), *Rehabilitation of the adult and child with traumatic brain injury* (pp. 8–16). Philadelphia: F.A. Davis.

Rohe, D.E., & DePompolo, R.W. (1985). Substance abuse policies in rehabilitation medicine departments. *Archives of Physical Medicine and Rehabilitation, 66,* 701–703.

Roy-Byrne, P.P., Weingartner, H., Bierer, L.M., Thompson, K., & Post, R.M. (1986). Effortful and automatic cognitive processes in depression. *Archives of General Psychiatry, 43,* 265–267.

Ryan, C., & Butters, N. (1986). The neuropsychology of alcoholism. In D. Wedding, A.M. Horton, & J. Webster (Eds.), *The neuropsychology handbook* (pp. 376–409). New York: Springer.

Safer, D.J. (1973). A familial factor in minimal brain dysfunction. *Behavior Genetics, 3,* 175–186.

Schonhaut, S., & Satz, P. (1983). Prognosis for children with learning disabilities: A review of follow-up studies. In M.P. Rutter (Ed.), *Developmental neuropsychiatry* (pp. 542–563). New York: Guilford Press.

Scott, J. (1988). Chronic depression. *British Journal of Psychiatry, 153*, 287–297.

Taylor, E.M. (1959). *The appraisal of children with cerebral deficits.* Cambridge, MA: Harvard University Press.

Wechsler, D. (1981). *Wechsler Adult Intelligence Scale–Revised manual.* New York: Psychological Corporation.

Weiss, G., Hechtman, L., Perlman, T., Hopkins, J., & Wener, A. (1979). Hyperactives as young adults: A controlled prospective 10-year follow-up of 75 children. *Archives of General Psychiatry, 36*, 675–681.

Wender, P.H. (1987). *The hyperactive child, adolescent, and adult: Attention deficit disorder through the lifespan.* New York: Oxford University Press.

Wender, P.H., Reimherr, F.W., Wood, D., & Ward, M. (1985). A controlled study of methylphenidate in the treatment of attention deficit disorder, residual type, in adults. *American Journal of Psychiatry, 142*, 547–552.

CHAPTER 9

Overcoming Obstacles in Cognitive Rehabilitation of Persons with Severe Traumatic Brain Injury

ROBERT J. SBORDONE

Approximately 9.75 million people in the United States sustain some form of head trauma each year. Approximately one quarter of these injuries include skull fractures and intracranial injuries, resulting in long-lasting and often permanent alterations in cognitive, emotional, and behavioral functioning (Cooper, 1982). While rehabilitation programs for persons with traumatic brain injury have traditionally been geared toward physical recovery, there has been a growing effort to improve cognitive functioning through what has often been rather loosely referred to as *cognitive rehabilitation*. Unfortunately, cognitive rehabilitation is a difficult process that involves overcoming a number of difficult obstacles. This chapter examines these obstacles and discusses techniques to overcome them.

POOR UNDERSTANDING OF BRAIN-BEHAVIOR RELATIONSHIPS

The first obstacle is that the relationship between damage to specific brain sites and alterations in behavior has not been well understood among rehabilitation professionals. Alexander (1984) reported that postmortem computerized axial tomography (CT) studies of cerebral contusions show a strong predilection for the orbital frontal and inferior temporal areas of the brain. He emphasized that injury to the orbital frontal lobe produced powerful effects on personality, and on social and emotional functioning. Cummings

(1985) reported that injury to the orbital frontal regions will typically result in a pattern of disinhibition in which the following problems will frequently be exhibited: inappropriate social comments, inappropriate or antisocial behaviors, evidence of marked personality change, poor judgment and insight, and an inability to regulate his or her emotions. Injury to the frontal convexity region will typically produce a pattern of apathy that is often accompanied by brief angry or aggressive outbursts. Injury to the medial regions of the frontal lobe will often typically result in an akinetic mute state, characterized by a lack of spontaneous movement, lack of verbalization, and failure to respond to orally presented commands. As a consequence, traumatically brain-injured individuals with frontal lobe disorder are often perceived as depressed or poorly motivated and are thus referred to mental health professionals, who often do not recognize their frontal lobe disorder and instead treat them with psychotherapy or psychotropic medications.

Lishman (1968) reviewed the relationship between the location of the brain injury and resulting psychiatric and emotional problems. He found that left hemisphere injuries are more likely to produce psychiatric disability than right hemisphere injuries, although persons with right frontal lobe injuries were more likely to have psychiatric problems than those with left frontal lobe injuries. He also pointed out that temporal lobe injuries are more likely to produce psychi-

Part of this paper was presented at a symposium on cognitive rehabilitation in Richmond, Virginia, on September 17, 1988.

atric disability than frontal, parietal, or occipital injuries. This association was greatest when injuries occurred to the left temporal lobe. Other investigators (e.g., Bach-Y-Rita, Lion, Climent, & Ervin, 1971) have reported that several months after injury, persons with prominent temporal lobe injuries will often develop brief, sudden, violent or destructive outbursts of temper after minor provocations, followed by emotional distress and remorse.

PESSIMISTIC PROGNOSIS OF RECOVERY

The second obstacle is the widely held belief that most of the recovery following head injury occurs within the first 6 months, and that virtually all the recovery occurs within 1–2 years postinjury. This belief is based on the conclusions of Bond (1975) and Bond and Brooks (1976), who assessed the recovery of persons who had sustained severe traumatic brain injury. Sbordone (1987) strongly criticized these studies and raised a number of methodological issues that were ignored by those authors. For example, neither study used a representative sample of persons with brain injury (i.e., the individuals used in both studies had been referred for neurosurgical treatment). Both studies based their findings entirely on the Wechsler Adult Intelligence Scale–Revised (WAIS-R) (Wechsler, 1981) IQ test scores. The authors did not report the premorbid IQ scores of their subjects and failed to utilize suitable control groups. They also ignored the possible influence of such factors as age, gender, education or employment status, medications, or physical disability. The authors also failed to consider the disruptive effects of depression or other psychiatric problems on the cognitive functioning of their subjects, which may have adversely affected their cognitive performance on the WAIS.

A number of investigators have reported data that strongly contradict the conclusions of Bond (1975) and Bond and Brooks (1976). For example, Miller and Stern (1965) followed 100 consecutive cases of head injury. Ninety-two persons with head injury were reexamined on an average of 11 years postinjury, and the quality of their recovery was assessed. Only 10 of the 92 showed evidence of persistent dementia, and only 5 of the 92 remained unemployed. Although the majority of these persons ($n = 77$) had sustained severe brain injury, half ($n = 38$) had returned to their previous occupational status. Of these individuals, 28 out of the 38 (73.7%) had returned to work, even though their physicians, who evaluated them on the average of 3 years postinjury, had expressed serious doubt that they would ever be able to work again. Klonoff, Low, and Clark (1977) reported that 76.3% of brain-injured children and adolescents made a marked recovery over a 5-year follow-up period. These investigators found a significant improvement between follow-up years 4 and 5. They also found that neurological measures, such as the electroencephalogram (EEG), improved throughout the entire 5-year follow-up study. Thomsen (1981) described a 44-year-old male who sustained a very severe brain injury that resulted in severe cognitive impairments at 2 years postinjury, including global aphasia, frontal lobe dysfunction, and disinhibition. She reported that at 12 years postinjury, her client exhibited only mild cognitive problems. More recently, Sbordone (1990) reported on 20 persons who had sustained severe traumatic brain injury an average of 9.8 years earlier. He found that detailed questionnaires and lengthy interviews held with at least two significant others and the brain-injured individuals revealed significant improvement in cognitive, motor, emotional, behavioral, and social functioning after 1 year postinjury, which continued at roughly the same rate over the next 8.8 years.

SECONDARY AFFECTIVE DISTURBANCES

The third obstacle is secondary affective disturbances. The author has found that at least two different types of affective disturbances can occur in persons who sustain brain injury. The first type was reported by Sbordone (1985), and is described as an "atypical bipolar depression" that frequently follows right frontotemporal lobe or diencephalic injuries and consists of a manic and a depressive phase, each lasting for 1–2 days, which alternate and tend to exacerbate in sever-

ity over time. However, most affective disturbances subsequent to brain injury fall under the
second type, which can be more directly ascribed
to a variety of psychosocial factors (Sbordone,
1987). Factors that affect the psychological functioning of persons with brain injury are:

Alcohol
Comparison to premorbid level of functioning
Condemnation of family
Depression
Drugs
Egocentricity
Failure
Family pressures
Fatigue
Frequent criticisms
Guilt
Inability to work
Infantilization by others
Limited awareness of deficits
Litigation
Loss of hope
Loss of mastery over environment
Loss of social contact
Nervousness
Overdependency on others
Pessimistic predictions of recovery
Poor self-image
Psychotropic medications
Social difficulties
Stress
Suicidal ideation
Unrealistic expectations
Use of disability to control others

As a consequence of brain injury, the problem-solving and emotional coping skills of the
individual are markedly diminished. Thus, persons with traumatic brain injury can become easily upset and frustrated. As a result of diminished
coping skills, they are more likely to become
nervous or depressed. As a result of frequent un-
fair comparisons between their present and premorbid levels of intellectual functioning, they
are likely to see themselves as impaired. As their
awareness of their cognitive deficits increases
with time, which parallels their improving cognitive functioning, they are likely to perceive

themselves as getting worse rather than improving. Unfortunately, very few brain-injured persons possess an adequate understanding of their
injury and the recovery process.

Many brain-injured persons set unrealisti-
cally high expectations of recovery. Some of
this, of course, may reflect the severity of their
brain injury, while in other cases it may also reflect the unrealistic expectations of their families
and significant others. Most persons with traumatic brain injury receive pressure from their
families and significant others to behave at their
premorbid level of functioning. Their failure to
behave at this level may invite harsh criticisms.
Because of a combination of pressure from families and significant others and limited awareness
of their cognitive deficits, these persons are
likely to return to work or school prematurely.
The author has found that approximately 95% of
the brain-injured persons who return prematurely to school or work encounter significant
problems, which often result in their termination
from work or in severe academic difficulties.
When this occurs, they will frequently lose status within their families and the respect of others
(Sbordone, 1987).

The overwhelming majority of brain-injured
individuals have been told by their physicians
and/or rehabilitation professionals that they will
continue to recover for up to 1 or 2 years postinjury. While this prospect may sound encouraging during the acute stages of recovery, it has a
devastating impact when the "recovery period"
elapses. Many traumatically brain-injured individuals become severely depressed when the 1-
or 2-year period of recovery lapses, and often experience suicidal thoughts.

RELATIONSHIP
BETWEEN COGNITIVE
AND EMOTIONAL FUNCTIONING

The fourth obstacle is the assumption that cognitive and emotional functioning are unrelated.
Rehabilitation professionals working with traumatically brain-injured clients must understand the
principles of a conditional neurological lesion
(Sbordone, 1987, 1988). This principle argues

that the behavioral manifestations of a neurological insult, such as a brain injury, are a function of the degree to which the individual is under stress, fatigue, emotional distress, or excessive metabolic demands. This principle predicts that the cognitive functioning of persons with brain injury is likely to diminish significantly whenever they become depressed, anxious, or exposed to stress. For example, a number of authors have reported that depression can exaggerate or even introduce cognitive impairment on a variety of neuropsychological tests (e.g., Fisher, Sweet, & Pfaelzer-Smith, 1986). Since the majority of persons with traumatic brain injury become significantly depressed and anxious between 6 and 12 months postinjury (Lezak, 1987; Sbordone, 1987, 1988), it is important to recognize factors that can significantly interfere with their functioning.

Psychometric tests such as the Wechsler Adult Intelligence Scale–Revised (Wechsler, 1981) tend to be, in this author's experience, particularly sensitive to emotional factors. Other psychometric tests, however, may be less sensitive. For example, Sbordone (1987) described a 51-year-old male who sustained a closed head injury that resulted in 3 days of coma and a post-traumatic amnesia of 12 days. When the client was tested at 6 months postinjury, he obtained a Full Scale WAIS-R IQ of 97 with a Verbal IQ of 106 and a Performance IQ of 78. When retested at 1 year postinjury, the client's Full Scale IQ dropped to 90. Most of this was due to a 13-point drop from his previous Verbal IQ score and more specifically on subtests that tended to be particularly sensitive to emotional factors, such as Digit Span, Arithmetic, and Comprehension. Little change was seen on Performance subtests. On the basis of these test results, one might conclude that this client's cognitive functioning had worsened or failed to improve. However, when his performance on neuropsychological tests such as the Wisconsin Card Sorting Test (Heaton, 1981) and the Luria-Nebraska Neuropsychological Battery (Golden, Hammeke, & Purisch, 1985) was examined, evidence of significant improvement in his cognitive functioning was found between 6 and 12 months postinjury. While these findings may appear somewhat contradictory to many psychologists, they can best be explained in terms of the relationship between the individual's emotional and cognitive functioning. For example, this client was also administered the Minnesota Multiphasic Personality Inventory (MMPI) (Hathway & McKinley, 1970) to evaluate his emotional functioning. His profile at 6 months postinjury revealed evidence of only mild depression and anxiety. However, when tested 1 year postinjury, his MMPI profile, particularly the Depression and Psychasthenia scales, had dramatically elevated. Thus, the client was reporting considerably more depression and anxiety at 1 year postinjury. This is commonly found since, as traumatically brain-injured clients' cognitive functioning improves, one typically expects greater awareness of their shortcomings and frequent comparisons to their premorbid levels of functioning and concomitant increases in depression and anxiety.

Clients typically exhibit significant improvement in their cognitive functioning when their secondary depression begins to remit. Sbordone (1987) described a 58-year-old male who sustained a brain injury that resulted in a coma of 2 days and a post-traumatic amnesia of 7 days. The client had completed only 8 years of formal education and was employed as a truck driver at the time of his injury. When tested at 3 years postinjury, he obtained an IQ of 81 on the Standard Progressive Matrices Test (Raven, 1958). When tested on the Sbordone-Hall Memory Battery (Sbordone & Hall, 1990), his immediate and delayed visual and verbal memory was found to be severely impaired. When tested 1 year later, his IQ improved to 108. Improvements in cognitive functioning were also observed on other neuropsychological tests. A comparison of his profile on the MMPI at both 3 and 4 years postinjury revealed that his scores on the Depression, Psychoasthenia, and Schizophrenia scales had significantly decreased. The major reason for this improvement is that this client had been referred to a clinical psychologist for weekly supportive psychotherapy. After 1 year of psychotherapy, the client was considerably less depressed and anxious.

OVER-RELIANCE ON NEUROPSYCHOLOGICAL TEST DATA

The fifth obstacle is over-reliance on the results of neuropsychological test data. While neuropsychological tests have traditionally been utilized to evaluate cognitive functioning, the conditions of formal testing may compensate for or mask many of the client's functional impairments (Baxter, Cohen, & Ylvisaker, 1985; Szekeres, Ylvisaker, & Holland, 1985). For example, the quiet and structured testing environment may help the client compensate for problems of attention and concentration; frequent breaks and rest periods may compensate for the client's problems of endurance, perseverance, and fatigue. The use of clear and repetitive instructions masks the client's difficulty in task orientation, flexible reorientation of new tasks, and problem-solving skills; the interactive style of the examiner may mask the client's motivational difficulties, problems with initiation, and response inhibition (Sbordone, 1988).

The results of neuropsychological testing are often heavily influenced by a number of extraneous factors that may have little relationship to brain dysfunction. Factors such as sensory (e.g., diplopia) and peripheral impairments (e.g., fractures or radiculopathies), fatigue, anxiety, medications, medical diseases (e.g., hypothyroidism), pain, motor difficulties, motivation, or linguistic and cultural issues can adversely affect the client's performance on neuropsychological testing. For example, a traumatically brain-injured client during the relatively early stages of recovery may only tolerate 10 minutes of cognitive activity before becoming extremely lethargic, confused, and antagonistic toward the examiner. Thus, the administration of a comprehensive neuropsychological battery, such as the Halstead-Reitan Neuropsychological Battery (Halstead & Reitan, 1951) (which usually takes 6–8 hours to complete), during the early stages of recovery will typically produce an inaccurate description of the client's cognitive skills and abilities. Similarly, the administration of the WAIS-R (Wechsler, 1981), which tends to be culturally and linguistically biased, to a Mexican-

born male whose education and understanding of English and the American culture are limited, would most likely result in spuriously poor scores (Sbordone, in press).

For example, how should we interpret the performance of a 20-year-old client who completes only two out of six possible categories on the Wisconsin Card Sorting Test (Heaton, 1981) and makes 63 errors, whose preexisting IQ was 78? Conversely, how should we interpret the performance of an individual with a preinjury IQ of 148, whose scores on neuropsychological tests fall within the normal range? It is obvious that the psychologist examining these data must formulate a different set of expectations based on what would have been expected of this client's performance prior to the injury.

The actual test scores may not actually provide us with the best index of the severity of cognitive and behavioral dysfunction. Persons with orbital frontal lobe injury tend to exhibit little or no evidence of neuropsychological impairment during formal testing. Yet, their family and significant others will typically report a wide range of significant behavioral and emotional problems. The author has found, from his own experience, that the best single indicator of the severity of behavioral and cognitive dysfunction following traumatic brain injury is the magnitude of the discrepancy between the client's complaints and those of significant others. For example, persons with extensive frontal lobe damage will typically deny having any cognitive or behavioral difficulties, while their family will identify as many as 25 to 30 problems. The author has also found that as clients improve in their functioning, the discrepancy between their complaints and those of the significant others will diminish.

Neuropsychological tests also have a number of shortcomings (Sbordone, 1988). For example, the test items may have insufficient ecological validity, in the sense that they do not adequately test the client in real-world situations: The tests may assess preinjury skills, abilities, or knowledge, rather than cognitive functions sensitive to brain injury, and may fail to measure the client's ability to generalize newly acquired skills or compensatory behaviors. As a consequence, many neuropsychological test reports tend to be "test bound," since they only report test data and omit information from significant others and behavioral observations of the client during and outside of the testing situation. They tend to be acollateral, in that they rarely contain interviews with significant others, and ahistorical, in that they fail to provide a chronological history of the client's injury and obtain an inadequate history of the client prior to the injury. Most neuropsychological reports tend to focus on the client's deficits and presumed site of brain injury rather than discuss the individual's strengths, coping strategies, and compensatory behaviors. The tests tend to be aprescriptive, in that they offer little in the way of specific therapy recommendations. As a consequence, the overwhelming majority of neuropsychological test reports are often of limited value in planning cognitive rehabilitation.

Qualitative Approach

A qualitative approach that examines how the client goes about taking a specific test or the process of how the client obtained the score, rather than the level of performance, is helpful in identifying the client's compensatory behavioral strategies or the client's failure to utilize appropriate strategies in therapy. A qualitative approach looks at all factors that influence the client's test-taking behavior. It examines the types of errors made by the client; the client's motivation to perform the task; the client's ability to recognize and correct errors; the effect of cues or prompting on the client's performance; and the possible influences of such factors as anxiety, depression, bizarre thinking, fatigue, and inadequate motivation. The chief disadvantage to this approach is that it is highly subjective and thus may be influenced by the particular examiner-client interaction.

The choice of tests or type of evaluation should be determined by the type of neurological injury and the length of time since the injury. Psychologists assessing clients who have sustained cerebral contusions resulting in prominent orbital frontal lobe damage should avoid placing heavy emphasis on their neuropsycho-

logical test data; instead, they should rely heavily on the observations of significant others, the client's behavior in relatively unstructured situations, and a qualitative neuropsychological assessment approach. Psychologists assessing clients who have sustained diffuse axonal injuries can typically rely on quantitative neuropsychological test data, since the client's impairments are likely to be seen across a wide variety of different tests. However, lengthy test batteries should be avoided during the first 6 months postinjury, since the test results will be highly influenced by the client's rapid fatigue, confusion, and impaired attention skills. The use of briefer tests that focus more on the client's attention-concentration and recent memory skills are likely to be more useful, since marked impairment in these areas virtually guarantees severe impairments in the client's problem-solving, social, and behavioral functioning.

Test Interpretation Issues

Many psychologists assume that complex processes, such as attention-concentration skills, can be adequately assessed by administering one or two psychological tests to the client. For example, many psychologists frequently evaluate the client's attention-concentration skills by such tests as Digit Span (Wechsler, 1981), Trail Making (Parts A and B) (Reitan, 1958), or the Symbol Digit Modalities (Smith, 1968). In actuality, attention-concentration skills can be broken down into the following skills:

1. Alertness: general readiness of the individual to respond to the environment
2. Stimulus selectivity: ability to select specific stimuli
3. Concentration: ability to maintain attentional set
4. Freedom from distraction: ability to inhibit inappropriate set shifting
5. Vigilance: ability to detect changes in stimulus input
6. Flexibility: ability to initiate set shifting
7. Capacity: amount of information that can be effectively processed by the individual
8. Speed of processing: rate of speed at which attentional tasks can be processed

9. Resistance to fatigue: ability to prevent set deterioration
10. Resistance to emotional factors: ability to maintain attentional set when emotional
11. Resistance to interference from stimulus overload: ability to preserve set under conditions of stimulus overload
12. Resistance to contiguous stimuli: ability to maintain set when presented with contiguous stimuli

Tests such as the Digit Span, Trail Making, and Symbol Digit Modalities do not measure all of these various aspects of attention-concentration. Thus, "normal" scores on these tests may not rule out that a particular client may have a number of significant attentional impairments secondary to the traumatic brain injury (Sbordone, in press).

FAILURE TO UTILIZE NEUROBEHAVIORAL ASSESSMENT APPROACHES IN PLANNING COGNITIVE REHABILITATION

The sixth obstacle is the failure of rehabilitation professionals to utilize a neurobehavioral assessment approach in planning cognitive rehabilitation intervention programs. Neurobehavioral assessment (Sbordone, 1988) places considerable emphasis on gathering a detailed history that includes developmental, clinical, and social factors, and reviewing educational, medical, and rehabilitation records. Included should be information from the client's family, including the occupational, marital, and educational background of parents and siblings, as well as a history of substance abuse and marital, criminal, and psychiatric problems. A sexual history is important since it may shed light on marital strains (if the client is married). Information about the pattern of social relationships, including the history of the ability of the client both to make and to maintain friendships, and the quality of those relationships, should also be obtained.

Behavioral observation of the client across a variety of settings is an essential component of the neurobehavioral assessment process, and should include, but not be limited to, open-ended and structured conversations, structured and unstructured settings, familiar and unfamiliar settings, and rest breaks during formal testing procedures. The client's behavior under each of these circumstances conveys an enormous amount of information about the client's communication skills, compensatory behaviors, motivation, cognitive abilities, and ability to cope with the demands of the environment.

Neuropsychological testing is also an essential component of the neurobehavioral assessment process. Testing should permit evaluation of basic areas of cognitive-communicative functioning such as attention-concentration, memory, motor and sensory-perceptual abilities, problem-solving skills, executive functions, mental flexibility, reasoning, planning, categorization, sequential thinking, language abilities, intellectual functioning, abstract reasoning, conceptual skills, visuospatial and constructional skills, speed of information processing, freedom from distraction, and academic skills, as well as emotional and social functioning. The choice of specific tests to be administered should reflect the client's cultural, educational, and linguistic background; the particular complaints expressed by the client and/or family; the severity of the client's deficits; the length of time since the injury; specific referral questions; the client's cooperation and motivation; previous testing; and physical disabilities.

FAILURE TO UNDERSTAND THE STAGES OF RECOVERY FOLLOWING SEVERE HEAD TRAUMA

The seventh obstacle is our failure to understand the stages of recovery following severe head trauma. After an individual sustains a severe closed head injury, he or she passes through a set of qualitatively distinct stages of cognitive functioning. Recognition of such stages can be invaluable in planning treatment and management strategies, since each stage places different demands on the clinicians and family and/or significant others. The Rancho Los Amigos Scale of Cognitive Function (Hagen, 1981) has been widely used for this purpose (see Table 19.1, this volume, for a descriptive summary of the various levels of the Rancho Scale). Recently, Sbordone (1987) proposed a six-stage model of neurobehavioral recovery. Table 9.1 presents these six stages of cognitive recovery from severe head trauma.

During the first stage, the individual is in coma. The second stage begins when the person first opens his or her eyes. This stage is characterized by either severe agitation, confusion, or a persistent vegetative state. If the individual is not in the latter, he or she is typically disoriented to place and time but not to person. The third stage begins when the individual becomes oriented to place but continues to remain disoriented to time (e.g., day of the week). The most salient characteristic of this stage is the marked denial of cognitive deficits. When the individual becomes oriented to place and time and begins to complain of cognitive deficits, he or she has entered into the fourth stage. The fifth stage is characterized by an increase in depression and frequent comparisons to preinjury functioning. The sixth and final stage of recovery is characterized by an acceptance of residual cognitive deficits and the use of effective compensatory behaviors and coping strategies.

FAILURE TO TREAT CLIENTS ACCORDING TO THEIR STAGE OF NEUROBEHAVIORAL RECOVERY

The eighth obstacle is our failure to base our interventions for traumatically brain-injured clients on their stage of neurobehavioral recovery.

First Stage

During the first stage of recovery when the client is in coma, it is the family who must bear the emotional and psychological burden caused by the injury. While cognitive rehabilitation during this stage is implausible, family members should receive educational and family therapy to rectify their misperceptions and help them cope with their feelings of helplessness, shock, denial, and confusion.

Second and Third Stages

Neurobehavioral assessment typically indicates that traumatically brain-injured clients, during

Table 9.1. Stages of neurobehavioral recovery in traumatic brain injury

Stages of recovery	Characteristics
Stage 1	Injury In coma
Stage 2	Opens eyes Severe agitation-restlessness or vegetative state Severe confusion Disoriented to place and time
Stage 3	Oriented to place but not time Moderate confusion Denial of cognitive deficits May complain of somatic problems Fatigues very easily Poor judgment Marked to severe attention deficits Severe memory deficits Severe social difficulties Severe problem-solving difficulties
Stage 4	Oriented to place and time Becoming aware of cognitive deficits Mild confusion Mild to moderate attention difficulties Marked problem-solving difficulties Moderate to marked memory deficits Early onset of depression-nervousness Unsuccessful attempts to return to work or school Poor endurance May appear relatively normal Moderate to marked social difficulties
Stage 5	Significant depression-nervousness Mild to moderate memory deficits Mild to moderate problem-solving difficulties Frequent comparison to premorbid self Given little hope of further recovery Has returned to work or school Mild to moderate social difficulties

(continued)

Table 9.1. *(continued)*

Stages of recovery	Characteristics
Stage 6	Mild memory impairment Mild problem-solving difficulties Acceptance of residual deficits Improving social relationships Return of most premorbid responsibilities Generally positive self-image

From Sbordone, R.J. (1990). Psychotherapeutic treatment of the client with traumatic brain injury: A conceptual model. In J.S. Kreutzer & P. Wehman (Eds.), *Community integration following traumatic brain injury* (pp. 144–145). Baltimore: Paul H. Brookes Publishing Co.; reprinted with permission.

the second and third stages of the recovery process, have severe attentional problems and are unable to comprehend environmental or social cues or are unable to organize this information. As a consequence, their behavior is poorly organized, which results in frequent rambling and incoherent conversations, and they have a poorly organized semantic base, which typically results in unusual associations. Thus, clients lack self-awareness, and are unable to monitor their behavior or recognize or correct their errors. In addition, they frequently exhibit emotional outbursts that have been described as "catastrophic reactions" (Goldstein, 1942).

It is recommended that environmental modification techniques (e.g., modifying the client's environment to meet his or her needs and to reduce confusion and emotional distress) be utilized during the second and third stages of the recovery process to minimize emotional outbursts. This would include placing clients in a highly controlled and structured environment so that they will eventually learn its expectations. Activities should be selected so that clients will not exceed their impaired ability to encode and process information. The highly structured environment may also serve as an "ancillary cortex and brain stem," since it regulates the various environmental stimuli that impinge upon traumatically brain-injured clients and compensates for their impaired attentional and organizational skills (Sbordone, 1990).

The client should be encouraged to achieve success in this highly structured environment

since, with increasing successes, gradual increases can be made in the environment's demand characteristics. Unfortunately, many clients are transferred to another program or discharged home during this stage, which typically creates confusion and frequently precipitates catastrophic emotional behavior that typically alienates their family and/or significant others. This author recommends that the client not be discharged home or transferred to another program prior to entering the fourth stage of recovery—unless the home environment or new program is highly restructured.

Fourth Stage

While persons with traumatic brain injury may appear relatively "normal" during the fourth stage of recovery, their conceptual and problem-solving skills are markedly impaired. Their ability to encode, store, and retrieve information, particularly after delays of 30 minutes or longer, is also markedly impaired. Increases in the rate of encoding, the complexity of material, or the abstractness of language are likely to produce a disproportionate number of errors of cognitive processing (Hagen, 1981). Although the clients' ability to monitor their behavior has improved, they are only partially aware of the errors they are making. Since clients lack the cognitive resources to correct or rectify these errors, they experience a sense of frustration that often leads to depression, catastrophic reactions, or socially inappropriate behavior. In addition, clients are frequently pressured by family members to return to work, school, or household responsibilities. Unfortunately, since clients with traumatic brain injury are only minimally aware of their cognitive impairments during this stage of recovery, they frequently attempt to return to work, school, or household responsibilities, but are likely to fail or perform poorly. Such outcomes are poorly tolerated by the client and family. Recently, there has been a growing awareness that clients during this stage of recovery may also develop an "atypical bipolar depression" or affective disorder characterized by rapid mood swings, irritability, grandiose thinking, impulsive and often violent behavior, pressured speech, hyperactivity and hypersexuality, as well as exhibit behavioral manifestations of temporal lobe epilepsy (Sbordone, 1988; Shukla, Cook, Mukherjee, Godwin, & Miller, 1987). This author has found that Tegretol is often quite helpful when treating these conditions. (For further discussion of pharmacological intervention, the reader is referred to Chapter 7, this volume.)

Therapy for clients during the fourth stage of recovery should utilize environmental and behavioral modification techniques. Environmental modification within this stage should attempt to maximize the client's functioning in relatively structured or familiar environments. Activities during this stage of recovery should be neither overwhelming nor boring, and should be familiar and liked by the client. Clinicians should be flexible in scheduling time with the client in order to fit in therapy when the client is alert and not fatigued. Frequent rest periods and naps, as well as keeping the demands of the client within his or her fluctuating capabilities throughout the course of the day, are frequently effective in preventing such outcomes as agitation, irritability, combative outbursts, lethargy, and foul language.

Compensatory assistive devices (e.g., notebooks, charts, calendars, watches, microcomputers, tape recorders) should be utilized to improve the client's sense of mastery over his or her environment (see also Chapter 12, this volume). When angry outbursts or socially inappropriate behaviors occur, the client's attention should be directed to innocuous tasks. Restraints should be kept to a minimum at all times, allowing as much freedom of movement as possible within the well-defined boundaries of the environment. In the absence of such boundaries, clients are likely to become confused, agitated, and disoriented (Howard, 1988).

The use of behavior modification strategies during the fourth stage of recovery is highly recommended since the client's improved level of cognitive functioning permits such techniques to be utilized to diminish the frequency of inappropriate behavior and increase the frequency of positive behavior. During this stage, behavior modification can be utilized to increase independent ambulation (Eames & Wood, 1985) and reduce maladaptive social behavior (Burke &

Lewis, 1986). Unfortunately, while behavior analysis procedures have been gaining acceptance as a viable treatment for traumatically brain-injured individuals, behavior analysis procedures are frequently misunderstood and are often applied incorrectly by many therapists (Jacobs, 1988).

Fifth Stage

During the fifth stage of recovery, clients are typically characterized by mild to moderate memory, problem-solving, and emotional difficulties. They may also exhibit mild word-finding, fluency, and word-retrieval problems, as well as a number of subtle, nonverbal communication problems. While their ability to self-monitor their behavior and to generalize their behavior to new situations and environments has improved, it is still impaired. During this stage, clients become more aware of their cognitive-communicative impairments. While their ability to engage in reasoning tasks is generally good in concrete or structured settings, these skills are likely to be poor in either stressful or unstructured settings. When presented with complex communications or materials, they are likely to become lost in details and fail to grasp the main idea or underlying concept. Their ability to encode and organize new information is frequently related to its rate of presentation, quantity, and complexity (Sbordone, 1988).

During the fifth stage of recovery, clients should continue to receive behavior modification therapy. A token economy program is likely to be most effective because of improved cognitive functioning, particularly with respect to recent memory. Eames and Wood (1985) stressed the importance of the relative preparedness of clients when considering token economy programs. They reported that token economy programs were often ineffective when traumatically brain-injured clients were placed in the program prior to reaching a sufficient level of recovery. However, when these clients were placed in the program after they had achieved a higher level of recovery (6–12 months later), they derived considerable benefit and demonstrated significant improvement in their behavioral functioning.

Sixth Stage

Traumatically brain-injured clients in the sixth and final stage of recovery are typically left with mild residual cognitive problems. If they acquired compensatory skills and strategies during the previous stages of recovery, they will usually be capable of functioning at a relatively effective level within their environment—providing it has not reinforced their disability, has not made unrealistic demands, and has not rejected them. Many clients will have returned to their preinjury vocational and social responsibilities. As a consequence, their self-esteem has become generally positive. The cognitive impairments of these clients during this stage are rarely apparent to casual acquaintances. During this stage, traumatically brain-injured clients typically rely heavily on their mastery of compensatory behaviors and strategies to cope with new situations or crises. When these clients become fatigued or are placed under excessive environmental demands and emotional stresses, they typically regress and exhibit cognitive and emotional behaviors that were seen during stages four and five (Sbordone, 1988, 1990).

SUMMARY

Within the past few years, there has been a growing realization that effective cognitive rehabilitation of clients with traumatic brain injury is a difficult task that involves overcoming such obstacles as: a poor understanding of brain-behavior relationships; the myth that most, if not all, of the recovery occurs within the first year postinjury; secondary affective and psychiatric problems; the myth that clients' cognitive and emotional functioning are unrelated; reliance on traditional methods of intervention; over-reliance on neuropsychological test data in planning cognitive rehabilitation; failure to utilize neurobehavioral methods; and failure to recognize the stages of recovery and provide appropriate intervention during each stage of recovery. When an individual sustains a severe traumatic brain injury, he or she will pass through six discrete stages of recovery. It is important for the clinician to recognize these stages and plan rehabilitation and intervention according to the client's stage of recovery.

It cannot be stressed enough that clinicians who work with brain-injured clients must possess a thorough understanding of the principle of a conditional neurological lesion, which argues that the behavioral manifestations of a brain injury vary as a function of the degree to which the client is under stress, fatigue, emotional distress, or excessive metabolic demands. Understanding this principle will afford clinicians with a better appreciation of the devastating impact that emotional factors and environmental stressors can have on the client's functioning.

REFERENCES

Alexander, M.P. (1984). Neurobehavioral consequences of closed head injury. *Neurology and Neurosurgery, Update Series 20,* 1–8.

Bach-Y-Rita, G., Lion, J., Climent, C., & Ervin, F.R. (1971). Episodic dyscontrol: A study of 130 violent patients. *American Journal of Psychiatry, 127,* 49–54.

Baxter, R., Cohen, S.B., & Ylvisaker, M. (1985). Comprehensive cognitive assessment. In M. Ylvisaker (Ed.), *Head injury rehabilitation: Children and adolescents* (pp. 247–274). San Diego: College-Hill Press.

Bond, M.R. (1975). Assessment of the psychosocial outcome after severe head injury. In *CIBA Foundation Symposium 34, Outcome of severe damage to the central nervous system* (pp. 141–157). Amsterdam: Elsevier/Excerpta Medica.

Bond, M.R., & Brooks, D.N. (1976). Understanding

the process of recovery as a basis for the investigation of rehabilitation for the brain-injured. *Scandinavian Journal of Rehabilitation Medicine, 8,* 127–133.

Burke, W.H., & Lewis, F.D. (1986). Management of maladaptive social behavior in the brain-injured adult. *International Journal of Rehabilitation Research, 9,* 335–342.

Cooper, P.R. (1982). Epidemiology of head trauma. In P.R. Cooper (Ed.), *Head injury* (pp. 1–14). Baltimore: Williams & Wilkins.

Cummings, J.L. (1985). *Clinical neuropsychiatry.* New York: Grune & Stratton.

Eames, P., & Wood, R. (1985). Rehabilitation after severe brain injury: A follow-up study of a behavior modification approach. *Journal of Neurology, Neurosurgery, and Psychiatry, 48,* 613–619.

Fisher, D.G., Sweet, J.J., & Pfaelzer-Smith, E.A.

(1986). Influence of depression on repeated neuro-psychological testing. *International Journal of Clinical Neuropsychology, 8,* 14–18.

Golden, C.C., Hammeke, T.A., & Purisch, A.D. (1985). *Luria-Nebraska Neuropsychological Battery.* Los Angeles: Western Psychological Services.

Goldstein, H. (1942). *After effects of brain injuries in man.* New York: Grune & Stratton.

Hagen, C. (1981). Language disorders secondary to closed head injury: Diagnosis and treatment. *Topics in Language Disorders, 1*(4), 73–83.

Halstead, W., & Reitan, R.M. (1951). *Halstead-Reitan Neuropsychological Battery and allied procedures.* Tucson, AZ: Reitan Neuropsychological Laboratory.

Hathway, S., & McKinley, J.C. (1970). *Minnesota Multiphasic Personality Inventory.* Minneapolis: University of Minnesota Press.

Heaton, R. (1981). *Wisconsin Card Sorting Test.* Odessa, FL: Psychological Assessment Resources.

Howard, M.E. (1988). Behavior management in the acute care rehabilitation setting. *Journal of Head Trauma Rehabilitation, 3*(3), 114–22.

Jacobs, H.E. (1988). Yes, behavioral analysis can help, but do you know how to harness it? *Brain Injury, 2*(4), 339–346.

Klonoff, H., Low, M.D., & Clark, C. (1977). Head injuries in children: A prospective five year follow-up. *Journal of Neurology, Neurosurgery, and Psychiatry, 40,* 1211–1219.

Lezak, M.D. (1987). Relationships between personality disorders, social disturbances, and physical disability following traumatic brain injury. *Journal of Head Trauma Rehabilitation, 2*(1), 57–69.

Lishman, W.A. (1968). Brain damage in relation to psychiatric disability after head injury. *British Journal of Psychiatry, 114,* 373–410.

Miller, H., & Stern, G. (1965). The long-term prognosis of severe head injury. *Lancet, 1,* 225–229.

Raven, J.C. (1958). *Standard Progressive Matrices Test.* Cambridge, England: H.K. Lewis & Co.

Reitan, R.M. (1958). Validity of the Trail Making Test as an indication of organic brain damage. *Perceptual and Motor Skills, 8,* 271–276.

Sbordone, R.J. (1985, March). *Atypical bipolar de-pressive disorder following right diencephalic brain injury.* Paper presented at the International Conference on Traumatic Brain Injury, San Jose, CA.

Sbordone, R.J. (1987). A conceptual model of neuro-psychologically based cognitive rehabilitation. In J.M. Williams & C.J. Long (Eds.), *The rehabilitation of cognitive disabilities* (pp. 1–25). New York: Plenum.

Sbordone, R.J. (1988). Assessment and treatment of cognitive communicative impairments in the closed-head injury patient: A neurobehavioral-systems approach. *Journal of Head Trauma Rehabilitation, 3*(2), 55–62.

Sbordone, R.J. (1990). Psychotherapeutic treatment of the client with traumatic brain injury: A conceptual model. In J.S. Kreutzer & P. Wehman (Eds.), *Community integration following traumatic brain injury* (pp. 139–153). Baltimore: Paul H. Brookes Publishing Co.

Sbordone, R.J. (in press). Neuropsychological assessment of the traumatically brain-injured client. *Psychotherapy in private practice.*

Sbordone, R.J., & Hall, S. (1990). *Sbordone-Hall Memory Battery* (rev. ed.). Irvine, CA: Robert J. Sbordone, Ph.D., Inc.

Shukla, S., Cook, B.L., Mukherjee, S., Godwin, C., & Miller, M.G. (1987). Mania following head trauma. *American Journal of Psychiatry, 144*(1), 93–96.

Smith, A. (1968). The Symbol Digit Modalities Test: A neuropsychologic test for screening of learning and other cerebral disorders. *Learning Disorders, 3,* 83–91.

Szekeres, S.F., Ylvisaker, M., & Holland, A.L. (1985). Cognitive rehabilitation therapy: A framework for intervention. In M. Ylvisaker (Ed.), *Head injury rehabilitation: Children and adolescents* (pp. 219–246). San Diego: College-Hill Press.

Thomsen, I.V. (1981). Neuropsychological treatment and long-time follow-up in an aphasic patient with very severe head trauma. *Journal of Clinical Neuropsychology, 3*(1), 43–51.

Wechsler, D. (1981). *Wechsler Adult Intelligence Scale–Revised.* New York: Psychological Corporation.

CHAPTER 10

Management of Psychosocial and Behavior Problems in Cognitive Rehabilitation

CATHERINE A. MATEER AND DENNIS WILLIAMS

Intensive study of the physical, cognitive, behavioral, and emotional problems of persons with head injury has taken place over the last decade. It has become apparent that the deficits in human functioning that routinely cause the greatest problems for both clients and their families are those affecting social behavior or conduct and underlying emotional functioning. Social behavior is critical to effective involvement in family, community, and work environments. Impaired interpersonal behavior and instability of mood can be devastating to social and vocational reintegration and can limit the capacity to learn or use spared or recovered physical and cognitive functions. It is in the area of behavior disorders following traumatic brain injury, however, that our assessment and interventions are perhaps least mature and their efficacy most poorly documented.

ASSESSMENT OF BEHAVIORAL/AFFECTIVE DISORDERS FOLLOWING TRAUMATIC BRAIN INJURY

At this time, cognitive rehabilitation specialists are still struggling with effective assessment of behavior and behavior change following traumatic brain injury. Indeed, we are often still at the stage of listing and labeling specific problem behaviors and/or "personality changes." Information concerning behavior change has tended to rely on observations by professionals, or on self- or family-report. Those researchers with a more "behavioral bent" tend to restrict themselves to observable actions, while others speculate on alterations in the client's underlying mood state or psychological perceptions.

Eames (1988), who has written extensively about behavioral modification approaches, provided a descriptive classification of behavior disorders after brain injury. He divided them into *active* behaviors, *passive* behaviors, and *syndromal* behaviors. Active behavior disorders included aggressive, impulsive, disinhibited, and antisocial actions. Passive behaviors were described by the terms "insightless," "driveless," "abulic (lacking in motivation)," "slow," and "anhedonic." Syndromal behaviors included the categories of "manipulative," "hysterical," "ritualistic" or "obsessive-compulsive," "cyclothymic," "confabulatory," and "paranoid." Although he stressed that the client's behavior must be "observed, measured, recorded and analyzed" (p. 2), it was not clear exactly what behaviors might be targeted for analysis in each of his classifications. Eames also stressed that clinicians must be aware of the complexity of causation: the interaction between the brain disorder, the person, and the context. Equally as important as the injury is "the head it happened to."

Some of these same concepts, particularly the importance of context and individual history, were incorporated into the schema that Prigatano and his colleagues (1986) proposed for classifying personality and behavior disorders after brain injury. They described three overlapping and broad categories that encompass most of the behavioral problems frequently encountered in the clinical setting. Reactionary problems are those the person experiences as a response to injury and include manifestations of frustration, depression, and anxiety. They represent an understandable response to loss and to changed abilities and circumstances. Neuropsychologically based problems referred to those mental and behavioral disturbances directly associated with tissue damage and neurological/physiological abnormalities. They include irritability, explosive anger, impulsivity, and denial. This schema also includes what were termed characterological problems, dysfunctional behaviors the person may have manifested prior to injury or those arising from premorbid personality dispositions (Prigatano et al., 1986).

Lezak and O'Brien (1988) summarized the most frequent personality changes reported after brain injury according to a survey of nine studies. The most frequently reported changes included irritability, apathy, depression, anxiety, impatience, impulsivity, lability, paranoia, and phobic responses. The difficulty with such listings is they treat each problem behavior or area of concern in isolation from the others and do not seek to see trends or patterns of response. They also provide little or no direction for specific assessment or intervention techniques.

A number of specific scales or inventories have been proposed to deal with the behavioral consequences of traumatic brain injury. They have attempted to avoid the potential biases of other objective tests that typically have been standardized on normal or psychiatric samples. One of these is the Neurobehavioral Rating Scale (NRS) (Levin et al., 1987). This 27-item, 7-point rating scale is to be completed by staff members working with the brain-injured individual. A study of 101 persons with head injury, ranging widely in severity of injury, yielded four factors on the NRS:

Factor 1 consisted of items evaluating coherence of cognition and efficiency of memory, motor retardation (slowing), and emotional withdrawal.

Factor 2 included items reflecting inaccurate self-appraisal, unrealistic planning, and disinhibition—features frequently ascribed to frontal lobe function.

Factor 3 reflected physical complaints, anxiety, depression, and irritability.

Factor 4 included ratings for expressive and receptive language deficits.

Results demonstrated satisfactory interrater reliability and reflected both the chronicity and severity of closed head injury. Use of such a standardized rating tool should prove helpful in the analysis and consistent conceptualization of such changes both in individuals and in large-scale head injury population studies.

The Portland Adaptability Inventory (PAI) (Lezak, 1987) was another tool designed to provide a systematic framework for recording psychosocial problems arising from personality alterations and social maladaptations following traumatic brain injury. This instrument was found useful in tracing the course of psychosocial problems over time. The scale involves ratings of 21 items: 7 dealing with Temperament and Personality, 8 with Activities of Social Behavior, and 6 with Physical Competence. In addition, interrelations among personality dimensions, social consequences, and some cognitive competencies were seen to emerge. In this way, the PAI has contributed to the elucidation of neurocognitive-behavioral patterns.

Corey (1987), of the authors' Center for Cognitive Rehabilition, in Puyallup, Washington, developed a model of psychosocial assessment composed of 10 major areas. Five involve symptoms that are related directly to the effects of head injury: interpersonal skills, social comprehension and judgment, self-regulation, context dependency, and adjustment to disability. The other five areas involve psychosocial factors that are partially or totally independent of the injury but that affect psychosocial functioning. These areas are substance abuse, significant preinjury psychological or psychiatric problems, endogenous clinical depression, relationship stressors, and situational stressors. This assessment is notable in its appreciation of the degree to which variables apart from the head injury itself may be influential in psychosocial/emotional functioning. Corey argued that psychosocial assessment is likely to be incomplete and quite misleading if these factors are not considered. Moreover, interventions may be inadequate or inappropriate.

MANAGEMENT OF BEHAVIORAL AND AFFECTIVE DISORDERS FOLLOWING TRAUMATIC BRAIN INJURY

Currently, behavioral management following traumatic brain injury may be generally grouped in terms of five categories: 1) pharmacological interventions, 2) behavior modification techniques, 3) cognitive/metacognitive training, 4) psychotherapeutic interventions, and 5) environmental management/accommodation. In clinical practice, these approaches are applied in combination, though preference for one approach over another is influenced by the characteristics of the particular client, and by the background and discipline of the clinician, as well as by the context in which therapy is delivered. Interventions of choice are also influenced by the behaviors receiving clinical focus. All may be effectively employed in a "what works" or multimodality regime, or they may be employed separately following identification of specific target behaviors.

1. Pharmacological approaches to management of behaviors following traumatic brain injury are attractive for a number of reasons, both rational and practical. Pharmacological agents are useful in stabilizing patients during the acute stages of traumatic brain injury, and may help prevent additional central nervous system damage from secondary degenerative events (Sutton, Weaver, & Feeney, 1987). In addition, some patients have identifiable organic damage, which may contribute to neurotransmitter imbalance or dysregulation (Mysiw & Jackson, 1987).

Unfortunately, though drugs may be useful in the acute stages of head injury, postacute problems may not yield to pharmacological approaches, or drugs may produce paradoxical effects that result in amplification of the problem. Moreover, some drugs have the potential to interfere with rehabilitation by compromising cognitive function. For example, use of sedative medicines (benzodiazapines, neuroleptics) in persons who are disinhibited or who appear confused should be resisted since they may have the effect of depressing arousal and often have amnestic properties. Problems of overactivity and especially of explosive, impulsive aggression in the postacute stage are perhaps most problematic of the active disorders. Currently, the most frequently used pharmacological agents for management of dyscontrol or dramatic behavioral swings are anticonvulsants (particularly Tegretol), Lithium, and psychostimulants (Ritalin). Additional experimental work focusing on improving cognitive efficiency has involved the use of nootropics (Piracetam), levodopa, and opium antagonists (Naloxone). Antidepressants, particularly Prozac, have been found useful for stabilization of mood. In spite of the reported clinical usefulness of pharmacological agents, careful, controlled studies of drug effectiveness in persons with head injury have only recently begun to appear in the literature. (For further discussion of pharmacological intervention for persons with traumatic brain injury, the reader is referred to Chapter 7, this volume.)

2. Behavior modification employs well-known and well-established technologies that are primarily designed to shape desirable behaviors or to extinguish undesirable ones. Behavior modification programs typically employ measurements of baseline frequency of the targeted behavior, followed by intervention that positively rewards (reinforces) desirable behaviors while ignoring or punishing (e.g., by use of aversive stimuli, cost-response) undesired behaviors.

Undoubtedly, the largest series of case examples and the strongest underlying rationale for this approach has been that provided by Rodger Wood, based on work at the Kemsley Unit at St. Andrew's Hospital, Northampton (1987). He described institutionally based token economy systems and provided clear case-by-case data documenting the efficacy of this approach. There is little doubt that behaviors can be modified using these powerful techniques. What remains less clear is the degree to which more adaptive behaviors will need to remain under strict stimulus/response control outside the environment in which they are shaped and modified. The other long-standing criticism of strict behavioral approaches to intervention is that they only address symptoms, not the underlying causes, and that alternate symptoms/behaviors may emerge if behavioral antecedents are not modified. Other potential problems in a rehabilitation setting include problems with staff noncompliance with behavior plans due to time constraints and insufficient stimulus control, particularly in outpatient or day treatment settings (Mateer & Ruff, in press).

Some of the greatest problems with "behavior management" may be reflected in the attitudes it reinforces for some clinicians. These include assuming any of the following: 1) "bad" behaviors are associated with a "bad" person; 2) problem behaviors are volitional on the part of the head-injured person; 3) "bad" behaviors should be punished, without developing strategies for differential reinforcement of other behaviors, or training of more appropriate behaviors.

3. Cognitive/metacognitive training involves increasing the client's awareness of specific deficits, increasing self-awareness, and providing training in the use of structured routines (see Chapter 11, this volume). Self-management techniques, memory books, and personal organizers are all examples of metacognitive systems that may be incorporated into cognitive therapeutic approaches. There have been only a few reports, however, on how use of such techniques or tools should be trained in persons with traumatic brain injury (Sohlberg & Mateer, 1990). As with behavioral modification systems, metacognitive strategies have been found not to generalize readily to day-to-day contexts. Even well-practiced techniques may not be spontaneously employed outside of the training setting. For this reason, cognitive rehabilitation programs must incorporate provision for training in multiple settings in order to enhance generalization, and provision for periodic maintenance checks should be included in follow-up plans.

4. Psychotherapeutic interventions are also well known. Such approaches utilize insight-oriented therapy, enhancement of self-esteem, cognitive-behavioral approaches, and individual or group counseling support to facilitate the individual's adjustment to his or her disability. The approach covers a very broad range of therapeutic theories and applications, ranging from classical Freudian/Jungian/psychoanalytical approaches over extended periods of time to a variety of brief, even single-session therapeutic approaches to problems. Practitioners of psychotherapeutic techniques represent a mix of disciplines including analytical psychotherapy, hypnotherapy, and psychosocial counseling. There is widespread belief that these approaches will be most effective with the mildly to moderately impaired traumatically brain-injured client. In cases of individuals with more severe impairment, psychotherapeutic interventions may have their greatest usefulness with family members and caregivers.

5. Environmental management/accommodation involves *altering* the environment or the situation in such a way that the client may experience success in spite of his or her deficits. This approach usually focuses on the training of primary caregivers, employers, and/or educators and involves increasing awareness of the brain-injured individual's strengths and weaknesses, and demonstrating means to enhance the individual's level of independent function. Weaknesses of such an approach lie in the necessity to modify virtually every major environment in which the client functions; while modification of the school, home, and workplace might be possible, modification of all community contexts would not.

In a general sense, behavioral, social, and affective interventions following traumatic brain injury can be seen on a continuum. Judd and Segueira (personal communication, November 13, 1990) discussed this continuum in introducing the notion of "neuropsychotherapy." In the early postinjury stages, individuals may be least aware of changes in ability; thus, they are likely to play a smaller role in therapy, with caregivers/ therapists taking more responsibility. At that stage, pharmacological management, behavior modification, and environmental restructuring will likely be the interventions of choice. As the client recovers a level of insight and awareness, he or she can take more responsibility and control; at that point, the psychotherapeutic and metacognitive training will likely be more effective, and caregivers/therapists can and should relinquish some degree of control and structure. For clients with more severe injury, this transition may not be possible and caregivers will continue to play a major role in behavior management.

DEVELOPING THE INTERVENTION PLAN: FOCUS ON BEHAVIORAL PATTERNS, NOT BEHAVIORS

Although the literature, as well as the foregoing discussion of evaluation and intervention tends toward listing deficits or areas of behavioral concern, many of these behaviors do not seem to occur as independent variables. Rather, what one tends to see after traumatic brain injury are *clusters* of behavioral abnormalities that appear to emerge in concert. These clusters or patterns of behavior are likely related to the site, mechanism, and severity of injury as well as to preexisting personality, temperament, and coping styles.

Increasingly, the cognitive neuropsychology literature is providing a foundation on which to delineate and describe cognitive losses. For example, it is no longer appropriate to speak of someone as having a memory impairment, but rather to describe the underlying reason for a memory failure. Two clients may get the same score on a memory test for two vastly different reasons—one due to failure of attentional processes or encoding mechanisms, the other due to a failure of retrieval mechanisms or of storage (see Chapter 12, this volume). These two types of memory loss need to be treated very differently. Similarly, two clients may exhibit anger outbursts, but for two very different reasons. Anger may be an expression of frustration (psychogenic) or a manifestation of dyscontrol secondary to organic injury of self-regulatory mechanisms (neurogenic). Just as there are problems with viewing a specific behavior as the same in all cases, there are problems with a blanket management approach to a specific behavior.

In the authors' clinical experience with head-injured clients, they have come to recognize readily identifiable and repeatedly encountered clusters of behavioral features. While there are insufficient data to speak of behavioral patterns as typical of behavioral subtypes, the authors believe that exploring the possibility of behavioral subgroups or subtypes may contribute

to the clinical assessment and therapy of a very troublesome aspect of traumatic brain injury.

Subgrouping or subtyping has been shown to be a valid means of conceptualizing patterns of behavior that appear to cluster within larger heterogeneous groups. Porter and Rourke (1985), for example, reported four distinct socioemotional patterns in children with learning disabilities. They found that approximately 44% of their sample were functioning adequately (subtype 1); 26% had marked internalized psychological disturbance (subtype 2); 13% showed disproportional pervasiveness or intensity of somatic concerns (subtype 3); and 17% demonstrated overactivity, distractibility, interpersonal sensitivity, and antisocial behavior (subtype 4). On the basis of these groupings, appropriate intervention approaches were discussed.

Subtype profiles have been shown to be reliable and, as such, predictive of deficit patterns over time (Knights & Stoddart, 1981). Furthermore, subtyping would facilitate prediction of behavioral response in specific contexts and would allow tailoring of intervention plans that consider patterns of behavior in relation to their bases, rather than behaviors as singular entities.

A series of heuristically derived "cases" that capture some of the behavioral constellations the authors have frequently seen are discussed next, along with therapy recommendations for each.

Case A

Description

Case A clients will have sustained moderate to severe cerebral trauma of a diffuse nature. They demonstrate moderate to severe attention deficits and memory disturbances. Such clients are able to initiate behavior that is appropriate, but are unable to remember or to maintain focus on initial goals. Therefore, activity is often tangential, appearing directionless or purposeless. Awareness of changes in cognitive function is usually situationally generated, and situational "reminders" can result in sudden and surprising revelations of deficit. This may trigger brief but powerful emotional responses and develop task or situational aversion that, though not clearly recalled by the client, may generate avoidance mechanisms. Avoidance behaviors and withdrawal from challenge would be typical. As such clients recognize that problems are associated with cognitive abilities, repeated confrontation with frustration and numerous failures may increase self-criticism and decrease self-esteem. Characteristically, Case A clients are readily frustrated, hesitant to try new things, and labile in mood and affect. Lability may be directly associated with immediate experience, and is primarily psychogenic in nature.

Because such individuals may not recall deficits on a moment-to-moment basis, they are often initially confused by problems encountered in everyday situations. In this state of bewilderment, helpless or dependent behaviors may develop, which are resented both by the client and by the supporting caregiver. Often such clients are irritable and defensive when faced with their dependency; this may be particularly true for men who perceived themselves as self-reliant individualists or who, prior to their injury, perceived themselves in terms of dominant-male roles. However, resentment may be just as fierce in women who have striven hard for independence or for professional standing.

Intervention Strategies

A variety of strategies might be used to address the irritability and anger in such clients. Since it is situationally generated, the first step might be to identify circumstances or situations that produce the responses and then to avoid them. Exposure to those situations can be reintroduced later in recovery. The client, family, and staff can be taught the use of time-outs, during which they can briefly back off from situations producing irritation. These clients can often benefit from training in relaxation and calming self-talk. Both therapeutic and functional task hierarchies should be carefully arranged and incremented so that the potential is increased for successes and minimized for failures. External reminders of the aims of therapy and progress in specific areas of function may be extremely beneficial. Repeated acknowledgment that the kinds of feelings they are having are normal and expected

may be immediately valuable, as are support and reassurance.

Case B

Description

Case B clients manifest attention and memory disturbances similar to Case A clients, but the nature of underlying cognitive problems is quite different. Essential abilities associated with the frontal lobes, and so with self-perception and social awareness, are disturbed. Thus, there is little or no recognition of newly acquired deficits. For this reason, the client does not see any reason not to resume former activities and becomes suspicious of family members or caregivers who attempt to control or regulate participation in home, work, or community contexts. Responses often appear childish or impulsive; they may lack modulation or may be exaggerated. Dyscontrol in the form of tantrums, rage, and physical and/or verbal aggressiveness is often seen in response to apparently trivial or innocuous trigger events. Problems with modulation of behavior may be manifested in appetite disorders or in disturbances of sleep-wake patterns. Such clients' emotional reactions are shallow and surprisingly fleeting. Behaviors are inconsistent, yet often appear volitional. Although frustration is recognized, the reasons for frustration are not. There is, therefore, a tendency to blame others for problems, particularly since others are usually actively involved in immediate interventions in problematic contexts.

Intervention Strategies

It would be particularly important with a client with this level of impulsivity and lack of self-monitoring to restrict access to dangerous situations—including vehicles, sharp or otherwise dangerous tools, and weapons. Case B clients may benefit from very direct, clear, and repeated messages about their problems. Reeducation might be facilitated by having clients make judgments about the quality of their performance immediately before and after doing a task, and giving firm feedback to them about their judgments. Both staff and family can be trained in this technique. Clients can be trained to check out their judgment with others. Messages need to be simple, and a common terminology should be agreed upon by staff and family for describing the problems and behaviors of interest.

Clients with this profile may respond to behavioral approaches for increasing desired behaviors and decreasing undesirable ones. Learning will probably take longer than in other clients, however, and generalization will be minimal to other contexts or environments. Therefore, careful selection of key target behaviors for modification will be essential, and active training in different contexts will probably be necessary.

These clients will often do best with structure and consistency. The environmental manipulations and control and institution of routines discussed earlier as a therapy approach may be valuable here. Case A and B clients may also benefit from metacognitive strategy training that provides a consistent structure for approaching particular kinds of tasks or dealing with particular problems.

Clients with frontal lobe injury who display this kind of self-regulatory difficulty and lack of awareness probably benefit minimally from traditional, insight-oriented, psychotherapeutic approaches. Neural mechanisms necessary for inferential reasoning, insight, and generalization of concepts may not be available, so input needs to be clear, consistent, and unambiguous. Since affective disorders require active and prolonged rumination, neither Case A nor Case B clients are likely to demonstrate full-blown anxiety or depression—although they may demonstrate blunted or restricted affect. More likely, they will demonstrate acute and fleeting sadness and agitation, which may be rapidly dissipated by redirection of attention to other activities, tasks, or ideas.

Finally, clients represented by both Cases A and B may temporarily benefit from medications aimed at reducing agitation while other, more lasting management techniques are put into place. Case B clients may also benefit from psychostimulant medication, which has been found to reduce distractibility and impulsivity in some cases, just as Ritalin and dextroamphetamines

reduce negative symptoms associated with attention deficit hyperactivity disorder. Tegretol has been found to be of some use in cases of organic dyscontrol.

Case C

Description

Case C clients may demonstrate "mild" cognitive deficits after sustaining a severe whiplash injury and/or concussion. Deficits are seen in attention, memory, and organizationl skills. Unlike Case A and Case B clients, often these clients are acutely aware of their deficits. The result of this hyperawareness is sometimes striking in its disabling potential. These clients have adequate memory and attention to sustain rumination over real and perceived cognitive changes. As a consequence, anxiety and depression, propensity for panic attacks or agoraphobic responses, and low self-esteem are frequently manifested. Case C clients often isolate themselves from social settings. Anxiety may generate speech dysfluency, sleeplessness, and appetite problems. In addition, heightened anxiety may result in inertia or in restless, nonproductive activities.

Intervention Strategies

Case C individuals are frequently characterized by a history of being high achievers and/or high-risk takers. They tend to have good insight into their problems and often excellent analytical abilities. In these clients in particular, a focus on behavior is a primary symptom of their disorder, and attempts to modify behavior while ignoring its underlying causes are generally ineffective. Rather, use of insight-oriented analytical approaches can often allow these clients to modify their behavior through an understanding of their own disorder and the reasons behind their behavior. Case C clients do not respond well to the conventional brief therapies and behavior modification techniques. In fact, these techniques tend in many cases to worsen their condition. Therefore, the approach to these clients must be particularly cautious and well planned. Therapies should avoid punishment for "bad" or negative behaviors; rather, subtle regard for what may be thought of as more appropriate or positive behavior should be provided.

For some of these clients, a supportive group milieu may be very beneficial. Group exchange may reduce isolation, a sense that they are "the only one" experiencing the problems, or that they are going crazy. Some clients with this profile may, however, consider themselves to be superior to their fellow participants or become so anxious in a group that they are unable to participate meaningfully. Such responses may negate any effective group therapeutic methods, as such Case C clients cannot or will not relate to their peers' problems. In general, these types of individuals are probably the least appropriate for highly structured rehabilitation regimes and probably will respond best to individual therapeutic approaches. They may not be good candidates for the more recognized programs, but may respond well on an individual basis to psychosocial, cognitive, and vocational therapies.

At some point, these clients may recognize that the therapist is attempting to produce changes in their lives and thought processes. As a consequence, what may be perceived as willful resistance is frequently encountered. Over time, their responses and behaviors may have become adaptive, so change and new responses may make them feel more uncomfortable. Some of the more classical cognitive-behavioral approaches to stress, pain, and/or anger management may be helpful in these individuals. They usually have the cognitive capacity to learn and use imagery, self-talk, and metacognitive and other self-management approaches. Also, the authors have found that Case C clients are often very amenable to and make powerful gains in cognitive functioning through attention and executive function training and training in use of memory and organizational aids (Mateer, Sohlberg, & Youngman, 1990). Mild tranquilizing or anti-anxiety compounds may be of initial benefit, but should be tapered and discontinued as early as possible during the course of therapy.

Case D

Description

Case D clients have severe sensory motor impairments. They cannot ambulate independently, so are wheelchair dependent. Communication is often severely limited by dysarthria and sometimes by varying degrees of aphasia. In spite of these limitations, however, they have sufficient awareness of their deficits to experience frustration when obstructions are encountered. Restlessness, agitation, and anger are commonly observed. These are associated with inappropriate interactions. Some actions appear intentionally aimed at hurting others, particularly caregivers, and involve verbal or physical assault. In addition, behaviors intended to elicit guilt in caregivers may be seen. Additional behavioral problems include uncooperativeness in dressing, grooming, and activities of daily living; refusal of responsibility for any aspect of their immediate situation; and verbalization of self-defeating thoughts or demonstration of self-defeating actions.

Intervention Strategies

These individuals are probably expressing anger, grief, frustration, and severe depression in the only way they can, given their limited repertoire of responses and restricted communication. Mixed with these emotions are probably fear and anxiousness about physical function (e.g., potential for falling, choking, being left unattended). Case D clients may despise the dependence they feel and the assistance they genuinely need from others.

It may help to acknowledge the depression and the frustration, and provide verbal or physical support and reassurance. As antidepressants usually further compromise cognitive function in these clients, they should be avoided in all but the most severely depressed individuals (i.e., those at risk for self-destructive behavior or those who have progressed toward a vegetative state). It will often be critical to maximize to the extent possible feelings of independence and self-determination. To the extent they are cognitively able, Case D persons should be allowed and encouraged to make choices. They should be given as much control over their environment as possible by providing adaptive methods of environmental control (e.g., for light switches, door openings and closures, entertainment devices, telephones). If safe, they should be provided with a means for privacy. Case D clients may benefit from being encouraged to make choices about scheduling, diet, and so on. If choice is offered, however, it will be important to truly honor and respect that choice.

Although their independent action should be encouraged, it should be made clear that some behaviors are not acceptable and will not be tolerated. Physical aggression, in particular, should never be allowed or excused. Messages about responsibility for basic mutual respect need to be clear, and consequences for aggression must be fair, immediate, and consistent. Family and friends can often be either tremendously helpful or tremendously harmful with such clients. Close monitoring of behavioral response to visitors and to the visit should be undertaken. Family education and training in wheelchair etiquette and social implications, as well as wheelchair "operation," will be important.

Relaxation training and anger and pain management techniques may be helpful for Case D clients. Sleep patterns should be monitored and good sleep/wake cycles should be maintained by providing stimulation and activity during the day and decreasing distractions at night. Such individuals should not be offered unrealistic expectations for future recovery, but hope concerning future options and choices should be expressed.

SUMMARY AND CONCLUSIONS

In spite of significant and exciting developments in cognitive rehabilitation over the past decade, the areas of behavioral assessment and intervention remain relatively underdeveloped. Currently, clinical assessments often consist of listing or labeling behaviors, and interventions are frequently nonspecific and sometimes inappropriate given the cognitive limitations of the client and the reality of the client's world.

The authors propose that it is probably more profitable to look at constellations of behaviors, perhaps behavioral subgroups or subtypes, because singular behaviors may have quite different antecedents. Table 10.1 shows those behaviors most often seen following traumatic brain injury. As may be seen, a number of behaviors appear to be shared by all four clinical types discussed in this chapter (Cases A, B, C,

Table 10.1. Constellations of behaviors most often seen after traumatic brain injury

Behavior	Cases			
	A	B	C	D
Anger	+	+	+	+
Impatience/frustration	+	+	+	+
Irritability	+	+	+	+
Lability	+	+	+	+
Restlessness	+	+	+	+
Withdrawal	+		+	+
Paranoial/delusional thinking		+		+
Anxiety			+	+
Depression			+	+
Hopelessness			+	+
Phobias			+	
Suspiciousness/distrust		+		+
Childishness		+		+
Aggressiveness		+		+
Decreased self-awareness	+	+		
Misperceptions of others	+	+		
Impulsivity	+	+		
Helplessness/social dependency	+			+
Agitation		+		
Apathy		+		
Blunted intellect		+		
Disinhibition		+		
Indifference		+		

Adapted from Lezak and O'Brien (1988).
Note: See text discussion for description of Cases A, B, C, & D.

and D), yet each case may be identified by a particular pattern of behaviors. A particular behavioral manifestation may derive from quite different neurological or psychological origins. Different behavioral subgroups, given their differing underlying origins, may be expected to respond quite differently to selective management approaches.

The use of a checklist of "typical" head injury behaviors, while having some face validity, does not allow selective discriminative approaches to therapy and may lead the clinician into a false sense of diagnostic security. The cases described in this chapter emerged only from their salience in clinical experience. It could be very bene- ficial, however, to undertake more formal investigation of constellations of behavior to determine whether reliable traumatic brain injury subtypes may be identified.

REFERENCES

Corey, M. (1987). A comprehensive model for psychosocial assessment of individuals with closed head injury. *Cognitive Rehabilitation, 5,* 28–33.

Eames, P. (1988). Behavior disorders after severe head injury: Their nature and causes and strategies for management. *Journal of Head Trauma Rehabilitation, 3,* 1–6.

Knights, R., & Stoddart, C. (1981). Profile approaches to neuropsychological diagnosis in children. In G. Hynd & J. Obrzut (Eds.), *Neuropsychological assessment and the school-aged child* (pp. 335–351). New York: Grune & Stratton.

Levin, H.S., High, W.M., Goethe, K.E., Sisson, R.A., Overall, J.E., Rhoades, H.M., Eisenberg, H.M., Kalisky, Z., & Gary, H.E. (1987). The Neurobehavioral Rating Scale: Assessment of the behavioral sequelae of head injury by the clinician. *Journal of Neurology, Neurosurgery, and Psychiatry, 50,* 183–193.

Lezak, M.D. (1987). Relationships between personality disorders, social disturbances, and physical disability following traumatic brain injury. *Journal of Head Trauma Rehabilitation, 2,* 57–69.

Lezak, M.D., & O'Brien, K.P. (1988). Longitudinal study of emotional, social, and physical changes after head injury. *Journal of Learning Disabilities, 21,* 456–463.

Mateer, C.A., & Ruff, R.M. (in press). Effectiveness of behavior management procedures in the rehabilitation of head-injured patients. In R.U. Wood (Ed.), *Neurobehavioral sequelae of traumatic brain injury.* London: Lawrence Erlbaum Associates.

Mateer, C.A., Sohlberg, M.M., & Youngman, P.K. (1990). The management of acquired attention and memory deficits. In R.L. Wood & I. Fussey (Eds.), *Cognitive rehabilitation in perspective* (pp. 68–95). London: Taylor and Francis.

Mysiw, W.J., & Jackson, R.D. (1987). Tricyclic antidepressant therapy after traumatic brain injury. *Journal of Head Trauma Rehabilitation, 2,* 34–42.

Porter, J., & Rourke, B. (1985). Socioemotional functioning of learning disabled children: A subtypal analysis of personality patterns. In B. Rourke (Ed.), *Neuropsychology of learning disabilities: Essentials of subtype analysis* (pp. 257–280). New York: Guilford Press.

Prigatano, G.P., Fordyce, D.J., Pepping, M., Roueche, J.R., Wood, B.C., & Zeiner, H.K. (1986). *Neuropsychological rehabilitation after brain injury.* Baltimore: Johns Hopkins University Press.

Sohlberg, M.M., & Mateer, C.A. (1990). Training use of compensatory memory aids: A three stage behavioral program. *Journal of Clinical and Experimental Neuropsychology, 11,* 871–891.

Sutton, R.L., Weaver, M.S., & Feeney, D.M. (1987). Drug-induced modifications of behavioral recovery following cortical trauma. *Journal of Head Trauma Rehabilitation, 2,* 50–58.

Wood, R.L. (1987). *Brain injury rehabilitation: A neurobehavioral approach.* Rockville, MD: Aspen.

INTERDISCIPLINARY APPROACHES TO COGNITIVE REHABILITATION

There is little doubt that brain injury rehabilitation professionals are strong advocates for interdisciplinary intervention. The complexity of cognition and behavior may account for the fact that responsibilities for cognitive rehabilitation are often shared among members of several disciplines. Speech-language pathologists, psychologists, and occupational therapists often have a primary role in therapy. However, practitioners in nursing, therapeutic recreation, psychiatry, social work, and special education are likely to play a role in the therapy process as well.

This section is intended to provide readers with practical information regarding methods of practice in cognitive rehabilitation. Professionals have suggested that a variety of therapy techniques and modalities are effective. Practitioners have worked effectively with groups as well as individuals. Therapy goals have been directed toward improved self-awareness, social skills, memory, attention, perception, and other primary cognitive skills. Therapy approaches include the use of computers, games, role-playing exercises, compensatory techniques, and workbook activities.

Although the incidence of traumatic brain injury for children and adolescents is less than that for adults, the problems of children and adolescents are perhaps more serious. Unfortunately, there is relatively little information available to help guide practitioners who work with this population. A chapter within this section is thus devoted to the special needs of children and adolescents with traumatic brain injury.

CHAPTER 11

Training Awareness and Compensation in Postacute Head Injury Rehabilitation

PEGGY P. BARCO, BRUCE CROSSON,
M. MELINDA BOLESTA, DIANE WERTS, AND ROBERT STOUT

Problems in awareness after head injury might be best understood by first discussing varying facets of awareness in non-brain-injured persons. Not everyone is completely aware of their individual strengths and weaknesses. It is impossible, for example, to be aware of every instance in which an error is made, or when a negative impact on others has resulted. Our levels of awareness probably vary from one area of our lives to another. What becomes important, however, is that our level of awareness in most areas of our lives is adequate so as to be able to maintain the ability to function at home, in the community, and/or at work.

Lack of awareness of one's own difficulties can result in repeated failures and adverse consequences in functioning in daily life in non-brain-injured persons as well as those with brain injury. Etiology can be varied and can include social-cultural factors and environmental stressors, as well as brain dysfunction. In severe cases, the result is that individuals possess a level of awareness lower than the accepted norm, and functioning in daily life becomes disturbed. Intervention of one form or another, depending on the etiology, is thus required.

This chapter, however, is devoted to the understanding and treatment of awareness deficits that have resulted from the neurological changes that can follow head trauma. In persons with traumatic brain injury, there is often a reported dramatic change from premorbid functioning. It is not uncommon that individuals who have sustained a head injury appear to lack awareness of their functioning at home, in the community, and/or at work. Frequently, the nature and degree of brain injury or the pattern of cognitive deficits are diagnostic clues to the existence of an awareness deficit, telling us that this problem is not simply a "normal" individual fluctuation in awareness ability, or solely the result of psychological denial.

In the literature on head injury rehabilitation, the term *denial* has been used to describe a varying scope of phenomena. In some places, denial is used to refer to any circumstance in which head-injured clients state they have no deficit, when one indeed exists. This definition can be confusing because it fails to distinguish between psychological and neurological causes. Making this distinction with respect to cause is extremely important because it will determine what treatment is used to address a client's decreased awareness. The authors of this chapter agree with those who reserve the word denial for a reluctance (either conscious or unconscious) to recognize deficits, based upon psychological factors (Deaton, 1986; Lezak, 1978; Nockelby & Deaton, 1987; Prigatano et al., 1986). In this chapter, the term *awareness deficit* is used to refer to an inability to recognize deficits or problem circumstances caused by neurological injury. Conversely, the preservation of clients' ability to recognize their own problem areas is a

The authors' work in head injury rehabilitation and the development of this model were made possible by gifts from the late Dorothy C. Danforth, Carolyn and Donald Danforth, Jr., and Dorothy and Jefferson Miller. The authors are indebted for their support.

strength that can be used in rehabilitation. The focus of this chapter is to define awareness deficits and explore related interventions.

Psychological denial and awareness deficits due to brain dysfunction can coexist. Often denial and awareness difficulties may present initially with similar behavioral manifestations; however, it is important to differentiate the two clinically. This is best accomplished by a professional trained in both the neurological and the psychological manifestations of brain injury. Additionally, the therapy emphasis and prognosis of a client with denial will likely differ from one with an organic awareness deficit. For clients without premorbid personality disturbance, denial is frequently addressed most effectively when the future cost of maintaining the denial is seen as greater than the emotional cost of accepting the injury. In some instances, this involves letting clients experience the fact that they cannot perform a certain activity (e.g., going to college); thus, it may require a significant amount of time to resolve acceptance issues. Psychotherapy may also be effective in treating denial. Deaton (1986) discussed the measurement and intervention strategies specific to dealing with denial as a psychological defense.

Neurologically based awareness deficits must be understood in the context of damage to the neurological substrates that support self-awareness. Numerous authors have made reference to lack of progress in rehabilitation and difficulties in achieving productive living due, at least partially, to poor awareness of deficit areas (e.g., Askenasy & Rahmani, 1988; Ben-Yishay, Silver, Piasetsky, & Rattock, 1987; Cicerone & Tupper, 1986; Kreutzer, Wehman, Morton, & Stonnington, 1988). Our ability to address awareness deficits successfully as clinicians depends upon our ability to understand the types of awareness deficits and their relationship to other neurological problems, as well as corresponding therapy applications.

Recently, there has been more written regarding the late stages of cognitive rehabilitation and training in compensatory strategies (e.g., Ben-Yishay, 1988; Haarbauer-Krupa, Henry, Szekeres, & Ylvisaker, 1985; Kreutzer et al., 1988; Lam, McMahon, Priddy, & Gehred-Schultz,

1988; Prigatano et al., 1986; Szekeres, Ylvisaker, & Cohen, 1987; Szekeres, Ylvisaker, & Holland, 1985; Ylvisaker & Szekeres, 1989). These sources contain valuable information in the use of specific techniques to train compensatory strategies, as well as some general techniques to facilitate awareness in head-injured clients. They do not, however, explore the different types of awareness deficits commonly observed in clients with head injury, and how the various interventions relate to the level of awareness at which the client is functioning. Ylvisaker, Szekeres, Henry, Sullivan, and Wheeler (1987) began to discuss the relationship between various therapy techniques and clients' level of awareness:

> Patients who lack an awareness of their deficits or the functional implications of these deficits may, if compliant, go through the motions of rehearsing a strategy but are clearly not engaged in the process. Consequently, the likelihood of the patient's learning or putting the strategy to functional use is minimal. For these patients, treatment that focuses on self awareness of strengths and weaknesses, emphasizing the relation these have to patients' goals, is a necessary first stage in the rehabilitation plan. (pp. 140, 142)

Varying types of awareness deficits that guide interventions have been discussed by Crosson et al. (1989).

The purpose of this chapter is to delineate specifically the types of awareness deficits, as well as assessment and facilitation techniques appropriate to each type. Further, as with many other neurological changes after brain injury, awareness deficits may have to be accepted as a rather permanent change in functioning. Considering this proposition, one must ask how awareness deficits affect a client's ability to compensate for other deficit areas. Thus, the final portion of this chapter explores different approaches to compensation based on a client's level of awareness.

TYPES OF AWARENESS DEFICITS

Dealing with awareness deficits in therapy can be a confusing experience for therapists, clients, and families. Most therapists with at least some experience in head injury rehabilitation have treated clients who can describe their deficits with a fair degree of accuracy, may even be able to state what compensations they should apply in specific circumstances, and yet are unable to initiate compensations to avoid serious difficulties. Frequently, such difficulties in initiating compensations are attributed to lack of motivation or to psychological denial. Thus, therapists often see the clients as having greater control over their behavior than is actually the case. Although motivation and denial can be important factors in head injury rehabilitation, the key to intervening in situations such as the one just described is understanding the different types of awareness that can be disrupted by head injury.

Crosson et al. (1989) described a model of awareness that consists of three interdependent levels (Figure 11.1). At the bottom of the pyramid is intellectual awareness, which provides the foundation for the other types of awareness. The succeeding levels are emergent and anticipatory awareness, respectively.

Intellectual Awareness

Intellectual awareness is the cognitive capacity of the client to understand to some degree that a particular function is diminished from premorbid levels. At the most basic level, intellectual awareness involves clients' understanding that they are having difficulty with some specific activities. For example, clients might discern that they did not understand what a relative tried to tell them on some occasion. A higher level of intellectual awareness is required to recognize that the activities with which one has trouble have something in common. For example, clients might realize that they have trouble understanding others in many circumstances, not simply on a specific occasion. The highest level of intellectual awareness is recognizing the implications of one's deficits; for example, that difficulty with auditory comprehension could interfere with receiving instructions from one's boss in the workplace.

Intervention strategies for problems in intellectual awareness are discussed later in this chapter, but it is important here to note that a client's neurological injury may cause enduring limitations in intellectual awareness, particularly when significant deficits in abstract reasoning or memory exist. Some degree of intellectual awareness is a prerequisite for emergent and anticipatory awareness.

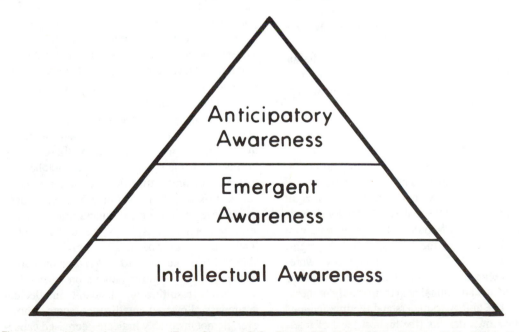

Figure 11.1.   Model of awareness. (From Crosson, B.C., Barco, P.P., Velozo, C.A., Bolesta, M.M., Werts, D., & Brobeck, T. [1989]. Awareness and compensation in post-acute head injury rehabilitation. *Journal of Head Trauma Rehabilitation, 4*[3], 47; reprinted with permission of Aspen Publishers, Inc., © 1989.)

Emergent Awareness

Emergent awareness refers to the ability of clients to recognize a problem when it is actually occurring. It is necessary for clients to realize that a deficit exists in order to recognize problems related to the deficit when they occur. This is why some degree of intellectual awareness is necessary to support emergent awareness. Implicit in the concept of emergent awareness is the client's ability to recognize the occurrence of problems without unusual feedback from friends, relatives, and therapists. For example, clients who consistently require relatives or therapists to make them aware of their socially inappropriate behavior do not possess emergent awareness.

Clients with intellectual but not emergent awareness may be confusing to therapists. The ability to apply compensations is usually dependent on being able to recognize that a problem is occurring. In such cases, clients with emergent awareness problems may be able to describe their deficits or even appropriate compensations—but because they do not recognize that a problem is occurring, they cannot initiate compensations when needed. In other words, if the client cannot recognize that a problem is occurring, the client does not see a reason to compensate. It is particularly common for an emergent awareness deficit to be mistaken for problems in motivation or even denial. Effective remediation requires that more permanent deficits in emergent awareness be recognized and dealt with in the intervention program.

Anticipatory Awareness

Anticipatory awareness is the ability to anticipate that a problem is going to happen because of some deficit. For example, clients with a right visual neglect might realize that they will have trouble reading inventory numbers because of a tendency to omit the last digits on the right. Once again, the concept of anticipatory awareness implies that clients can anticipate problems without any additional help from family or therapists. The ability to understand the implications of one's own deficits (the highest level of intellectual awareness) is closely linked to anticipatory awareness. If clients do not understand that

deficits are likely to cause certain practical problems, they will not be able to anticipate such problems. Further, if they are unable to recognize problems when they are occurring, they are unlikely to anticipate that such problems might happen with respect to specific future events.

Pure deficits in anticipatory awareness may be more rare than deficits in intellectual or emergent awareness. However, when the former do occur, they also can be mistaken for poor motivation. Family members or therapists may exhort such clients to apply compensations to avoid certain problems. Yet often clients must be in the midst of a problem before recognizing that a compensation is needed. Frustration on the part of therapists, family members, and clients can be avoided if anticipatory awareness deficits and their implications can be recognized.

ASSESSMENT OF AND INTERVENTION FOR AWARENESS DEFICITS

The first step in developing an approach to increasing awareness and developing appropriate compensatory training is to assess the client's current level of functioning. To do this, it is important to determine the client's current ability to be aware of the deficit areas. This includes an assessment of cognitive and intellectual deficits that may affect awareness, as well as the client's present level of awareness of the problem areas and their implications.

Certain types of brain lesions affect awareness at each of the different levels, and can result in enduring limitations at any of these levels. Diffuse white matter injury and frontal lobe contusion are common after closed head injury (Jennett & Teasdale, 1981), and may frequently cause a decrease in intellectual functioning and abstract reasoning. Thus, low scores on basic intelligence testing may be an indicator of a questionable ability of the client to understand the nature of the specific cognitive deficits on an intellectual level, resulting in deficient intellectual awareness. Lowered intelligence scores, however, do not invariably indicate decreased capacity for intellectual awareness. There are clients with significant decreases in intellectual functioning who nonetheless have attained adequate levels of intellectual awareness. Also, severe and global deficits on memory tests may foreshadow deficits in intellectual awareness. Injuries to the midline diencephalon, basal forebrain, or deep temporal lobe, which can seriously affect memory, may be an indicator that a client will have difficulty remembering and, therefore, integrating experiences. For intellectual awareness, clients must remember and integrate past experiences to draw conclusions about the commonalities between these experiences.

Disturbances in sensory and perceptual mechanisms, particularly common in posterior right hemisphere injury, may affect a client's ability to perceive relationships between self and environment accurately. These types of deficits would likely affect emergent awareness by influencing the ability to realize a problem is currently happening. Upon neuropsychological evaluation, such clients frequently have deficits in the perception and/or integration of visuospatial material.

Finally, difficulties in disinhibition, impulsiveness, or inability to project/plan into the future would affect a client's ability to anticipate adequately that a particular deficit will lead to problems in the future, resulting in defective anticipatory awareness. Ingvar (1985) pointed out that such difficulties projecting into the future can be a product of frontal lobe dysfunction. Neuropsychological tests sensitive to frontal lobe functions may be predictive of deficient anticipatory awareness if intellectual and emergent awareness are intact. This is particularly true if such frontal lobe deficits are relatively isolated on testing.

Assessment of awareness, and deficits that have the potential of affecting awareness, can be done both formally and informally. Background data provided by computerized axial tomography (CT) and magnetic resonance imaging (MRI) scans will provide the necessary information related to structural brain damage. Formal neuropsychological and related health professional evaluations will provide further information regarding localization and, also, specific information regarding sensory, perceptual, and cognitive processes affected by the injury. How-

ever, a very important part of evaluation of awareness deficits is the assessment gained by interview and skilled observation of the client in a variety of less structured situations. While these observations are not formally standardized, there are guidelines that assist in specifying a client's level of awareness. These guidelines for observation, informal assessment, and intervention are discussed next, in relationship to level of awareness.

Intellectual Awareness

Assessment

Assessment of intellectual awareness is often accomplished in an informal interview where the client is asked to describe what difficulties have occurred since the head injury. Intellectual awareness is most readily apparent when a client is able to describe accurately in some detail the problems that have resulted since the brain injury. Variable levels of intellectual awareness can be present. Self-rating scales, of which the purpose is to determine the congruence between the client's awareness of limitations with either a family member or professional, have been discussed by several authors (e.g., Crewe & Athelstan, 1984; Prigatano et al., 1986; Wachter, Fawber, & Scott, 1987; Ylvisaker & Szekeres, 1989). For example, clients may actually feel that they have not changed at all since the injury and may not be able to identify any problem areas, which can be in sharp contrast to family members' opinions. This type of response would indicate a significant lack of intellectual awareness.

In many cases, however, "borderline" intellectual awareness exists. Such cases may include clients who can state their problem areas, but may preface their statements with expressions like: "My family says I have memory problems." This would lead one to question the client's true belief and intellectual awareness of the problems; however, it is indicative of a higher awareness than a client who cannot even report any "suspected" problem areas. A further example of "borderline" intellectual awareness is the client who can clearly explain some problem areas, but is not aware of other deficit areas. A common example is the client who is able to describe physical limitations accurately and wants to focus therapy solely on improving the physical deficits, without an awareness of the less "tangible" cognitive deficits. It is also possible for clients to be intellectually aware of some cognitive deficits, and not others. For example, a client may be aware of memory problems, but not difficulties with problem solving.

Finally, the highest level of intellectual awareness is assessed by whether or not a client can describe the functional implications the deficits have on his or her life. This can often be determined by interviewing clients about their goals and expectations. Due to the inherent levels within intellectual awareness itself, reassessment of status is often necessary throughout the course of rehabilitation. It is not uncommon for a subacute head-injured person to be lacking in at least some aspects of intellectual awareness. If this is found to be true, it becomes the therapist's role to facilitate intellectual awareness, as this type of awareness becomes the foundation for more advanced skills and abilities.

Facilitation

Facilitating intellectual awareness can be achieved through repetitive education with both the client and family. Of course, the client must have the underlying skills and abilities to be capable of new learning and of understanding the deficit at some level to profit from such education. The role of education in the therapy of awareness deficits has been previously discussed (Lam et al., 1988; Szekeres et al., 1987; Ylvisaker et al., 1987). Emphasis is placed on explaining deficit areas to both the client and family, as well as explaining what the functional implications could be. For some clients, the initial lack of intellectual awareness can be related to a lack of accurate information about how the brain works relative to their deficits. For this reason, the Brain Education Unit is one method used to provide this information to clients and family members at the Head Injury Resource Center in St. Louis, Missouri. The purpose of this unit is to educate clients and families about brain function and the types of damage that can occur after head injury, as well as recovery patterns. Clients' specific deficit areas are reviewed with them and com-

pared to the area(s) of damage unique to their own brain. This is accomplished with supplementary material, including understandable diagrams, workbooks, and visual models. The Brain Education Unit appears to be an important initial step in acceptance for many clients. Clients learn that deficits are related to the brain injury, and not due to any specific fault of their own.

Providing feedback to the client during times that the deficit area is affecting performance is another method with which to facilitate intellectual awareness. Feedback, a common therapeutic intervention, is used at this stage to point out to the client that a problem exists. Consistent feedback helps identify to the client what the deficit actually is and how it may be affecting functional performance. When possible, one common and effective method for doing this is videotaping. Videotaping has been utilized as a mode to increase self-awareness of strengths and weaknesses (e.g., Alexy, Foster, Baker, 1983; Haarbauer-Krupa et al., 1985; Prigatano et al., 1986; Ylvisaker et al., 1987). Feedback through videotaping is immediate, concrete, and objective. Thus, it allows clients to see what the deficit is, concurrent with the feedback being provided.

When discussing deficit areas with the client, intellectual awareness can best be facilitated by using the same terminology across various team members. Occasionally, if there is a specific deficit with an individual client that is going to be addressed by the intervention team and for which frequent feedback will be provided, the client will assist in "labeling" the problem. This allows the client to associate the problem with a specific term, and helps the client to recognize the same deficit across varied situations. If different terminology is applied to the same problem behavior, the client may begin to think different problems exist as opposed to one.

One important factor in a client's ability to benefit from feedback is the client's capacity to establish trust in relationships. Difficulties with establishing trust affect a client's ability to accept feedback from others that problems exist, as opposed to relying on his or her own impression that there are no problems. It can become necessary to allow clients to "fail" at a task, in order for them actually to see the effects of a deficit area on their lives (e.g., Lam et al., 1988; Ylvisaker et al., 1987). This may involve simply failing at a task within the therapy environment before attempting a goal outside of therapy (e.g., returning to college). If such a "planned failure" is anticipated, it is necessary that the client be provided with emotional support, counseling, and education after the "failure" in order to profit from the experience and minimize the likelihood for unproductive emotional reaction or repetition of the failure.

To assess and reinforce further the facilitation of intellectual awareness, clients can participate with therapists in formulating a strength-and-weakness list (H.K. Zeiner, personal communication, 1986). When formulating the strength-and-weakness list, the therapist should make careful observation of what the client views as personal strengths and weaknesses since the head injury. This can also be an assessment of intellectual awareness of the client. The therapist needs to observe how much cuing is needed for the client to identify pertinent areas. The therapist's role then focuses on assisting the client to identify omitted areas to be added to the list, as well as providing the client with education and functional examples to supplement the awareness. Of course, the list can be altered as necessary throughout the program. Interestingly, another important aspect of the strength-and-weakness list is that it can also be useful for self-esteem. In some cases, individuals can be so focused on the "negative" problem areas that they lose sight of their positive qualities. Psychological intervention may be necessary for these clients. Throughout therapy, it is important to continue to emphasize and build upon a client's areas of strength while facilitating awareness of deficit areas.

Once the client has at least some intellectual awareness, intervention can focus on continuing to increase this intellectual awareness, if appropriate. It also can advance to evaluating whether the client is capable of a higher level of awareness, specifically the next level in the hierarchy—emergent awareness. It is possible, however, that the client will not be able to achieve even a minimal level of intellectual awareness. This could be due to many different factors, some of which were mentioned earlier.

For example, severe deficits in abstract reasoning or severe memory disorders will limit the client's capacity to learn about and understand deficit areas. Without at least minimal intellectual awareness, it is not appropriate to pursue facilitation of more advanced levels of awareness. For the head-injured client without intellectual awareness, there are only very limited options of compensations appropriate to be utilized.

Compensation

Compensations become an emphasis of intervention after attempts at facilitating intellectual awareness are not effective. If the client does not realize the existence of problem areas, it is unlikely that the motivation and ability to apply compensations will exist. Therefore, the type of compensation most appropriate for the client without intellectual awareness is known as *external compensation*. External compensation is the most structured and least versatile form of compensation. External compensation is the application of a technique to compensate for a deficit that is initiated by an agent in the environment other than the client, or by modification of the environment itself. In essence, external compensations include all forms of compensation that exist outside of the client's own initiation.

Environmental modifications or restructuring consist of modifying any aspect of the client's environment to facilitate effective functioning despite significant cognitive deficits (Deaton, 1987; Grimm & Bleiberg, 1986; Szekeres et al., 1985; Ylvisaker et al., 1987). In addition to environmental compensations, external compensations include strategies that are elicited by someone other than the client (e.g., cuing provided to the client by a family member or job coach). If external compensation is going to be the main emphasis from a therapeutic standpoint, it becomes the therapist's role to assess realistically the ability and willingness of a significant other to participate in the implementation of the compensations, and/or the extent that the environment can be modified or adapted.

It is important to remember that the purpose of any compensation is to maximize the independence of the client. If a member in the support system (often a family member) is going to serve as an agent to assist the client in compensating, then this member first needs to be willing to assume this role. This person must also have the type of relationship with the client that will facilitate the use of compensation. For example, negative indicators for use of an external agent would include the presence of significant interpersonal conflict between the client and the significant other, or the need of the significant other to have the client more dependent on him or her. If it appears that a support system exists that is able to serve as a mode of external compensation, intervention then focuses on providing education regarding deficit areas and training so that the key members of the support system have adequate knowledge in the implementation of specified strategies. Intervention from a support system can involve a range of assistance based on the client's abilities. For example, it may range from the support system providing regular cues to the client, to actually performing an activity for the client. Ylvisaker et al. (1987) discussed general guidelines specific to training and working with family members. It is equally important for clients to be given as much information about the compensation plan as they are capable of understanding, including information about the role their support system will have. Cooperation and agreement from both the client and the support system are necessary for this type of compensation to be successful in the long term. If they are not successful in working together, this may not be a feasible type of compensation. In such circumstances, family therapy may be beneficial; however, since family dynamics rarely change rapidly, this would involve long-term intervention.

As previously stated, if altering or modifying the environment is going to be done as part of external compensation, the therapist needs to have access to this environment and the agreement of others in the environment to alter it. This is most commonly done in work settings, where a therapist works closely with a job supervisor in adapting and modifying job responsibilities to meet the client's strengths and skills. To do this, a therapist needs to have a strong background in job and task analysis, and a good knowledge of the client's strengths and deficits, as well as a

flexible and willing employer with whom to work. Supported employment can also be an example of external compensation in the work setting. The purpose of supported employment includes providing ongoing support to the head-injured person at the employment site (Kreutzer et al., 1988). (For further discussion of supported employment for persons with traumatic brain injury, the reader is referred to Chapter 20, this volume.)

A stable environment is preferable for alterations and adaptations within the environment to be successful over the long term. In implementing external compensations, therapists must realize it is a mistake to depend on clients themselves who are lacking intellectual awareness to implement the necessary changes in their environment. Clients need to have some intellectual awareness in order to be capable of recognizing how the environment can best be modified to meet their individual needs, as well as to implement such modifications.

Emergent Awareness

Assessment

Prior to assessing the presence of emergent awareness, it is necessary for the client to have at least some degree of intellectual awareness. Problems in emergent awareness are indicated when clients are in the process of having difficulties due to some deficit area, are unable to recognize that the difficulties are occurring, and therefore cannot alter the course of these difficulties. Observation by a trained professional during a client's performance of a cognitive task or functional activity is the most readily available form of assessment of emergent awareness. For example, does the client attempt to correct problems as they occur? If so, this would be evidence of emergent awareness. If, however, the client continues to perform the task without noticing the occurrence of problems, this indicates deficient emergent awareness.

Like intellectual awareness, emergent awareness can be present to different degrees. For example, a client may show signs of frustration in performing an activity but be unable to associate the frustration to deficit areas resulting from the head injury. This would be indicative of at least some awareness that a problem is occurring, as compared to the client who continues to perform the activity without any indications that difficulties are occurring. The therapist may find it helpful to ask carefully timed questions of clients during task performance to gather further information about how clients themselves think they are doing. Additionally, it is possible a client may have a higher level of emergent awareness for one deficit area than another. For example, a client may be able to recognize difficulties with remembering events that happened an hour earlier, but not recognize difficulties with maintaining attention. Thus, in assessing emergent awareness, therapists must look for indications that the client is aware that a problem is occurring (e.g., signs of frustration, attempts made by the client to correct problems that are occurring), across all deficit areas addressed in therapy.

Facilitation

As with intellectual awareness, providing feedback to clients during and after task performance is an important method in facilitating emergent awareness. The goal of providing feedback in the facilitation of emergent awareness is for the clients to begin to recognize *when* problems are affecting them. In comparison, the goal of feedback in facilitating intellectual awareness is to inform and educate; that is, to make clients aware of the general existence of the deficits. The general principles for providing feedback to clients remain the same, including using consistent terminology and being direct and specific. Since the goal is now recognition of the problem when it is occurring, it becomes important for the therapist not only to specify the problem to the clients as it occurs, but also to specify the observable "signs" of how the problem is affecting the client. Even though sometimes these signs may seem quite obvious, it often takes repetition and practice for the client to be able to identify them consistently. For example, a client with a tendency to become tangential and talk in extensive detail about topics until others become bored or disinterested may also have difficulty recognizing this behavior when it occurs. Therapy could include cuing the client to observe

some of the signs that this problem was occurring (e.g., observing social feedback from listeners such as lack of eye contact, frequent yawning).

The amount and method of cuing should be individualized. One method for providing cuing includes beginning with a general cue and, if unsuccessful, providing a series of cues, increasing the specificity until the client is able to complete the activity appropriately (Cicerone & Tupper, 1986). The goal, of course, is for clients to require the fewest possible cues or, ideally, no cues to be able to recognize problems as they occur. Often, it is impossible to eliminate cuing completely, which means that a member of the support system must be available to perform the necessary cuing. This would then be considered a form of external compensation, which was discussed earlier.

Videotaping is not only useful in facilitating intellectual awareness, but emergent awareness as well. Videotape feedback is especially useful in facilitating awareness of interpersonal and communication difficulties. Initially, when viewing tapes, clients with emergent awareness difficulties may be unable to identify their problem areas independently. Therefore, cuing and specifying observable signs to the client are equally important tools of intervention to continue using when reviewing tapes. Additional structure can be provided to the client to help identify specific areas to evaluate (e.g., checklists of categories to evaluate). Videotape feedback is effective in a group context, where the individual must learn to evaluate others' performance as well as his or her own. It is not uncommon for clients first to be able to identify a similar problem in others prior to being able to recognize it in themselves. Videotape feedback allows the client to begin the process of developing emergent awareness in graduated steps, with structure and support as necessary. As with any form of feedback, it is equally important to acknowledge a client's strengths as well as deficit areas.

Another therapeutic method to facilitate emergent awareness is a technique developed and utilized at the Head Injury Resource Center, involving the use of a self-rating scale for specific problem areas (see Figure 11.2). Such a

DATE:

KEY:

	1	2	3	4	5
	poor attention-concentration		average attention-concentration		excellent attention-concentration

RATING

GROUP	Self Rating					Therapist				
Cognitive Group Task/Comments										
1.	1	2	3	4	5	1	2	3	4	5
2.	1	2	3	4	5	1	2	3	4	5
Specialized Therapy I Task/Comments:										
1.	1	2	3	4	5	1	2	3	4	5
2.	1	2	3	4	5	1	2	3	4	5
Specialized Therapy II Task/Comments:										
1.	1	2	3	4	5	1	2	3	4	5
2.	1	2	3	4	5	1	2	3	4	5
Adjustment/Communication Task/Comments:										
1.	1	2	3	4	5	1	2	3	4	5
2.	1	2	3	4	5	1	2	3	4	5
Life Skills Task/Comments:										
1.	1	2	3	4	5	1	2	3	4	5
2.	1	2	3	4	5	1	2	3	4	5

Figure 11.2.   Self-rating scale: Attention. (Copyright 1987 Head Injury Resource Center, St. John's Mercy Rehabilitation Center, St. Louis, MO; reprinted by permission.)

self-rating scale is used to assist the client in focusing on when a particular deficit area is affecting performance. This scale involves clients rating themselves on a Likert-type scale regarding the extent to which a particular problem affects them during a task or therapy session. A similar rating is done concurrently by the therapist. This method can be used for a variety of problem areas (e.g., maintaining attention, interpersonal difficulties, communication deficits). Thus, this self-rating scale can be readily adapted to meet an individual client's needs. It is especially useful for clients who benefit from concrete feedback. The goal of this method becomes that the client more closely approximates the therapist's ratings over time. It is important

for effectiveness that this tool be used consistently among team members throughout the intervention.

Essentially, all the methods of facilitating emergent awareness just described utilize feedback of some type. As with intellectual awareness, the client's ability to establish trust is a necessary component in order to benefit from the feedback. Similar to techniques utilized in facilitating intellectual awareness, "planned failure" may become necessary for the client to experience the implications of the deficit areas.

Once clients show some evidence of emergent awareness, the therapy plan can continue to further the extent of emergent awareness while beginning to assess their capacity for anticipa-

EMERGENT → ANTICIPATORY

tory awareness. If, however, clients show little or no evidence of emergent awareness over the course of therapy, it is possible that they may have a permanent deficit in this area. Intervention can then focus on compensations that can be utilized with limited or no emergent awareness.

Compensation

Situational compensation is the preferred type of compensation utilized with clients who show evidence of intellectual awareness, but lack adequate emergent awareness. This type of compensation does not require the client to recognize problems as they are occurring, because the client is trained to apply the compensation habitually in all situations that might be appropriate. However, it does require the client's general awareness of the existence of a problem (i.e., intellectual awareness) in order to see a need and be motivated to compensate. For example, clients may have memory difficulties that affect the ability to remember to perform specified routine household responsibilities. Because the clients do not recognize when they forget a duty, they are trained always to utilize a checklist as a memory compensation for their duties. This compensation is triggered by the situation (e.g., performing household duties), and is based on the premise that it must be habitually applied in this circumstance. Thus, it becomes the therapist's role to identify the situation, develop the appropriate compensation, and train the client through practice and repetition in use of the strategy.

Situational compensation is thus preferred over external compensation, because it is under the control and initiation of the client. It does not require alteration of the environment or another person to trigger the compensation. Yet, situational compensation is not considered a flexible type of compensation. Since the client is utilizing this compensation at all times in the identified situation, it is possible that the clients will occasionally use it when in fact it may not be needed. However, since the client cannot recognize when it is necessary to use the compensation, due to the emergent awareness deficit, it must be habitually applied as a "precautionary tool" at all times in the specified situation. Also,

it will be necessary for the client to have a limited number of these situational compensations, because the more compensations of this type that are given to the client, the less likely the client will be able to utilize them effectively and consistently. Therefore, it is important for the therapist and client to prioritize what is most needed, and develop compensations accordingly and in consideration of individual strengths and current abilities.

Anticipatory Awareness

Assessment

Anticipatory awareness, the highest level of awareness, refers to the ability to anticipate that a particular deficit could cause a problem in a specific situation. Anticipatory awareness is closely related to the ability to plan and project into a future circumstance, and it involves the ability to recognize the implications of one's own deficits. In head-injured clients, anticipatory awareness does not come easily because it relies on cognitive skills that are commonly affected in head injury (e.g., planning, initiating, abstraction, insight), as well as requiring some degree of intellectual and emergent awareness. To determine if a client is capable of anticipatory awareness, once again observation combined with timely questions is most appropriate. When assessing this level of awareness, a therapist might ask the client what types of problems, if any, the client might expect to have in a variety of situations and why. For those clients who have some evidence of anticipatory awareness, therapists most likely would observe them initiating compensation prior to the actual occurrence of the problem in an attempt to prevent or minimize the effect of the problem. If a client is able to anticipate the need for and implement a compensatory strategy prior to the occurrence of a problem, it is known as *anticipatory compensation* (this is discussed later). Clients with deficits in anticipatory awareness have difficulty anticipating when problems would likely affect them and under what circumstances. They would not be observed to initiate compensations in preparation for problems, due to their inability to anticipate the need. In such cases, clients have to be in the midst of a problem before recognizing the need to compensate. During the observational assessment of anticipatory awareness, it is important that the therapist not provide cuing or other forms of assistance to the client. It is necessary to observe what compensation clients initiate on their own, to determine if anticipatory awareness does exist.

Facilitation

Clients who are more readily capable of anticipatory awareness may first need to be educated in their deficits, and to experience at least some effects of their deficits. Then, they may rather naturally begin to anticipate when the deficits are likely to affect them. With other clients, anticipatory awareness may not appear so easily, and may require a greater degree of therapeutic intervention. Therapists can facilitate anticipatory awareness by guiding clients into planning for deficits. This can be accomplished by providing cues to clients to plan and anticipate what deficits may affect them prior to starting a task. Reduction of cuing over time is necessary for clients to develop true anticipatory awareness. The therapy environment can be utilized as an opportunity for the client to test out the ability to anticipate what problems may likely occur in a variety of situations. If situations are not actually available, the therapist can devise them or describe potential circumstances to clients, to see if they are capable of anticipating the occurrence of the problem areas. It should be noted that anticipatory awareness usually does not appear immediately. This type of awareness requires clients to experience a variety of situations and learn from their mistakes in order to begin to anticipate problems prior to their actual occurrence. It is likely that many head-injured clients will never be consistent in their ability to anticipate problems, and, therefore, will need to be trained in compensations to be implemented after the problem has already occurred.

Compensation

Recognition compensations are the preferred type of compensation to teach the client who has some capacity for recognizing problems as they occur (i.e., emergent awareness), but cannot anticipate problems prior to their actual occurrence. When clients recognize a problem is occurring, this recognition triggers them to initiate a compensation to reduce or correct the problem. For example, clients may be able to recognize nonverbal signals from others that they are becoming tangential. Once they are aware that the problem is occurring, they can implement an appropriate strategy (e.g., redirecting the focus of their discussion) to alter the course of the conversation. This type of compensation is more versatile than both situational and external compensations. Unlike situational compensations (which are applied habitually in all specified situations), recognition compensations are applied only in situations as they are needed.

After determining that recognition compensation will be the most appropriate form of compensation, a therapist's role is to assist in developing specific strategies appropriate for the client. As with any self-initiated compensation, it is important to observe what the client may already be doing to compensate and what the client's current strengths are. If the client is already applying strategies, it becomes the therapist's role to evaluate the effectiveness of these strategies and make recommendations regarding modifications to improve their effectiveness, when applicable. It is preferable to utilize a strategy with which the client is comfortable because that will increase the likelihood that the client will follow through with its use. In helping clients formulate strategies, it is also important to consider their areas of strength and utilize these strengths in the development of strategies. When teaching compensations to clients, it is important that different therapists be consistent with the type of strategy chosen for a particular deficit area. If different ways of compensating for the same problem are given, the client may become confused about which strategy to utilize and when. Extensive practice, under professional supervision, is required to improve the effectiveness of compensation and the willingness of the client to utilize strategies when needed. Ylvisaker et al. (1987) discussed factors in selecting and teaching strategies specific to individual needs.

The final and most advanced type of compensation is known as anticipatory compensation, and is utilized when clients demonstrate evidence of anticipatory awareness. These compensations are triggered by the anticipation that a problem is likely to occur. Anticipatory compensations are the most preferable type of compensation because a problem can be avoided or minimized if a compensation is used from the start. This is contrasted to recognition compensation, where the client must be in the midst of a problem to recognize the need for compensating, and after some undesirable consequences have occurred. Clients who are capable of anticipatory awareness and anticipatory compensation may also be more capable of tailoring compensations to a particular situation. Development and training in specific strategies is similar to what was described with recognition compensations, with the exception that these clients may be able to learn more types of strategies due to their ability to project and plan. Thus, anticipatory compensations are the most desirable and versatile form of compensation. A therapist's role is to provide clients with as much opportunity in a variety of situations to practice and develop these skills.

CASE STUDY

Background and Initial Assessment Data

The client described in this case study, a female in her early 20s, was involved in a motor vehicle accident resulting in a severe closed head injury. Prior to this head injury, the client had attended 15 years of school, and she had decided to postpone the completion of her final year of college. Prior to her accident, she was successfully employed full time in an office position. Acute CT scan indicated contusion in white matter underlying the left frontal lobe, the left medial frontal cortex, the posterior limb of the left internal capsule, and the right frontal lobe. An MRI scan also suggested bilateral temporal lobe contusion. This client was in a coma for 20 days, and had post-traumatic amnesia of approximately 6 weeks. After regaining consciousness, she received acute inpatient rehabilitation for about 2½–3 months. During the course of her inpatient treatment, she was noted to have a short attention span and to be prone to agitation. She did appear to make rapid progress. Decreases in inappropriate behavior and distractibility were noted. At times, she was noted to have difficulty maintaining the topic of conversation, and monitoring her own linguistic functions. She received outpatient therapy for an additional 2 months prior to being referred to an outpatient comprehensive day treatment program. Thus, it was approximately 5 months postinjury when she was referred for further evaluation and rehabilitation.

Pertinent neuropsychological evaluation findings 5 months postinjury indicated this clients's Verbal IQ was in the average range and her Performance IQ was in the low average range, which could be indicative of impairment in the functioning of the nondominant right hemisphere. Mild difficulties were noted in verbal memory, which appeared primarily related to distractibility. Nonverbal memory was in the above average range. A moderate decrease in motor speed existed for both hands, with impairment of the nondominant left hand being greater. Otherwise, this client was generally within normal range with basic language skills, perceptual functions, and problem-solving skills.

In addition to neuropsychological testing, a multidisciplinary team evaluation was performed. The pertinent findings related to this discussion on awareness are summarzied as follows: A speech-language evaluation revealed that she continued to have mild to moderate difficulties with topic maintenance, topic shifting, verbal organization, verbosity, and identification of main ideas on less structured tasks. These findings were, in part, related to attention. An occupational therapy evaluation revealed difficulty maintaining attention on less structured and functionally oriented tasks. It was noted that this client had a tendency to make more errors than would be expected normally. These errors were scattered and inconsistent, again indicating probable lapses of attention. For example, on one task where the client was required to follow directions to go somewhere outside the center (under supervision of the therapist), she was observed to become so distracted by her own conversation that she actually kept walking by the street where she was instructed to turn, three times. Even with cuing from the therapist, she continued to miss the street because she was distracted by her own conversation. During this occupational therapy evaluation, the therapist would point out the errors to the client, and afterward, the client was observed to make "excuses" for them.

Upon review of the evaluation results with the multidisciplinary team, it was obvious the client was not aware of the existence of these cognitive deficits, or the implications of these deficits to her functional life and future goals. In many ways, this client was high functioning; however, the attention difficulties were interfering with her abilities to utilize her skills fully. Thus, a main area of emphasis in the day treatment program was increasing her awareness of the attention difficulties, facilitating improvement in attention, and compensating for what deficits remained.

Intellectual Awareness

The first step in this process was to explore further the extent to which the client was capable of intellectual awareness. To determine if the client had any understanding of what types of problems she was having, a therapist informally interviewed her upon admission to the program. In spite of earlier discussions reviewing the evaluation results, the client was unable to be specific regarding her areas of difficulties, including the attention deficit. Essentially, she was not able to describe verbally any of the cognitive problems she was having. Although she remembered, with assistance from the therapist, the discussion of "attention problems," she was uncertain what this actually meant.

In an effort to increase intellectual awareness, the beginning portion of the program focused on educating the client regarding her deficit areas, and how these deficits affected her functionally. The emphasis throughout the team was placed on the attention difficulties, because these appeared to affect her performance in many situations. To assist in this education process, the client went through the Brain Education Unit (described earlier in this chapter) to explain further the relationships of her deficits to

the areas of her brain that were damaged, and also to understand the functioning and recovery process after brain injury.

The multidisciplinary team began specifying to the client examples of how "attention" was affecting her throughout the day and in a variety of therapeutic tasks. Since the team members were beginning to provide feedback to her, they developed common terminology so that the client could see that it was basically the same problem affecting her in a variety of situations. Collaboratively, the team and the client "labeled" two areas to be emphasized. *Rambling* was the term used when the client was having difficulty with topic maintenance and verbosity. *Difficulty paying attention* was used to describe the attention deficits. Throughout the treatment day, therapists would provide feedback (using the terminology agreed upon) to the client whenever these difficulties occurred. For example, difficulties in paying attention were pointed out to the client in a variety of situations, including cooking activities, checkbook tasks, and math equations. Likewise, she received feedback when rambling occurred. This difficulty could be easily pointed out with the use of videotaping during communication activities.

The goal was for the client to begin to acknowledge the existence of these problems, and to increase her understanding of them. After approximately 3–4 weeks, the client was reassessed regarding her intellectual awareness of these problems by having her formulate a strength-and-weakness list. The client was able to describe independently and accurately the majority of her strengths and problem areas on this list. Thus, she appeared to have an increased intellectual awareness of her cognitive difficulties. However, she was intellectually unable to recognize the implications of these deficits to her functioning and life goals.

Emergent Awareness

Because this client showed definite signs of increased intellectual awareness, the focus of therapy turned to evaluating the presence of emergent awareness. In other words, was the client able to recognize these cognitive deficits at the time of occurrence? To do this, the therapists reduced their cuing and feedback during task performance to see if the client was able to show signs of recognition when problems occurred. It was noted that although the client was intellectually aware of the deficits, she was not totally aware of them at the time they were affecting her. One of the most obvious examples emerged during a series of study skill tasks devoted to evaluating her ability to return to college, since that was one of her goals. During these tasks, the therapists noted that the client had difficulty maintaining her attention when reading/studying for longer than 10 minutes. The client would begin to yawn and stare around the room, become very inconsistent with highlighting main points, and not remember anything she read. The client did not recognize the difficulty she was having, and either continued with the task, which resulted in poor performance, or became frustrated and claimed she was extremely bored. The frustration was a sign of limited emergent awareness, however; the client was not able to relate it to the deficit area. When asked how she thought she was doing or if she was having any problems, she expressed she was doing fine and blamed any difficulties on the task itself. Thus, it appeared she was not able to recognize the attention difficulties when they were affecting her.

In order to facilitate emergent awareness, continued effort was put forth in providing feedback to her. This feedback was also expanded to have her family and other clients in the program provide similar feedback to her in less structured activities (e.g., during lunches, in home environment). Of course, this was done with the consent of the client, and other clients in the program were instructed in the proper method of providing feedback. To assist with structuring the feedback in a manner to facilitate emergent awareness, the self-rating tool (see Figure 11.2) was implemented so the client would first be able to rate herself on a behavior (in this case, attention), and then immediately compare her ratings to the therapist's rating. The therapist, when providing feedback, would specify to her the observable signs of the attention deficit. For example, observable signs of attention difficulties consisted of the client's yawning frequently throughout the task, staring, making more mistakes than anticipated, looking tired or distractible, or taking too much or too little time to do something. This allowed the client to begin to recognize these same signs. The goal was for the client to establish at least some recognition of the difficulty (i.e., maintaining attention) when it was actually occurring.

The self-rating form was used consistently after each task or therapy throughout the day. Initially, the client's rating was very different from the therapist's, but over time her rating began to approximate that of the therapists. The client even began to make notations such as "I was distracted by conversations in the other office." The use of the form yielded further diagnostic information. It was found that there were certain times and types of activities in which this client had more difficulty maintaining her attention, predisposing her to increased likelihood of attention problems. These activities were mainly those she was less interested in and/or those that did not emphasize physical movement or interaction with other people. Also, if this client was very emotional (either upset or excited), she would have more difficulty with maintaining attention, most likely being distracted by her internal thoughts. The self-rating tool seemed to help facilitate emergent awareness, as indicated by both her ratings becoming similar to the therapists' ratings and her verbal statements of recognition of the problems. Since the client was able to begin recognizing her problems at the time of their occurrence, the natural course of action was helping her to learn ways of compensating for the problems. For example, at times when she noticed difficulties paying attention, she was to take short breaks, double check her work, and/or put more effort into concentrating.

Anticipatory Awareness

Within the context of the day treatment program, the client was able to begin compensating adequately for attention problems by utilizing a recognition-based compensation. Essentially, the client was implementing the compensation triggered by recognition that the problem was occurring. Attempts at higher levels of awareness (i.e., anticipatory awareness) were not as successful. The client was very inconsistent in her ability to anticipate the likelihood of attention problems occurring. To evaluate this, the therapists began questioning the client to see if she could recognize days or activities that might predispose her to the likelihood of attention difficulties (e.g., emotional days, activities that were not physically active or were less interesting to her). What was observed was that this client was inconsistent in her ability to anticipate when and in what situations her attention problems were most likely to occur. She appeared to rely on the cues she received from therapists to anticipate problems. Thus, she appeared very inconsistent in her anticipatory awareness; therefore, recognition compensations were the compensations most appropriate to her level of awareness.

Conclusions

Although not discussed in detail in this chapter, the client was at a similar level of emergent awareness with her difficulty in topic maintenance and verbal conciseness. Interestingly, in the developing of her emergent awareness, she was first able to note a similar problem in another client in the program, prior to recognizing her own problem in this area. Videotaping also appeared to facilitate the development of emergent awareness. Recognizing the difficulty with topic maintenance on videotape preceded her ability to recognize it in actual conversations at the time of occurrence. Finally, she was able to utilize nonverbal cues from others as an observable indicator that she was not maintaining the topic of conversation appropriately (i.e., she was rambling). However, she was inconsistent in her ability to anticipate the likelihood that this problem was going to occur, prior to its actual occurrence.

One precaution should be noted: Even though the level of awareness of a particular deficit was determined within the structure of the day treatment program, when this client was moved to a job trial (volunteer work situation as part of the therapy program), a temporary regression was noted. She was placed in the medical school library in a position that involved some photocopying responsibilities. Initially, she was having significant attention problems and was not able to recognize them. For example, she would copy pages incorrectly, often cutting off half of the page without noticing it. It was not uncommon for her to have to copy a page two or three times. At this point, she benefited from "coaching" from a therapist, to refocus her on becoming aware of when the problem was occurring, and to facilitate the transfer of her skills and compensations more readily. With this assistance, the client was able to regain her emergent awareness and begin to initiate the appropriate compensations much more readily than she initially did within the day treatment program. Thus, clients may show some fluctuation in their awareness, especially in a more stressful or novel situation, and supportive services such as job coaching can help with generalization of abilities and skills.

SUMMARY AND CONCLUSIONS

Postacute head injury rehabilitation techniques vary depending on the level of awareness at which a client is functioning. Some clients may begin therapy with adequate awareness at all three levels in the hierarchy, and this strength can be readily used in their rehabilitation. However, most will require at least some intervention to attain their optimal level of awareness. Therefore, it is necessary to assess the client's level of awareness both before intervention planning and throughout the course of therapy in order to modify intervention approaches to coincide with changes in awareness level. The goal is for clients to reach the highest possible level of awareness for their deficit areas and, thereafter, to implement the most efficient form of compensation available.

Figure 11.3 summarizes the process of facilitating awareness and choosing the compensation appropriate to the ultimate level of awareness obtained. Basically, this approach begins with the evaluation of intellectual awareness. Facilitation of intellectual awareness is used if a deficit exists in this area. If adequate levels of intellectual awareness exist or can be established, similar procedures are applied to emergent awareness, the next level in the hierarchy, and so forth. When it becomes obvious that a

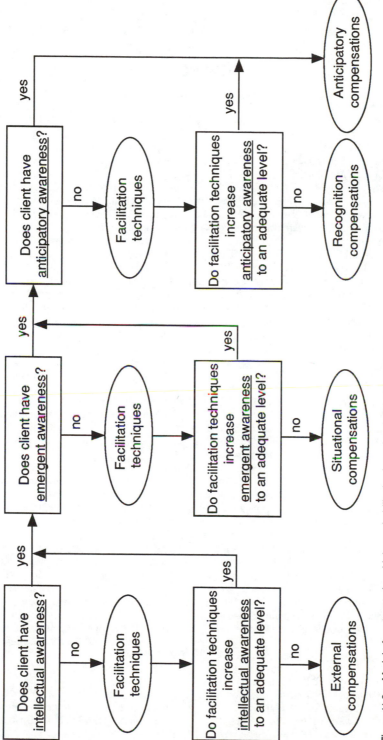

Figure 11.3. Model of postacute head injury rehabilitation based on level of awareness.

significant degree of awareness is unlikely to occur at a specified level in the hierarchy, then the appropriate type of compensation is designed.

Utilizing this approach is likely to result in increased organization, efficiency, and success of postacute head injury rehabilitation.

REFERENCES

Alexy, W.D., Foster, M., & Baker, A. (1983). Audiovisual feedback: An exercise in self-awareness for the head injured patient. *Cognitive Rehabilitation, 1*(6), 8–10.

Askenasy, J.J.M., & Rahmani, L. (1988). Neuropsycho-social rehabilitation of head injury. *American Journal of Physical Medicine, 66*(6), 315–327.

Ben-Yishay, Y. (1988, November). *What rehabilitation means in terms of real-world functions.* Paper presented at the seventh annual National Symposium, Head Injury Frontiers: Research, Rehabilitation, Re-entry, Atlanta.

Ben-Yishay, Y., Silver, S.M., Piasetsky, E.B., & Rattock, J. (1987). Relationship between employability and vocational outcome after intensive holistic cognitive rehabilitation. *Head Trauma Rehabilitation, 2*(1), 35–48.

Cicerone, K.D., & Tupper, D.E. (1986). Cognitive assessment in the neuropsychological rehabilitation of head-injured adults. In B.P. Uzzel & Y. Gross (Eds.), *Clinical neuropsychology of intervention* (pp. 59–83). Boston: Martinus Nijhoff.

Crewe, N.M., & Athelstan, G.T. (1984). *Functional Assessment Inventory manual.* Menomonie, WI: Materials Development Center.

Crosson, B.C., Barco, P.P., Velozo, C.A., Bolesta, M.M., Werts, D., & Brobeck, T. (1989). Awareness and compensation in post-acute head injury rehabilitation. *Journal of Head Trauma Rehabilitation, 4*(3), 46–54.

Deaton, A.V. (1986). Denial in the aftermath of traumatic head injury: Its manifestations, measurement, and treatment. *Rehabilitation Psychology, 31*(4), 231–240.

Deaton, A.V. (1987). Behavioral change strategies for children and adolescents with severe brain injury. *Journal of Learning Disabilities, 20*(10), 581–589.

Grimm, B.H., & Bleiberg, J. (1986). Psychological rehabilitation in traumatic brain injury. In S. Filskov & T. Boll (Eds.), *Handbook of clinical neuropsychology* (pp. 495–560). New York: John Wiley & Sons.

Haarbauer-Krupa, J.H., Henry, K., Szekeres, S.F., & Ylvisaker, M. (1985). Cognitive rehabilitation therapy: Late stages of recovery. In M. Ylvisaker (Ed.), *Head injury rehabilitation: Children and adolescents* (pp. 311–343). San Diego: College-Hill Press.

Ingvar, D.H. (1985). Memory of the future: An essay on the temporal organization of conscious awareness. *Human Neurobiology, 4,* 127–136.

Jennett, B., & Teasdale, G. (1981). *Management of head injuries.* Philadelphia: F.A. Davis.

Kreutzer, J.S., Wehman, P., Morton, M.V., & Stonnington, H.H. (1988). Supported employment and compensatory strategies for enhancing vocational outcome following traumatic brain injury. *Brain Injury, 2*(3), 205–223.

Lam, C.S., McMahon, B.T., Priddy, D.A., & Gehred-Schultz, A. (1988). Deficit awareness and treatment performance among traumatic head injury adults. *Brain Injury, 2*(3), 233–242.

Lezak, M.D. (1978). Living with the characterologically altered brain-injured patient. *Journal of Clinical Psychiatry, 39,* 592–598.

Nockelby, D.M., & Deaton, A.V. (1987). Denial versus distress: Coping patterns in post head trauma patients. *International Journal of Clinical Neuropsychology, IX*(4), 145–148.

Prigatano, G.P., Fordyce, D.J., Zeiner, H.K., Roueche, J.R., Pepping, M., & Wood, B.C. (Eds.). (1986). *Neuropsychological rehabilitation after brain injury.* Baltimore: Johns Hopkins University Press.

Szekeres, S.F., Ylvisaker, M., & Cohen, S.B. (1987). A framework for cognitive rehabilitation therapy. In M. Ylvisaker & E.M.R. Gobble (Eds.), *Community re-entry for head injured adults* (pp. 87–136). Boston: College-Hill Press.

Szekeres, S.F., Ylvisaker, M., & Holland, A.L. (1985). Cognitive rehabilitation therapy: A framework for intervention. In M. Ylvisaker (Ed.), *Head injury rehabilitation: Children and adolescents* (pp. 219–246). San Diego: College-Hill Press.

Wachter, J.F., Fawber, J.F., & Scott, M.B. (1987). Treatment aspects of vocational evaluation and placement for traumatically brain injured adults. In M. Ylvisaker & E.M.R. Gobble (Eds.), *Community re-entry for head injured adults* (pp. 259–299). Boston: College-Hill Press.

Ylvisaker, M., & Szekeres, S.F. (1989). Metacognitive and executive impairments in head-injured children and adults. *Topics in Language Disorders, 9*(2), 34–49.

Ylvisaker, M., Szekeres, S.F., Henry, K., Sullivan, D.M., & Wheeler, P. (1987). Topics in cognitive rehabilitation therapy. In M. Ylvisaker & E.M.R. Gobble (Eds.), *Community re-entry for head injured adults* (pp. 137–215). Boston: College-Hill Press.

CHAPTER 12

Retraining Memory
Theory, Evaluation, and Applications

RICK PARENTÉ AND ANTHONY DICESARE

Impaired memory is one of the most pervasive and persistent deficits after injury to the brain. Consequently, cognitive retraining programs usually emphasize retraining memory and attentional processes. Unfortunately, memory impairments may persist after months or years of intensive treatment. Indeed, persons with traumatic brain injury may never regain their former memory capacity.

Therapists are often frustrated by the lack of available literature that addresses the "hands-on" issues of cognitive rehabilitation and memory training. Intervention usually reduces to a form of stimulation therapy where the client is provided with structured activities to stimulate the mind. Although this approach may yield some improvement in the long term, the authors contend that considerably more benefit could be derived by first structuring the intervention so that it generalizes. Unfortunately, there are few published sources that illustrate how to plan a memory training program so that the effects are maximized or otherwise transfer to the client's job or activities of daily living (ADLs).

The purpose of this chapter is to explain how to plan an effective memory retraining program and to evaluate a variety of different memory training techniques. The chapter begins with a functional description of how memory works. Various theories of memory failure after head injury are also discussed. Generalization and transfer of learning principles are presented next, along with a discussion of how these principles can be used to predict the results of a variety of different memory training strategies. The chapter ends with a presentation of various prosthetic memory aids that have proven effective with several of the authors' clients with brain injury.

DYNAMICS OF MEMORY

A therapist cannot effectively retrain memory without first understanding how the memory system works. Figure 12.1 and Table 12.1 therefore present a functional memory model designed to help the therapist visualize the topology of memory dysfunction. The model is a simplified schematic of how the human information processing system functions; it is a very basic model that borrows heavily from early information processing theories of memory (Atkinson & Shriffrin, 1968). The reader should also review Baddeley and Hitch (1974) for a detailed explanation of how the working memory system and the long-term store interact. Also, as the neuropsychology of memory is not discussed here, the reader is referred to Kolb and Whishaw (1990, chap. 21) for a thorough and comprehensive treatment of this literature.

Sensory Memory Store

We are only briefly aware of the entirety of our experience before the brain and sensory system rearrange it into meaningful structures. The first stage of this transformation occurs in the sensory memory. This is an extremely large capacity system. Its function is to hold a virtual snapshot of experience so that we can select portions of it and process these fragments in the working memory. The system saves information as near-perfect replicas of experience. Most explorations of sensory memory have investigated the iconic (visual) and echoic (auditory) stores. There are virtually no investigations of the other systems: taste, smell, or touch. There has been only one investigation of sensory memory disruption after head injury (Parenté, Anderson-Parenté, & Shaw, 1989). The reader is referred to Dick (1974) for a

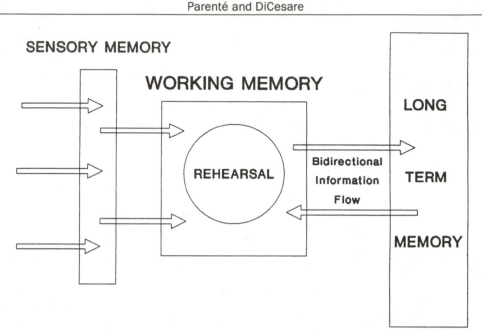

Figure 12.1. How memory works.

comprehensive review of the sensory memory literature.

Damage to the sensory register undermines information processing at the earliest stage. Because sensory memory precedes the later components of the system, damage can literally disrupt the formation of memories anywhere else. Clearly, if the sensory store is not functioning normally, then the working memory receives inaccurate information and distorted information may be stored in the long-term memory (LTM). It is therefore reasonable to suggest that memory retraining should begin with a comprehensive evaluation of the sensory register. Retraining any other system will be extremely difficult until the sensory store has been repaired.

Table 12.1. Summary of the memory system

Memory store	Function	Capacity
Sensory	Retention of sensory information for selection	Large
Working	Encoding	7 (+/−2) units
Long-term	Permanent storage	Infinite

Working Memory

Information is *encoded* or transformed in working memory for efficient storage and retrieval from LTM. However, a person must rehearse information to maintain it in working memory. Encoding is necessary because the working memory usually cannot store more than seven (plus or minus two) units of information. Information that has been stored in LTM is also retrieved and updated in the working memory. The arrow in Figure 12.1 that travels to the long-term memory from the working memory represents the storage process. The one that goes from the long-term memory to the working memory represents the retrieval process. Updating of information occurs in the working memory. Some types of information may never reach LTM. For example, we may need only remember certain phone numbers long enough to dial them. Similarly, we seldom recall shopping lists after we leave the store.

Figure 12.1 may give the mistaken impression that memory formation occurs in distinct stages, with working memory occupying the central position. It is more accurate to think of memory as a single process. Working memory is not synonymous with short-term memory

(STM). Short-term memory implies a "holding tank" where information is stored. The concept of working memory emphasizes the active processing of information as one experiences it.

Several authors have noted that working memory is a multidimensional system. Grafman (1984) developed a neuropsychological/human information processing integrative model of memory after working with Vietnam veterans with head injury. He proposed that people encode different types of information at different rates. Encoding may be rote rehearsal, rhyming, or various forms of semantic or imaginational transformations. He suggested that information is independently stored in long-term memory as either visual and/or linguistic-semantic codes, with all types of codes being integrated, if need be, to produce a response. His model identified three types of memory (immediate, short-term, and long-term) that can be selectively impaired by traumatic brain injury, depending upon the injury locus.

Baddeley and Hitch's (1974) discussion of the "articulatory loop" and the "visuospatial scratch pad" are especially interesting additions to the above discussion of working memory. They noted that the working memory processes both sequentially presented auditory verbal and visuospatial materials. In other words, a person with head injury may be able to remember one kind of material but not another. However, all persons with head injury may not suffer working memory impairments. Moreover, there is seldom a global impairment of memory after head injury. It is therefore necessary to determine which aspects are impaired and to plan intervention accordingly.

Long-Term Memory

Long-term memory stores information permanently after it is encoded in working memory. The capacity of LTM is virtually infinite. However, our ability to access information in the long-term store depends on whether or not we establish an appropriate access route. This difference between the availability and accessibility of information in LTM is clear to most therapists who note word-finding problems with their clients. Even though the client cannot retrieve the word unaided, when provided with an appropriate cue, he or she can then access the word or thought.

Both semantic and episodic memories are stored in LTM. Semantic memories are facts and acquired knowledge about our world, such as the memory that a dog is a mammal or that a bicycle is a means of transportation. Episodic memories are recordings of experiences that are unique to the individual (e.g., remembering what clothes one wore yesterday). These memories include information about the time, place, or context in which an event occurred. Episodic memories are the type most frequently disrupted after a traumatic brain injury, while semantic memories are relatively less affected.

THEORIES OF MEMORY FAILURE AFTER HEAD INJURY

Attention Deficit

Head injury typically disrupts the person's ability to attend and concentrate. An attention deficit theory of memory dysfunction assumes that information is not correctly perceived because the person does not effectively attend to the information at hand. We all know how difficult it is to understand what we see or hear when several things are competing for our attention. Memory span may be limited and the person with head injury may have difficulty allocating attention. Relative to Figure 12.1, the deficit resides in the initial stages of the model.

Sohlberg and Mateer (1986) developed an Attention Process Training (APT) program that has been proven effective for working with attention deficits after head injury. Presumably, training a person to allocate his or her attention or to perceive larger portions of available information would aid the encoding process. This type of training may therefore improve the ability of the person with head injury to learn and remember. Although the training does seem to improve memory for novel information after relatively mild head injury, it has never been tested with clients who demonstrate global anterograde amnesia. Nevertheless, this program is perhaps the best researched and efficacious attention training system available.

Encoding Deficit

An encoding deficit theory assumes that persons with head injury are unable to process information in the working memory. Huppert and Piercy (1978) suggested that head injury robs the person of the ability to encode information automatically. It is therefore reasonable to suggest that therapy should stress training conscious attention to reference tags, such as temporal aspects of what is seen or heard. It should also provide training with alternative encoding strategies such as imagery or mnemonic devices. Even though this type of training has been shown to improve memory (Parenté & Anderson, 1983; Wilson, 1987), persons with head injury still may not use the strategies spontaneously.

Storage Deficit

After head injury, information may not effectively traverse the path of the top arrow in Figure 12.1 that connects the working memory and LTM. In other words, the person with head injury either forgets more rapidly or never stores the information effectively. However, there is little published evidence to support this type of theory.

Retrieval Deficit

A retrieval deficit explanation of memory dysfunction after head injury concerns the lower arrow that connects the long-term memory and working memory portions of Figure 12.1. This notion assumes that persons with amnesia have difficulty accessing information in LTM. This logic implies that, after a head injury, new information is stored and is available in memory, but it is not readily accessible. Perhaps the person loses the ability to generate the appropriate cues. Perhaps he or she is distracted before an effective cue is formed. Although the deficit is not well understood, the concept of retrieval failure after head injury is difficult to deny.

Conclusions

Research findings on the relative impairment of storage versus retrieval mechanisms after post-traumatic amnesia are ambiguous. Measuring intrusion errors during free recall of word lists, Warrington and Weiskrantz (1986) suggested that clients who made more intrusion errors had a retrieval deficit. In a related study, Brooks (1975) suggested that fewer intrusion errors indicated a storage, as opposed to a retrieval, deficit. But Schacter and Crovitz (1977) disagreed, saying that there may be other ways of demonstrating the information has been stored, such as semantic or acoustic cuing. A reasonable conclusion is that memory deficits are far more complex than storage-retrieval or other dichotomous paradigms allow. Schacter and Crovitz believed that simple storage-retrieval explanations of memory deficits were not supported by Brooks (1972) or Levin and Peters (1976). Retention intervals and distractor activity may be involved to help explain contradictory findings.

None of the theories of memory dysfunction just discussed is universally accepted as the best. However, the diversity of explanation illustrates how memory deficits can occur in any portion of the model presented in Figure 12.1. In many cases, several areas will be affected and seldom will any one process be totally spared. Perhaps the major value of these theories is that they illustrate the utility of evaluating which systems are not functioning normally before planning therapy.

GENERALIZATION AND TRANSFER OF LEARNING PRINCIPLES

Memory rehabilitation therapies may not generalize or transfer to the person's activities of daily living. Unfortunately, there are few discussions of how to plan a generalizable memory retraining program. As a start, the authors distinguish between generalization and transfer of learning. Generalization is the ability to use a newly learned memory strategy in a novel situation. Many persons with head injury are unable to generalize. However, if the person demonstrates generalization, then he or she will benefit from therapy that teaches cognitive flexibility and strategies that apply in a variety of real-life circumstances. Transfer of learning involves training skills that are applicable in specific situations. If the ability to generalize has been lost, then therapy should focus on training skills that will transfer to job-related activities or ADLs. Indeed, training transferable skills may be the only available avenue to reemployment after head injury.

In some situations, the therapist may be unable to determine if he or she is training generalizable strategies or transferable skills. Fortunately, however, the transfer models presented next are applicable to a variety of training situations. The authors recommend that the therapist model the intervention regimen after one of the positive transfer paradigms described in this chapter.

While the principles of transfer of learning have been well researched (Ellis, 1969), their application to head injury rehabilitation has only recently been presented in the brain injury literature (Parenté & Anderson-Parenté, 1989). The following is a discussion of transfer of learning paradigms and how the therapist can use them to predict the results of various memory retraining therapies.

Six basic transfer of learning models are presented in Table 12.2. The characteristics of the therapy tasks are described by the first two columns of the table. Task elements are represented by one letter (e.g., A) in the far-left column. These are the physical characteristics of the task: actual training materials, color of the room, level of background noise, and so forth. The way the therapist trains the client to mentally organize, encode, or attend to the task elements is called a response set, and is abbreviated with another letter (e.g., B) in the second column. The goal of therapy is to replicate both the task elements (third column) and cognitive response sets (fourth column) in the client's ADLs

and job environment. To the extent that this is possible, the transfer models in Table 12.2 are capable of predicting the usefulness of most cognitive rehabilitation therapies (i.e., more pluses in the far-right column indicate positive transfer; more minuses indicate negative transfer).

The A-B:A-B model produces maximum transfer. This is because the task elements (A) and cognitive response sets (B) that the client learns in therapy are the same as those he or she will use on the job or at home. The therapy provides near-perfect domain-specific transfer of learning. Positive transfer also results from the A-B:A′-B′ and the A-B:C-B transfer models. The A-B:A′-B′ model provides training task elements and cognitive response sets similar to those the person with head injury will eventually encounter. With the A-B:C-B model, response sets are identical but the task elements differ. Nevertheless, both models predict positive transfer.

Table 12.2 indicates that only slight positive transfer will result from the A-B:C-D paradigm. This model is typical of many computerized therapy regimens. This type of training provides mental exercise under the assumption that "mental pushups" will strengthen memory. Since the task elements and response sets are dissimilar to the person's ADL or job requirements, the training may produce only negligible positive effects.

The A-B:A-D paradigm yields negative transfer. In this type of therapy, a client would learn a specific cognitive response set (B), but would have to learn a new response set for the same task elements later (D). For example, the therapist may train the client to put his or her

Table 12.2. Models of transfer

Therapy		Life		
Task element	Response set	Task element	Response set	Amount of transfer
A	B	A	B	+ + + +
A	B	A′	B′	+ + +
A	B	C	B	+ +
A	B	C	D	+
A	B	A	D	– – –
A	B	A	Br	– – – –

+ = positive transfer.
– = negative transfer.

personal belongings on a table in the front of the clinic on arrival. However, at home, the same client may misplace these items because the items are routinely stored on the dresser in his or her room.

Mental reorganization will be especially difficult in the A-B:A-Br model. Indeed, this model will usually produce the most negative transfer and should be avoided at all costs. This is because the client is forced to reassociate a cognitive response set to the same task elements. The lowercase r next to the second B indicates this repairing process. For example, confusion usually results when the client must find something in his or her room after a well-meaning person has reorganized the furniture or cleaned it up.

Maximizing the transferable quality of therapy is a matter of assuring that the training conforms to one of the above positive transfer models. Those therapies that conform to the first three designs will yield significant effects. However, those that force the client to learn new response sets later on or to reorganize will not be useful and, in the long term, may create more problems than they solve.

SURVEY OF TECHNIQUES AND STRATEGIES FOR RETRAINING MEMORY

Each of the cognitive rehabilitation training models discussed and evaluated next can be theoretically grounded to the basic memory model outlined in Figure 12.1. As therapy also conforms to one of the transfer paradigms, it is therefore possible to predict its relative effect.

Domain-Specific Training

Schacter and Glisky (1986) illustrated the value of matching the task demands in therapy to those of the real world. This involves creating a virtual simulation of what the person with head injury will encounter when he or she enters the work world. This type of training conforms to an A-B:A'-B' paradigm, which predicts maximum transfer.

Schacter and Glisky's (1986) reported successes training computer-related skills have been the most optimistic account of domain-specific training to date. The authors of this chapter have also found this type of training to be successful

with certain specific tasks. Two case histories are presented to illustrate the usefulness of this type of training.

In one case, the authors worked with a client who had been a claims processor at Blue Cross and Blue Shield. After an automobile accident, he was unable to return to his job due to memory loss. However, a simulation of his former job was constructed at the Maryland Rehabilitation Center and he trained on the simulator daily for over 6 months. He was then reintroduced into the workplace and, after 2 years, is still employed full time.

The second case involved a woman who was a legal secretary before her head injury. She was unable to return to her job at the law firm for about a year after leaving the hospital. She eventually returned to the law firm and worked as a typing pool manager and was responsible for distributing case reports and briefings to several word processors. She had to keep track of the reports' status and return the reports to the lawyers after completion. At any one time, there were about 50 documents in various stages of completion. Even though she kept lists of the various documents' status, it was clear that her system would have to improve before her performance would be considered adequate.

The authors trained domain-specific skills with a computer program that modeled her work environment. The training conformed to an A-B:A'-B' transfer model, because it required her to supply the secretaries with the case reports and to keep a mental record of their status. Moreover, the program included the names of the various lawyers and secretaries with whom she worked at the law firm. She practiced with the software after work for about 1 hour each day. Although this constituted only one portion of the total training program, the computer program was sufficient to retrain her memory for the job. She is still working full time and has not reported any difficulty with the job.

Sensory Memory Training

As mentioned earlier, a sensory memory deficit could potentially bottleneck processing in the rest of the system. Therefore, Parenté et al. (1989) developed a training program to improve processing in the iconic, or sensory, memory.

The person with head injury is taught to scan the iconic store in brief glimpses that are too fast to rely on eye muscle movements. If the training materials are similar to those in the real world, then the therapy conforms to an A-B:A′-B′ transfer model, which predicts positive transfer. The intervention conforms to an A-B:C-B model when the therapy and real-world materials differ.

This training program has proven useful for improving reading skill. Persons with head injury learned to scan arrays of letters that were viewed for only 50 milliseconds (Sperling, 1969). Eye muscle movements could therefore not be used to scan the letters. Performance on this task improved with practice, however. In addition, the training improved performance on later tests of reading comprehension and word recognition.

Attention-Concentration Training

Sohlberg and Mateer (1987) developed a systematic procedure for retraining attention and concentration. Their program deals with: 1) focused attention, 2) selective attention, 3) sustained attention, 4) alternating attention, and 5) divided attention. Although the training is not domain specific, it does teach a graded generalizable attentional response set. This is because attentional responses (B) trained in therapy are applicable in a variety of different life situations (A,C, etc.). The training therefore conforms to an A-B:C-B paradigm.

Attention-concentration training is functionally a hierarchy of therapy tasks at each of the above five levels. Sohlberg and Mateer's (1987) results clearly show that attention deficits in persons with brain injury can be improved by specific attention training. Prior to program entry, none of their subjects was living independently or was gainfully employed. The clinical goals for the subjects included independent living and employment; in each case, these vocational and independent living goals were accomplished, following 5–8 months of attention-concentration training.

Rehearsal

Simply training persons with head injury always to rehearse information subvocally yields remarkable improvement in memory functioning. Rehearsal improves memory because it sustains information in working memory, thereby facilitating encoding. Rehearsing improves memory for a variety of different types of information. Therefore, training the client always to rehearse new information (the B portion of the A-B:C-B model) at least 5–10 times will yield positive transfer in most new situations.

To demonstrate the power of rehearsal, the authors used a modification of the simple card game ace-to-king, described in detail by Craine and Gudeman (1982). This game involves showing a client three playing cards and placing them face down on the table. The person is then asked to arrange the cards in ascending order (ace to king). The number of times the cards are correctly ordered after exhausting the entire deck is the measure of performance. Persons with head injury usually score 8 out of 17 possible correct arrangements without any rehearsal instruction. When they are forced to rehearse the cards several times before arranging them, however, performance greatly improves. Indeed, two or three rehearsals are usually sufficient to produce perfect performance on this task. These results are presented in Figure 12.2.

Academic Therapy

Most academic therapy involves relearning functional skills. Often, the person with head injury learns new skills as a precursor to job training. For example, Minninger (1984) presented several examples of reading comprehension training that teach the person to encode text materials according to several different content patterns.

Wilson (1987) presented experimental evidence that the preview, question, read, state, and test (PQRST) system improves retention of text materials. Although the text (task elements) changes from therapy to the real world, the PQRST response set is still useful. Learning the technique produces positive transfer because it conforms to an A-B:C-B model.

The authors have found that simply training persons with head injury to translate mentally what they read into their own words is sufficient to improve recall of text materials. Figure 12.3 presents the results of a simple experiment performed at the Maryland Rehabilitation Center. Six clients with traumatic brain injury were asked to read a series of paragraphs on a standardized

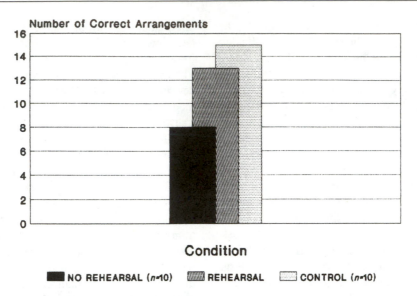

Figure 12.2.   Performance on rehearsal task (ace-to-king card game) before and after training.

reading comprehension test (Nelson-Denny Reading Test). They were then asked a series of multiple-choice questions about the content of the materials. Their scores are summarized in the before-training bar of Figure 12.3. The clients were then asked to read several more paragraphs, but to summarize the paragraphs in their own words. Each client was then tested with additional multiple-choice questions to assess knowledge of the second paragraph. Figure 12.3 indicates that performance on the test items clearly improved with the prior translation training. The improvement occurred with all 6 clients ($p < .05$ by sign test).

Stimulation Therapy

Exercising the mind is, perhaps, the oldest form of memory retraining. This therapy does not

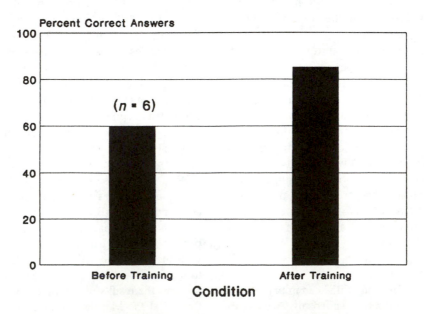

Figure 12.3.   Performance on Nelson-Denny Reading Test before and after training.

focus on any particular portion of the memory system. Since the task elements and cognitive response sets are unlike anything the person will encounter after leaving therapy, it conforms to an A-B:C-D model, which predicts a modicum of positive transfer.

A few studies have offered empirical evidence for the usefulness of stimulation therapy. Gianutsos and Gianutsos (1979) did show how improved performance on an information processing task was correlated with improved performance on a test of verbal recall. Ben-Yishay, Piasetsky, and Rattok (1987) demonstrated significant correlations between basic attention training exercises and performance on standardized tests. There is also a more recent report of improved performance on standardized tests with prior computer-based training relative to paper-and-pencil activities by Ruff et al. (1989). Bracy (1983) also reported success with computer training.

Despite these reports, the authors contend that there is little practical evidence that stimulation therapy produces functionally significant gains. Moreover, laboratory results may not generalize to real life, and the techniques and computer materials used in rehabilitation facilities, although face valid, may not be relevant to the demands of everyday living (Brooks, 1984; Gloag, 1985; Hart & Hayden, 1986).

Memory Strategy Training

Wilson (1987) showed that persons with head injury will benefit from learning to use imagery and mnemonics. Presumably, this is because they learn to encode more effectively, thereby improving storage and retrieval of information. Training persons with head injury to use memory strategies is an A-B:C-B transfer model. The B term represents the particular memory strategy. In essence, it is the cognitive response set. The A refers to specific things with which the person practices in therapy. The response set B should work just as effectively with the C items encountered in ADLs as it did with the A items in therapy.

However, while it is intuitively reasonable that training persons with brain injury to use memory strategies actually improves their mem-

ories, there are few quantitative evaluations of this question in the literature on head injury. Wilson (1987) presented data that demonstrate improved memory with a variety of different memory strategies. Patten (1972) reported success with 4 clients who were able to use imagery to compensate for poor verbal memory. Jones (1974) used imagery to improve memory deficits of clients who had undergone left temporal lobectomies.

Lewinsohn, Danaher, and Kikel (1977), however, found the effects of imagery-facilitated recall did not last beyond a 30-minute retention interval. These researchers were also disappointed with the results of an imagery-mediated name/face-learning training program. Glasgow, Zeiss, Barrera, and Lewinsohn (1977) were only able to train their subjects to use imagery with a small number of easily imaginable names.

Crovitz (1979) stressed the need for retrieval cues in imagery training. He noted the importance of giving persons with brain injury sufficient training time when instructing them in mnemonic techniques. He also found that plausible images were preferable to the traditional bizarre formations. Cutting (1978) failed to see improvement in clients with Korsakoff syndrome after imagery training, but Cermak (1976) found clients with Korsakoff syndrome did benefit from imagery, both in recognition and in free-recall tasks. Kovner, Mattis, and Pass (1983) taught clients with severe anterograde amnesia to use imaged stories to enhance their free recall of a list of words.

Moffat (1984) and O'Connor and Cermak (1987) emphasized that the practical applications of imagery training may be limited by the stress on encoding. Elaborate encoding demands, planning, and vigilance, all of which are necessary for effective imaginational encoding, are often beyond the capabilities of persons with brain injury. Other more serious limitations to imagery training as a rehabilitation technique concern maintenance and generalization. Schacter and Crovitz (1977) and Schacter and Glisky (1986) stated that empirical demonstrations of maintenance or generalization of mnemonic strategies are lacking. Their work with persons with amnesia and their interpretation of analogous findings in research with persons with mental retardation caused them to be pessimistic about the usefulness of mnemonic strategy training to achieve a general improvement in memory functioning. Lewinsohn et al. (1977) also were cautious about the practical efficacy of these techniques. In their study, the advantage of imagery training was not maintained after a delay interval. Thus, they declared, the practical utility of imagery and mnemonics remains to be validated.

Clearly, there have been few empirical investigations of exactly what effect memory strategy training has on the memory system after head injury. Therefore, the authors designed the following investigations to clarify this issue. Specifically, they were concerned with evaluating several memory strategies to determine which most improved memory. Also, they were concerned with how the various strategies affected the memory system as a whole. The authors evaluated embedded sentences, imagery, verbal labeling, and number chunking with several individuals with traumatic brain injury and amnesia.

Embedded Sentences and Imagery

The embedded sentence mnemonic strategy involves forming a sentence around a string of words or thoughts to integrate them into a functional unit that can be easily recalled. For example, to remember a list of words such as "gold, car, cattle, star, tree, blanket, and street," the person may form a bizarre sentence such as "The *gold car* drove down the *street* filled with *cattle* and *trees* under a *blanket* of *stars*." While this sentence makes little sense, it is easy to rehearse and easy to recall. It is also relatively easy to train a person with head injury to form such sentences.

Imagery instruction involves training the person to form mental pictures that integrate thoughts into a visual scene. The person then recalls the picture and uses it later to recall the required information. For example, when learning the above list of words, the person may learn to form a mental picture of a gold car driving down a street with cattle grazing beneath the trees on either side of the street. There is a thick blanket of stars twinkling in the sky. Clearly, embedded sentence mnemonics can involve an im-

agery component; however, the training differs in that the person is simply trained to rehearse the sentence rather than to imagine the scene. Imagery training was also evaluated to determine if it was useful for improving memory with persons who were traumatically brain injured.

In the first evaluation, 22 clients were given the Selective Reminding Test (Buschke, 1973). Each client recalled an unrelated word list that was repeated over 12 study-and-test trials. The examiner presented only those words that the person missed on the previous trial before their next recall. The scoring procedure yielded several indices of memory functioning. The recall performance (RECALL) score was simply the total number of words remembered after 12 study-and-test trials. Two measures of long-term retention were also calculated, long-term storage (LTS) and long-term recall (LTR). LTS is an index of how well the person stores words in long-term memory. LTR measures whether or not the word registers in LTM on any given trial. Consistent long-term recall (CLTR) measures the person's ability to recall consistently any given word over the test sequence.

Ten clients with head injury received no instruction before the examiner tested them with the Buschke Selective Reminding Test (1973). Six clients received imagery instruction before the test. These clients were simply told to form a mental picture around the words as they were read and to use the picture to help recall the words. The remaining 6 clients received embedded sentence training before they were tested. Forty college students were also tested (without imagery instruction) and their results were used as a no-injury control comparison condition.

Overall multivariate analysis of variance revealed differences among the four conditions ($F[5,58] = 12.25$, $p < .05$). Figure 12.4 indicates that the imagery instruction consistently improved memory relative to the no-training condition. Univariate analyses on the separate measures (imagery versus control conditions) indicated significant differences for the LTS, RECALL, and CLTR measures ($p < .05$). The effect of imagery was to improve long-term storage of the words, overall recall of the words, and consistent long-term recall. Univariate analyses

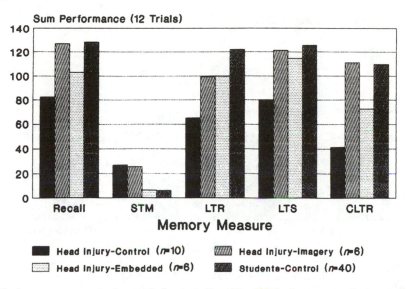

Figure 12.4. Performance on a selective reminding task (Buschke, 1973) after memory strategy training (STM = short-term memory, LTR = long-term recall, LTS = long-term storage, CLTR = consistent long-term recall, RECALL = recall performance).

performed on the embedded sentence versus control conditions did not yield any significant differences. Neither imagery nor embedded sentence training improved short-term memory.

Verbal Labeling

Verbal labeling is a technique of associating something new with something with which one is already familiar. For example, when the person must memorize an unfamiliar shape, it is useful to say that it "looks like" some familiar object. For example, the floor plan of the authors' psychology building is typically difficult for students to visualize until they are told that it is in the shape of an S. Once the floor plan is assigned a familiar label, the students can begin to picture where they are in relation to other offices and classrooms. After meeting a person for the first time, it may be useful for the client to choose a celebrity whom the new acquaintance looks like (e.g., a movie star), and then use the celebrity face as a cue to recall the name.

Figure 12.5 presents the results of an experiment that evaluated the effect of verbal labeling. All of the participants were persons with brain injury. Half the clients (n = 23) were tested with the visual paired association por-

tion of the Wechsler Memory Scale–Revised (Wechsler, 1987). Each client received three study-and-test trials to learn the associations. Each was tested again after a 30-minute delay. Another group of 23 clients received verbal labeling of the shapes as he or she learned them. Aside from this experimental manipulation, the test task was identical for both groups.

Multivariate analysis of variance revealed an overall significant difference between the groups ($F[4,41] = 3.966, p < .05$). Figure 12.5 illustrates quite clearly that clients who received verbal labeling of the shapes outperformed the control group across the study-and-test sequence. Individual analyses of variance performed on each of the study-and-test trials indicated a significant difference ($p < .05$). Another analysis of variance performed on the delayed recall data was not significant. This was probably due to the fact that the subjects in both conditions were brought to a criterion of perfect recall.

Figure 12.5 indicates that the group that received verbal-labeling instruction learned the paired associates after approximately three study-and-test trials. The group that received verbal-labeling instruction therefore performed as well (or slightly better) than the control group with only half the exposure to the study items.

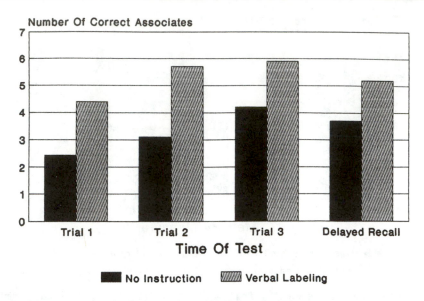

Figure 12.5.   Performance on visual paired associates (Wechsler, 1987) after verbal-labeling training.

Number Chunking

Number chunking is a simple technique for improving retention of number strings. It involves repeating individual digits as groups, which has the effect of increasing the number of total digits (the size of the number string) the person can recall. For example, most of us recall a telephone number as a series of separate digits. When we hear a phone number such as "494-9124," we say to ourselves, "four, nine, four, nine, one, two, four." Since the capacity of memory is usually restricted to seven plus or minus two digits, we will have a hard time recalling more than seven digits without extensive rehearsal. However, simply translating the information into larger chunks can have an immediate effect on memory. Rehearsing the same number string as "four ninety-four, ninety-one, twenty-four" will usually produce correct recall of a phone number without any additional rehearsal.

The number-chunking procedure was tested with 20 clients with head injury. Half were given a digit-span test without instruction, and the remaining half were taught how to chunk numbers before the test. The results are presented in Figure 12.6. The group that received number-chunking instructions outperformed the no-instruction group ($F[1,18] = 12.2, p < .05$). The level of recall in the instruction group was

close to the average level of recall for persons without head injury (seven digits).

Conclusions

Memory strategy training will not be effective with every person with head injury. A majority demonstrate diminished working memory span for various types of materials. However, to the extent that the client can attend initially, he or she will probably be helped by memory strategy training or other interventions designed to promote semantic encoding. A smaller minority of persons with head injury do not have the types of deficits described above, but do have impaired anterograde memory for most types of information. A very small percentage of persons with head injury are truly amnestic. That is, they have profound global anterograde memory disorders. There is little evidence that clients with global amnesia will benefit from this type of memory training.

PROSTHETIC MEMORY AIDS

Prosthetic memory aids are devices that obviate specific memory problems. They are usually designed to cue the person to some future activity. Some simply store personal information and organize it for convenient retrieval. These de-

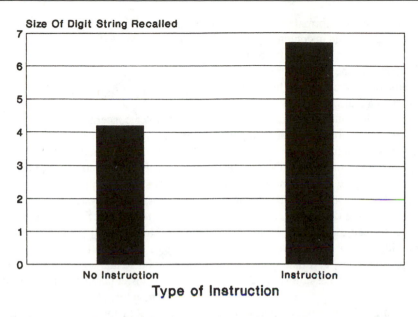

Figure 12.6.   Performance on digit-span task before and after number-chunking instruction.

vices are quite effective compensatory aids that work around the memory deficit but do not reduce its severity. Most are generally available in specialty catalogues or computer stores (e.g., Casio telememo watches; see Table 12.3)

Checklists are effective and simple-to-use prosthetic memory devices (Kreutzer, Wehman, Morton, & Stonnington, 1988). They are also easy to generate, inexpensive, and flexible. They ensure that a task is performed consistently and correctly. They also reduce the embarrassment and frustration that inevitably results from obsessive/compulsive behavior secondary to memory loss.

Electronic signaling devices can help a person with head injury locate keys, wallets, and purses. Others are available to help find cars in a parking lot. Some respond to hand claps or whis-

tles. That is, when the person whistles at a certain frequency or claps hands at 1-second intervals, the devices begin to beep. DAK sells a sounding device for finding cars. It mounts under the hood of the car and is activated by pressing a device that can be carried in a purse or on a key chain. When activated, the device blows the car's horn.

Telememo devices store personal information and phone numbers. They also signal appointments. Casio makes an entire line of "data bank" wrist watches that organize phone numbers alphabetically. The watches store as many as 50 phone numbers and corresponding names. One model (DB-50) is waterproof, and thus can be worn at all times, even in the shower.

Personal directories are devices that store message alarms and appointment reminders. At the appropriate time, the devices beep audibly. A reminder message then flashes on the screen. Some of these devices are as small as a credit card and are easily stored in a purse or wallet.

The authors recommend training the person with head injury to use *microcassette recorders* as immediate memory compensatory aids. These are especially useful for recording important messages, notes, or instructions. The person can usually speak into a recorder much faster than he

Table 12.3.   Vendors and toll-free numbers for prosthetic memory devices

Solutions Inc.: (800) 342-9888

Impact: (800) 345-4422

Danmark: (800) 533-3379

Sharper Image: (800) 344-4444

Hammacher/Schlemmer: (800) 543-3666

Syntronics: (800) 972-5855

or she can write the same information on paper. The cuing watch can be used in conjunction with the recorder because it can be set to beep every hour. This feature cues the head-injured person to rewind the tape recorder and listen to the messages. Recorders can also be used to record phone messages. This feature spares the person with head injury the embarrassment of having to ask for repetition of the information.

Although external memory aids can be quite useful, their efficacy is frequently limited because the client does not fully utilize the aid, often forgetting it is there (Harris, 1978; Moffat, 1984). Harris described the features of an optimal memory aid, noting that active cues are preferable to passive ones, and that specificity, temporal contiguity, and accessibility were also important.

Systems using an electronic digital watch that beeps to remind the client to review a daily schedule have been successful. Such external aids may help not only the client with amnesia, but also those relating to or interacting with the client. Fowler, Hart, and Sheahan (1972) used a broadly behavioral approach that relied on external memory aids—a printed schedule of daily activities and a portable hour timer. Hospital staff noted that the patient was able to keep daily appointments after implementing a schedule whereby he was praised for arriving on time and ignored if he arrived more than 10 minutes late.

The authors of this chapter contend that external aids are especially effective as therapeutic interventions. They offer an instant solution to nagging problems, and can often result in immediate return to work.

SUMMARY

This chapter concerned the theoretical development and evaluation of a model for retraining memory after traumatic brain injury. The authors presented a theoretical model of memory that allows the therapist to focus intervention on the defects in the system. The effects of most memory training techniques are shown to be predictable from well-known transfer of learning principles. Ideally, the therapist will structure intervention so that it conforms to one of several positive transfer paradigms and avoids those that produce negative transfer.

Several memory retraining techniques were also evaluated. The literature has indicated that attention-concentration training and domain-specific training can be highly effective training procedures after head injury. Persons with head injury have been shown to benefit from rehearsal, imagery, translation of verbal text, verbal labeling, and number chunking.

A variety of prosthetic devices were also discussed that may be useful for persons with head injury. The authors have found checklists, cuing/signaling devices, telememo watches, and personal data storage devices to be especially effective. As a general rule, the simpler the device, the greater the likelihood that the person with head injury will use it.

REFERENCES

Atkinson, R.C., & Shiffrin, R.M. (1968). Human memory: A proposed system and its control process. In K.W. Spence & J.K. Spence (Eds.), *The psychology of learning and motivation* (Vol. 2, pp. 418–420). New York: Academic Press.

Baddeley, A.D., & Hitch, G. (1974). Working memory. In G.H. Bower (Ed.), *The psychology of learning and motivation* (Vol. 8, pp. 320–342). New York: Academic Press.

Ben-Yishay, Y., Piasetsky, E.B., & Rattok, J. (1987). A systematic method for ameliorating disorders in basic attention. In M.J. Meir, A.L. Benton, & L. Diller (Eds.), *Neuropsychological rehabilitation* (pp. 165–181). New York: Guilford Press.

Bracy, O. (1983). Computer based cognitive rehabilitation. *Cognitive Rehabilitation, 1*(1), 7–8.

Brooks, D.N. (1972). Memory and head injury. *Journal of Nervous Mental Disorders, 155*, 350–355.

Brooks, D.N. (1975). Long and short term memory in head injured patients. *Cortex, 11*, 329–340.

Brooks, D.N. (1984). Cognitive deficits after head injury. In N. Brooks (Ed.), *Closed head injury: Psychological social and family consequences* (pp. 44–73). London: Oxford University Press.

Buschke, H. (1973). Selective reminding for analysis of memory and learning. *Journal of Verbal Learning and Verbal Behavior, 12*, 543–550.

Cermak, L.S. (1976). The encoding capacity of a

patient with amnesia due to encephalitis. *Neuropsychologia, 19,* 311–326.

Craine, G., & Gudeman, C. (1982). *Rehabilitation of brain functions.* Springfield, IL: Charles C Thomas.

Crovitz, L.S. (1979). Memory retraining in brain-damaged patients: The airplane list. *Cortex, 15,* 131–134.

Cutting, J. (1978). A cognitive approach to Korsakoff's syndrome. *Cortex, 14,* 485–495.

Dick, A.O. (1974). Iconic memory and its relation to perceptual processing and other memory mechanisms. *Perception and Psychophysics, 16,* 575–596.

Ellis, H.C. (1969). Transfer and retention. In M.H. Marx (Ed.), *Learning processes* (pp. 381–478). New York: Macmillan.

Fowler, R., Hart, J., & Sheahan, M. (1972). A prosthetic: An application of the prosthetic environment concept. *Rehabilitation Counseling Bulletin, 15,* 80–85.

Gianutsos, R., & Gianutsos, J. (1979). Rehabilitating the verbal recall of brain-injured patients by mnemonic training: An experimental demonstration using single-case methodology. *Journal of Clinical Neuropsychology, 1*(2), 117–135.

Glasgow, R.E., Zeiss, R.A., Barrera, M., & Lewinsohn, P.M. (1977). Case studies on remediating memory deficits in brain damaged individuals. *Journal of Clinical Psychology, 33*(4), 1049–1054.

Gloag, D. (1985). Rehabilitation after head injury: Cognitive problems. *British Medical Journal, 290,* 834–837.

Grafman, J. (1984). Memory assessment and remediation in brain-injured patients. In B.A. Edelstein & E.T. Couture (Eds.), *Behavioral assessment and rehabilitation of the traumatically brain-damaged* (pp. 151–189). London: Oxford University Press.

Harris, J. (1978). External memory aids. In M. Gruneberg, P. Morris, & R. Sykes (Eds.), *Practical aspects of memory* (pp. 172–179). London: Academic Press.

Hart, T., & Hayden, M.E. (1986). The ecological validity of neuropsychological assessment and remediation. In B.P. Uzzell & Y. Gross (Eds.), *Clinical neuropsychology of intervention* (pp. 21–50). Boston: Martinus Nijhoff.

Huppert, F.A., & Piercy, M. (1978). The role of trace strength in recency and frequency judgements by amnestic and control subjects. *Quarterly Journal of Experimental Psychology, 30,* 346–354.

Jones, M.K. (1974). Imagery as a mnemonic aid after left temporal lobectomy: Contrast between material specific and generalized memory disorders. *Neuropsychologia, 12,* 21–30.

Kolb, B., & Whishaw, I. (1990). *Fundamentals of human neuropsychology.* New York: W. H. Freeman.

Kovner, R., Mattis, S., & Pass, K. (1983). *Some amnestic patients can freely recall large amounts of in-formation in new contexts.* Paper presented at the meeting of the International Neuropsychological Society, Mexico City.

Kreutzer, J.S., Wehman, P., Morton, M.V., & Stonnington, H.H. (1988). Supported employment and compensatory strategies for enhancing vocational outcome following traumatic brain injury. *Brain Injury, 2,* 203–223.

Levin, H.S., & Peters, B.H. (1976). Neuropsychological testing for prosopagnosia without visual field defect. *Diseases of the Nervous System, 37*(2), 68–71.

Lewinsohn, P.M., Danaher, B.G., & Kikel, S. (1977). Visual imagery as a mnemonic aid for brain-injured persons. *Journal of Consulting and Clinical Psychology, 45,* 717–723.

Minninger, J. (1984). *Total recall.* Northhampshire: Thorsons.

Moffat, N. (1984). Strategies of memory therapy. In B.A. Wilson & N. Moffat (Eds.), *Clinical management of memory problems* (pp. 63–88). Rockville, MD: Aspen.

O'Connor, M., & Cermak, L.S. (1987). In M.J. Meier, A.L. Benton, & L. Diller (Eds.), *Neuropsychological rehabilitation* (pp. 260–279). New York: Guilford Press.

Parenté, R., & Anderson, J.K. (1983). Techniques for improving cognitive rehabilitation: Teaching organizational and encoding skills. *Cognitive Rehabilitation, 1*(4), 20–22.

Parenté, F.J., & Anderson-Parenté, J.K. (1989). Retraining memory: Theory and application. *Journal of Head Trauma Rehabilitation, 4*(3), 55–65.

Parenté, F.J., Anderson-Parenté, J.K., & Shaw, B. (1989). Retraining the mind's eye. *Journal of Head Trauma Rehabilitation, 4*(2), 53–62.

Patten, B.M. (1972). The ancient art of memory: Usefulness in treatment. *Archives of Neurology, 26,* 28–31.

Prigatano, G.P., Fordyce, D.J., Zeiner, H.K., Roueche, J.R., Pepping, M., & Wood, B.C. (1984). Neuropsychological rehabilitation after closed head injury in young adults. *Journal of Neurology, Neurosurgery, and Psychiatry, 47,* 505–513.

Ruff, R.M., Baser, C., Johnston, J., Marshall, L.F., Klauber, S.K., Klauber, M.R., & Minteer, M. (1989). Neuropsychological rehabilitation: An experimental study with head-injured patients. *Journal of Head Trauma Rehabilitation, 4*(3), 20–36.

Schacter, D.L., & Crovitz, H.F. (1977). Memory function after closed head injury: A review of quantitative research. *Cortex, 13,* 150–176.

Schacter, D.L., & Glisky, E.L. (1986). Memory remediation: Restoration, alleviation, and the acquisition of domain-specific knowledge. In Y. Gross & B.P. Uzzell (Eds.), *Clinical neuropsychology of intervention* (pp. 257–282). Boston: Martinus Nijhoff.

Sohlberg, M.M., & Mateer, C.A. (1986). *Attention Process Training (APT)*. Puyallup, WA: Association for Neuropsychological Research and Development.

Sohlberg, M.M., & Mateer, C.A. (1987). Effectiveness of an attention training program. *Journal of Clinical and Experimental Neuropsychology, 9,* 117–130.

Sperling, G.A. (1969). A model for visual memory tasks. In R.N. Haber (Ed.), *Information processing* *approaches to visual perception* (pp. 18–31). New York: Holt, Rinehart, & Winston.

Warrington, E.K., & Weiskrantz, L. (1986). A study of learning and retention in amnestic patients. *Neuropsychologia, 6,* 238–291,

Wechsler, D. (1987). *Wechsler Memory Scale–Revised*. New York: Psychological Corporation.

Wilson, B.A. (1987). *Rehabilitation of memory*. New York: Guilford Press.

CHAPTER 13

Computer Applications in Cognitive Rehabilitation

WILL LEVIN

Computer-assisted cognitive rehabilitation (CACR) has lately fallen into disfavor. After an initial period of fervor in the early and mid-1980s, the pendulum of opinion has more recently swung toward skepticism. The pioneers of cognitive rehabilitation were rightfully enthused about the possibilities the new technology offered for their emerging craft. The advent of affordable microcomputers brought promise of simple data collection, standard task presentation, and a potentially motivating environment for practicing cognitive activities. More recently, however, doubters have questioned the generalizability of computer-acquired skills to the everyday tasks of survival at home and at work (Gordon, Hibbard, & Kreutzer, 1989; Chapter 2, this volume). Clients of cognitive rehabilitation, striving to recover newly compromised intellectual abilities, are literally trying to relearn how to think productively. The question, then is: Are clients who are engaged with computerized tasks truly advancing toward self-reliance—or are they simply mastering functionally irrelevant keyboard responses?

There is a danger of polarizing the two positions. Proponents of CACR claim that it "works"; opponents say it does not. It is one of the precepts of this chapter that no useful purpose is served by formulating the debate in these stark terms. The computer, or more precisely, CACR software, is not an intervention method. Rather, it is a tool to be applied within the context of an intervention method. We do not ask whether a scalpel is or is not effective in surgery. Whether it is useful or not depends upon how it is used, under which conditions. A hammer and nails can help build a house, or can ruin it. Similarly, computer software may or may not aug-ment the rehabilitation endeavor, depending on how it is applied. While it is certainly appropriate, and necessary, to question the cost-effectiveness of current cognitive rehabilitation methods, it is a diversion to focus on the worth of the tools of the method. If the method is sound, computer technology can undoubtedly help the practitioner. If the method is unsound, no computer can rescue it from irrelevance. The appropriate issue, therefore, is not whether, but *how* computer technology can be effectively applied.

The first goal of this chapter is to develop a conceptual foundation for addressing this question. An overall theme is that the efficacy of CACR derives from the power of the rehabilitation model it implements. Whether CACR stands or falls depends on the practical value of the cognitive rehabilitation approach within which it is applied. The bulk of the chapter accordingly develops a particular intervention model, which the author hopes will be seen as a useful addition to the existing repertoire of cognitive rehabilitation methods. Just as important, it is offered as an example, demonstrating how CACR is appropriately applied strictly as an extension of a conceptually coherent model of cognitive rehabilitation.

The second goal of the chapter is to suggest specific ways in which computers can be applied in cognitive rehabilitation. Given the stated theme that CACR is best applied only within the context of a specified model, it stands to reason that the computer applications most emphasized in this chapter extend the model that is developed here. Still, it is hoped that the presented approaches may prove of interest to practitioners working from alternative intervention models.

The chapter is organized around three topics that are preliminary to the issue of computer applications: 1) the objectives of CACR, and of cognitive rehabilitation in general; 2) a theoretical framework that helps explain the link between cognitive impairment and the behaviors that impede self-sufficiency; and 3) an intervention model that derives from the training objectives and theory of impairment. The possibilities for computer applications are examined after these three discussions are presented.

OBJECTIVES OF CACR
AND COGNITIVE REHABILITATION

The list of possible deficits resulting from brain injury is long. It potentially includes impairments in motor skills, balance, bowel and bladder function, perceptual processing, communication, memory, and a host of other problems associated with physical or cognitive dysfunction. Rehabilitation specialists attempt to address all of these impairments, and more. However, if the rehabilitation mission is to help the client attain self-sufficiency, the primary barriers to that goal must be identified. Services are justifiably under scrutiny for cost-effectiveness, especially cognitive rehabilitation services. The urgent challenge, therefore, is to find the most direct route to the destination, and to dispense with wasteful detours.

Practically speaking, the twin objectives of controlling costs and enhancing the client's autonomy are accomplished in the same way: by reducing the individual's dependence upon others. Ultimately, this means that the efforts of rehabilitation specialists are most efficiently directed toward returning the client to work, school, or independent living. Every service provided must be accountable to these objectives.

Long-term outcome data suggest that deficits with behavioral self-regulation, particularly with regard to interpersonal behavior, are the most debilitating in maintaining employment and family integrity (Lezak, 1987). The burden, therefore, rests on practitioners of cognitive rehabilitation to demonstrate that their interventions significantly affect these outcomes. The case has been made that direct behavioral intervention in the settings of home and work are the most efficient means of facilitating self-

sufficiency (Kreutzer, Conder, Wehman, & Morrison, 1989). Specific behaviors in these settings are identified and trained, and environmental adaptations are designed to help the client compensate for residual deficits.

Why, then, invest time and money on "cognitive" interventions, particularly at computer screens, if one can directly affect target outcomes in their natural setting? The answer stems from the importance of enhancing the ultimate autonomy of the individual. Certainly behavioral interventions such as job coaching and family interaction training are powerful and worthwhile rehabilitation methods. It is hoped that more resources will be allocated to them. But fundamentally, these are approaches that emphasize compensatory rather than remedial objectives. Interventions are developed to adapt environments, especially social environments, to the limits of the individual's capacities. Although specific target behaviors are shaped, the focus is more on working within or around deficits than on ameliorating them.

The rationale for cognitive intervention has focused on empowering individuals to manage their own lives rather than have their behavior managed by helpers. To the extent that this is achieved, long-range costs, psychological as well as financial, are ultimately reduced.

INFORMATION PROCESSING
VERSUS BEHAVIORAL PERSPECTIVES

The principles of self-management are essentially the same as those applied in managing the behavior of others. A psychotherapist assists a client to refine his or her behavior by applying a variety of complex cognitive skills. In self-management, one does the same. Examples of such skills include: pinpointing problems; generating alternative intervention plans (usually by rearranging external circumstances); and selecting, implementing, evaluating, and revising plans as needed. Doing all of these things, for oneself or for another, requires the ability to think with discipline, clarity, and skill.

In training persons with head injury to do this kind of thinking, practitioners of cognitive rehabilitation have traditionally broken down the necessary skills into "building blocks" (Ben-Yishay & Diller, 1983; Bracy, 1986; Sohlberg & Mateer, 1989). The component parts are then practiced intensively and independently, each in stepwise fashion until mastery across building blocks is demonstrated. The success or failure of this approach ultimately depends on the accuracy of the analysis that identifies the building blocks, or cognitive components, of competent self-management.

The model presented in this chapter departs from tradition in one significant way. For the most part, intervention methods have been drawn from cognitive science, particularly from information processing models of cognition. The metaphor that originally inspired such models is the computer. Human cognition is seen to function in an analogous manner to the way information is processed by computer. Informational input is entered, coded, sorted, stored, retrieved, and directed to appropriate output modalities.

The metaphor, while elegant and appealing in many respects, yields a heuristic model of cognition that ultimately compels a fundamentally flawed intervention model. Specifically, it suggests a hierarchy of training tasks based on what is perceived to be occurring within the "black box" of the mind.

The information processing paradigm speculates on internal, unobservable mental processes based on the easily explainable electronic workings of the computer. The assumption is that one best determines the appropriate "building block" component cognitive skills by constructing models derived from assumptions about unobservable, private events. Traditional instructional practice is then followed by ordering these building blocks into a hierarchical pattern, from most basic or simple to most advanced and complex. Thus, the familiar cognitive rehabilitation paradigm emerges: first provide drills in attention (vigilance, selective attention, divided attention, etc.), then perceptual-motor integration, followed perhaps by memory drills, and eventually, by problem-solving tasks. The client moves up the ladder, through a hierarchy of modules derived from a logical analysis of what occurs inside the mind, from basic to complex. The expectation is that the client will come

closer to approximating fully competent self-management as he or she sequentially progresses through drills, often presented via computer, along the hierarchy of modules.

The proposed alternative to the information processing paradigm is a biological metaphor, specifically a model drawn from behavioral rather than cognitive science. Behavioral theory departs from information processing theory primarily in its adherence to the biological imperative of natural selection. More specifically, behavior, including self-management behavior, is ultimately selected by the environment rather than generated by internal, cognitive sources. Cognitive events realistically occur, but they are best understood not as causative events but as concurrent behaviors, determined by the same environmental contingencies that govern overt behavior.

The implication is that therapists best arrange training hierarchies according to observable interactions of the client with his or her external environment. In essence, one approaches the analysis from the outside in, rather than by emphasizing operations occurring within the mind of the individual. From the behavioral perspective, internal (or covert) cognitive operations evolve from prior overt actions performed in the natural environment. Put more simply, covert behavior originates in overt form. In this sense, the behavioral outlook is consistent with Piaget's evidence that concrete operations necessarily precede formal operations in the development of cognitive competence (Phillips, 1969).

The eventual outcome of this behavioral approach to training may not at first glance appear to be particularly radical or different. Certainly the familiar deficits of attention, memory, perceptual-motor functioning, and problem solving are not magically transcended. The tasks selected for training are in many ways familiar and similar. The difference is that the behavioral orientation leads to a more parsimonious, prescriptive training paradigm that is consistent with how behavioral skills are acquired and generalized.

To apply this outlook to the training of self-management skills, one begins by observing overt, behavioral demonstrations of self-management operations. Earlier in this chapter, these operations were presented as: pinpointing the problem; generating alternative plans for intervening (usually by rearranging external circumstances); and selecting, implementing, evaluating, and revising plans as needed. Each of these operations can be observed in overt form in various ways. For example, a mechanic pinpoints a problem by systematically testing each individual mechanical component in a complex system of parts. A scientist goes through a similar process in attempting to identify independent variables as they affect a dependent variable. Alternative solutions may be generated by creating lists or by engaging in other forms of verbal behavior (conversation) or nonverbal behavior (drawings or object manipulation). Selecting occurs through comparing alternatives according to some specified criterion. In similar ways, one can formulate concrete examples of overt implementation, evaluation, and revision of observable activities. Training hierarchies are constructed by breaking these observed behavioral operations into their essential, simplest forms.

The result is not necessarily a chain of small steps linked in sequence by their occurrence in time. A more effective approach might be to begin training in the middle of a behavior chain, working outward—only later to incorporate the initial and final steps. For example, in teaching piano playing, practice begins with simple scales, not with the first eight measures of "Concerto in F." In teaching throwing, one starts with the grip and simple wrist movements, not with drawing the whole arm back. Similarly, in teaching self-management skills, it is advantageous to start with the central component skill upon which more complex forms are eventually modeled, extended, and refined. The challenge, then, is to identify among the complex constellation of exchanges between person and environment the central component skill that lies at the core of self-management competence. The following section presents a theoretical construct that may be helpful in guiding that effort.

ZOOM NAVIGATION CONSTRUCT

Offering theoretical constructs in the arena of cognitive psychology can be seen as dangerous

business. As Claxton (1988) observed, "psychologists generate and discard new models at a rate that the motor trade would envy" (p. 4). This chapter has already challenged the utility of constructing hypothetical models of internal cognitive systems. It is perhaps appropriate to precede the introduction of a new construct with a brief explanation.

The criticism expressed in this chapter is not directed at theory building in general, but at the subject domain that information processing proponents have claimed for their analyses. Baddeley's (1982) view is sensible: "a theoretical concept should be evaluated . . . by the extent to which it performs the useful function of interpreting what we already know while facilitating further discovery" (in Claxton, 1988, p. 7). The position of this chapter, already described, is that behavior, including covert, cognitive events, is explained by environmental selection. A useful theory or construct from this perspective addresses the interaction of the individual with the external environment. It seeks to explain and organize events that are potentially observable and measurable, occurring as the individual behaves overtly in the context of environmental contingencies.

Ideally, such a theory would also shed light on the covert behaviors that are similarly shaped by environmental factors. It may lead to reasonable speculation regarding how internal processes are organized. There are two fundamental points, however: 1) the theory is based upon a biological rather than computational framework; and 2) it derives from observable data involving the individual's overt interaction with the environment, rather than hypothetical, logically inferred internal processes.

The author has selected behavioral self-management as a particularly productive focus for cognitive rehabilitation efforts, and has described the component skills as including: problem identification; generation of alternative solutions; and the selection, initiation, evaluation, and revision of solutions according to environmental consequences. These behaviors are familiar to many rehabilitation professionals as equivalent to the skills originally coined as "executive functions" by Lezak (1982). These are the abilities that are typically compromised following the diffuse injury resulting from head trauma, particularly if frontal lobe damage is sustained. Increasingly, attention is being drawn to their critical role in all forms of social and vocational pursuits (Boyd, Sautter, Bailey, Echols, & Douglas, 1987; Cicerone, 1989; Cicerone & Wood, 1987; Lawson & Rice, 1989; Sohlberg & Mateer, 1989).

In understanding executive functions, it may be helpful to envision a continuum of human behavior, with highly specialized neural events at one extreme, and complex, overt functional skills at the other. Along this "neurobehavioral continuum" one might place such activities as simple visual discriminations (such as reaction time tasks), or motor tasks (such as reaching for an object), or expert skills (such as neurosurgery). It is proposed here that the very midpoint of this continuum is where one might reasonably place executive function activities. These are the actions that define the border between covert cognitive behavior and overt self-management skills. These are the actions that are shaped as individuals study the subtle and delicate interaction between their behavior and the external world. The developing discovery of this interaction is at the core of what is typically referred to as competence, self-responsibility, or maturity. How does this discovery occur?

The author has coined the term *zoom navigation* to denote the process by which individuals observe their impact upon the environment and its effect upon their own behavior and subjective world. The process is defined as maintaining near simultaneous, conscious awareness of: 1) the immediate detail of a behavioral task, and 2) the larger environmental context in which the detailed task is executed. This concept is now further explained, with examples, and is then applied to a model of cognitive intervention.

Zoom navigation draws its name from the metaphor of a zoom lens on a camera. Cognitive psychologist Charles W. Eriksen (Eriksen & St. James, 1986) suggested the zoom lens metaphor as an appropriate analogy for characterizing the operation of the human visual attention system:

With a zoom lens at a low power setting there is a wide field of view with no magnification of the objects within that field. There is, therefore, little discrimination of detail. As the power of the lens increases, the field of view constricts, with a con-comitant increase in the resolving power for detail of the objects still remaining within the field. With a perfect lens system, there would be a complete tradeoff in terms of the loss of field of view with the corresponding increase of magnification or accessibility of detail for objects remaining within the field. (pp. 226–227)

Here the metaphor is applied to clarify the more general attentional process of changing one's conceptual (not just visual) focus from "close-up" detail to "wide-angle" context. In the arts of photography, film, and video, the concept of *zoom axis* applies to the continuum of visual depth, from close-up (foreground) to long shot (background). The individual more generally shifts attention along a similar continuum, by "zooming in" to focus intensively on immediate detail, and "zooming out" to bring into perspective the broad overview of a complex set of circumstances. One may zoom out from present to past or future, or from this action to its effect on the physical or social environment. Zoom navigation refers to the "navigation" of the zoom axes that extend from the individual's behavior to the world outside. It describes the process used to learn the relationship between one's actions and their outcome, for oneself, for others, or for the physical environment.

Zoom Navigation: Examples and Applications

Both overt and covert examples of zoom navigation can be considered. A small child learning to walk experiments with movements and observes their consequences for maintaining balance. The child strives toward simultaneous awareness of his or her actions and the external world. Ultimately, these relationships are learned, and walking becomes automatic, unconscious.

Similarly, one may observe a cocktail party–goer who studies the nonverbal reaction of his or her conversational partner before expressing an accommodating or provocative bit of repartee. Or, one may observe an executive who orchestrates a business meeting, urging the discussion toward consensus and closure while tracking both the agenda and the clock.

These are practical examples of overt activities requiring zoom navigation. In each case, the individual simultaneously maintains awareness of his or her own behavior and the context in which it is occurs. The examples also illustrate different types of contextual or environmental contingencies. The child explores the particular constraints of the physical context, the conversationalist observes social contingencies, and the executive focuses on time contingencies. All are navigating zoom axes by observing the mutual interplay between initiated action and the environmental context.

The zoom navigation construct is also helpful in suggesting explanations of covert cognitive behavior. The process, as applied to cognitive activity, is akin to the familiar constructs of induction and deduction (Sidman, 1960), or convergent and divergent thinking (Guilford, 1973). Zoom navigation, however, implies the execution of both complementary processes simultaneously, or near simultaneously. In solving an abstract problem, one may analyze a single case in the context of the general rule, or vice versa. By contrast, in determining how an apple and a banana are alike, one observes the specific properties that distinguish the objects from each other while simultaneously noticing the properties they share in common. In other words, one zoom navigates the axes between sameness and differentness. More precisely, one examines the details of each object, either covertly or overtly (if the objects are physically present) while also seeing both objects at once in comparison to one another. If either factor (differentness or sameness) is observed in isolation, without reference to the factor at the other pole of the axis, it is unlikely that the best response will be brought into focus. An apple and a banana are both smaller than a truck; they are both sweet tasting; they both grow on trees, and have skins . . . they are both fruits!

Mental arithmetic is another example. "If two apples cost 31¢, how much do a dozen apples cost?" The solution involves several steps, each of which must be performed while simultaneously accounting for specific values and the overall context. While attending to setting up the strategy, one must not lose awareness of the number values. While calculating the multiplication, one must maintain awareness of monetary units (cents, not dollars). In essence, one

must zoom one's attention back and forth, in and out, from detail to context, from strategy to operations to data.

Zoom navigation applies particularly nicely to scientific inquiry. Science is, after all, the discovery of contingencies, not obviously discernible, that determine the behavior of natural phenomena. In discovering a general rule, the expert scientist must consider the single case in the context of the universe of all possible cases. Norman (1980) stated:

> The study of cognition requires the consideration of all different aspects of an entire system. . . . Of course no one can study everything all at the same time, but I argue that we cannot ignore these things, either, else the individual pieces that we study in such detail will not fit together in the absence of some thought about the whole. (in Claxton, 1988, p. 9)

As zoom navigation is applied to the study of cognition, it may become more clear that little is to be gained by considering covert cognitive processes without reference to their environmental context. For example, in explaining the "behavior" of an automobile, should one diagram the relation of the carburetor to the pistons; or describe the effects of traffic, signs, and stoplights on the driver?

Zoom Navigation and Neuroanatomy

Links can be established between the zoom navigation construct and neural events. Posner and Petersen (1990) studied the relationship of covert attentional processes to brain structures. They identified three discrete attentional processes occurring at different locations within the brain. The subject disengages attention from a stimulus (posterior parietal cortex), shifts attention toward a new target stimulus (superior colliculus), and engages attention at the target stimulus (posterolateral thalamus). Summarizing these and other findings, they concluded:

> The attention system of the brain is anatomically separate from the data processing systems that perform operations on specific inputs. . . . In this sense the attention system is like other sensory and motor systems. It interacts with other parts of the brain, but maintains its own identity. . . . Attention is carried out by a network of anatomical areas. It is neither the property of a single center, nor a general

function of the brain operating as a whole (Mesulam, 1981; Rizzolatti, Gentilucci, & Matelli, 1985). (Posner & Petersen, 1990, p. 6)

These findings support the notion of a distinct and unified structural system that is involved in the processes of attentional shifting, including zooming out (disengaging) and zooming in (engaging).

From analyses of both visual and language attentional tasks, Posner (1990) speculated that a general attentional control system will be localized in the frontal cortex. This general system is seen to be involved in the selection of priority attentional targets, presumably in response to shifting environmental contingencies:

> We do not yet have definitive studies that have localized the different computations that are performed within the control structures found in the frontal areas. The relation of computational models of executive function to the complex anatomy of the frontal lobes still remains in the future. (Posner, 1990, p. 194)

Still, there is increasing evidence from neuropsychology and neuroscience research to inspire confidence that the neural structures accounting for executive attentional control (i.e., zoom navigation) will eventually be identified and localized in the frontal cortex.

Zoom Navigation and Psychometric Measures

Recently reported head trauma outcome data also support the centrality of zoom navigation in effective self-management. Bayless, Varney, and Roberts (1989) found that Lezak's (1982) Tinker Toy Test successfully discriminated between a group of 25 persons with head injury who had achieved successful vocational outcomes from a group of 25 who had not. Bayless et al. concluded: "The test seems particularly well suited for demonstrating the presence of deficits in executive functioning" (p. 917). Cicerone (1989) also conducted an extensive study linking, among other factors, psychometric test scores to long-term vocational outcome among persons with traumatic brain injury. The two highest correlations between test scores and outcome ($p < .001$) were demonstrated by the Trail Making Test: Part B (Reitan, 1958) and the Tinker Toy Test Complexity score.

Cicerone designated these specific tests as comprising the psychometric cluster measuring executive function. He concluded that the executive function factor is the most powerful predictor of vocational success. The scores on these two tests successfully discriminated those clients who were unemployed, and therefore dependent, from the rest of the research population.

A closer look at these two critical tasks reveals their sensitivity to the zoom navigation attentional act. The Trail Making Test: Part B (Reitan, 1958), long a familiar and instructive psychometric tool in brain injury assessment, requires simultaneous management of two alternating sequences. The client must switch between numerical and alphabetical sequencing tasks, requiring rapid disengagement, shifting, and engagement, from one to the other. In essence, the client tracks two simultaneous, separate tasks, focusing on the detail within each while also maintaining awareness of the broader context of which both tasks are a part.

The Tinker Toy Test (Lezak, 1982) is a more open-ended environment that requires the client to generate planful activity in an ambiguous setting. Specifically, the client must create a structure from traditional children's Tinker Toys, and is scored for such factors as symmetry and organization. This task requires continual simultaneous awareness of each immediate placement and its impact on the form of the whole structure. Each specific action is interpreted in light of its effect on the larger context. As with the Trail Making Test: Part B, the Tinker Toy Test primarily requires the types of attentional processes that exemplify the zoom navigation construct.

MULTITASKING MODEL

The chapter thus far has developed the zoom navigation construct as a conceptual tool linking external environmental contingencies to executive function skills and to covert cognitive behavior. The next challenge is to provide a practical training environment in which the crucial zoom navigation skill is systematically shaped and generalized. A model of cognitive rehabilitation is needed that not only specifically targets the development of zoom navigation, but also meets the following criteria:

A single, coherent *conceptual framework* is provided, allowing specialists from diverse disciplines to organize their collaborative efforts.

Prescriptive evaluation information is generated, and specific therapy paradigms are derived directly from standard assessment procedures.

Flexibility is assured, enabling each rehabilitation specialist the latitude to focus intensively within his or her own content area.

Individualization of services is provided to allow for clients with diverse patterns of cognitive strengths and deficits.

Quantifiable data are generated, enabling efficient program evaluation.

Ecological validity is demonstrated by providing for the generalization of functional skills to everyday, practical settings.

In Eugene, the Oregon Rehabilitation Center is developing a model, termed *Multitasking*, designed with these criteria in mind (Levin, Rawlings-Boyd, & Clapper, 1990). Still in the experimental stage, it is described here briefly as one example of executive function training based on the construct of zoom navigation. The model is termed Multitasking because it focuses on the cognitive skills required to manage multiple simultaneous tasks.

In order to train zoom navigation, a means of defining such skills in operational terms must be devised. Ways of measuring degrees of successful approximations of the skills are needed. For the purposes of Multitasking, zoom navigation is operationalized by embedding tasks within tasks (see also Mayer, Keating, & Rapp, 1986). A focused, detailed task demand may be embedded within a broader context of multiple similar tasks, which may in turn be embedded within a still broader environmental context. A functional example of such a paradigm is cooking a meal. The cook must follow the specific measurements within a given recipe, while coordinating the recipe requirements of two or three other dishes prepared concurrently, all within the demands of a time deadline (the arrival of hungry guests). Driving offers another familiar example. The driver must shift attention from

traffic to the dashboard gauges, while switching radio stations and conversing with passengers, all without losing track of the destination route and time deadline.

Everyday life is full of such requirements. In fact, one may argue that competent self-management consists primarily of managing these multiple task demands. Each of us, throughout our daily activities, must continually prioritize and select our next focus of attention by maintaining awareness of each detail within the context of the overall environmental contingencies. It might even be said that to the extent one consciously directs one's focus of attention, rather than submitting to distractions beyond the scope of conscious awareness, one is exercising "free will." Zoom navigation thus lies at the core of self-determination and autonomous functioning.

The means of task analyzing such recurring situations for training is presented in the work of Engelmann and his colleagues (Becker, Engelmann, & Thomas, 1975; Engelmann & Carnine, 1982). Engelmann is a designer of instructional curricula who for years has innovated and evaluated training paradigms developed primarily (although not exclusively) for persons with learning disabilities. The Multitasking model is drawn in large part from his concepts of training and generalizing behavioral operations.

The model embeds layers of training tasks within one another by presenting a basic paradigm comprising three task requirements:

1. The client must attend to instructions for executing a specific action, or *command*.

2. The client must monitor a specific *environmental contingency* before executing the command. The command to be executed may be event contingent or time contingent.

3. The client must manage distractions, or *interfering tasks,* before initiating the task execution according to the specified contingency.

The power of the paradigm lies in its parsimony, and in the possibility for varying the complexity of any or all of the three component task demands. The latter allows for extensive flexibility and individualization of the training environment.

Zoom navigation is practiced by repetition of the three-factor paradigm across therapy environments and across diverse task content and scope. Data are collected and fed back to the client, encouraging heightened self-monitoring of performance on this critical executive function skill.

Multitasking Training Formats

Multitasking is presented in three separate but operationally linked training formats. The first format, Warmup, presents brief tasks requiring focused concentration. These tasks are analogous to the repetitive cognitive drills that are most typically presented via computer. In the Warmup format, the subject is presented with a relatively simple command (e.g., recall a sentence, or imitate a sequence of motor actions). The command is not to be executed until a specific number of seconds have elapsed (i.e., 5–30 seconds). The time span must be estimated, within a 20% error tolerance. During the time span, a separate task demand is presented as attentional interference.

This example is quite difficult. The Warmup task can be expanded or contracted depending upon the demonstrated performance of the individual. For example, a simpler task would present a briefer command, perhaps omit or shorten the time span, and omit or simplify the interfering task. At the simplest level, the client may be required only to follow a simple, immediate command. A slightly more difficult example might be to estimate a 5-second interval by initiating a motor or verbal signal. A critical point is that an extremely complex task can also be constructed from the original three-factor paradigm, still requiring less than a minute for a completion cycle. The brief completion cycle enables the client to practice many repetitions of the required complex attentional shifting (zoom navigating) within a contained therapy time block. The possibility for multiple repetitions is critical, given the compromised acquisition rate among brain-injured individuals. With each repetition, the client gains practice attending to detailed task demands while maintaining simultaneous awareness of the contextual demands in which the task is performed. The obtained data can be analyzed over trials to determine whether errors occur with quality of task performance, perseveration on interfering tasks, or recall and initiation of the target task. The results prescribe the design of further tasks, allowing precise adjustment of any or all of the component task demands.

Whether the training is administered in an inpatient, outpatient, home, or vocational setting, the specific content of the tasks may vary. The physical therapist may present motor tasks; the speech-language pathologist may present language or numerical tasks; the job coach may present vocationally related practical tasks; and the parent, spouse, or caregiver may present home management tasks.

While the tasks vary, the paradigm and related cognitive requirements remain constant. This constancy of the cognitive process, as distinct from the content of the tasks, is paramount for achieving generalization of training. The probabilities for skill generalization increase as the specificity of the skill definition increases, and the diversity of settings increases. One difficulty in achieving generalization encountered in training modules may well be due to the multiplicity and diversity of cognitive processes practiced. The Multitasking model offers the advantage of providing practice on an identified single cognitive skill, within a single, constant training paradigm, even while tasks and settings vary.

The second training format, Agenda, applies the same functionally equivalent paradigm to a longer time contingency. The term Agenda exemplifies the training process in everyday terms. The client works with the clinician or caregiver to develop an agreed-upon agenda for action over the ensuing work session, which may range from a few minutes to an hour. Tasks relevant to the client's overall goals are listed and referred to as the work session unfolds. The client is given responsibility for and control over the completion of tasks on the agenda. Depending upon the skill level of the client, task shifting can be contingent upon completion of earlier tasks (event-contingent shift), time schedules (time-contingent shift), or a combination (task completion occurs within a time limit). The client must remain aware of the contingencies described on the written agenda, while still attending to the specifics of each task on the agenda list. As the client progresses, the prompt of the list can be faded, further challenging the limits of the memory system. In this way, the paradigm replicates that of the Warmup format: Specified actions are initiated after a delay, during which attention is distracted by interfering tasks (where each agenda task potentially interferes with the appropriate initiation of the next task).

It is important to reemphasize two points already mentioned. First, the client participates in setting the agenda. Second, the tasks are chosen for their relevance to the client's own explicitly identified personal goals. These two points increase the probability that the client is motivated by natural rather than artificial or coercive contingencies. This attention to the context within which the cognitive training tasks are performed is fundamental to Multitasking, and is another critical factor in promoting the generalization of acquired skills. Luria (1979) emphasized the critical influence of the context or motivating circumstances in shaping the learning process:

> We adopted the fundamental proposition that a change in the goal of a task inevitably leads to a significant change in the structure of the psychological processes which carry it out. A change in the structure of activity, in other words, implies a change in the brain organization of activity. (p. 172)

Simply providing repetitive drills on tasks that are isolated from the client's expressed purposes ignores the essential factor in fostering learning and generalization.

The third training format, Homework, requires the client to delay initiation of activities over still longer time frames. In this format, the client demonstrates follow through with assigned tasks over periods ranging from hours to days. This critical self-management skill is, of course, necessary for all autonomous adults, and represents a high level of recovery among individuals with traumatic brain injury. The commonsense familiarity of the Homework format need not obscure that it retains the constant, three-factor paradigm practiced in the prior formats: command execution, contingency monitoring, and interfering task completion. The client practices the same cognitive skills across task con-

tent, training discipline, time-unit demands, and settings.

Multitasking Training Hierarchies

In practice, Multitasking is first introduced to the more severely impaired client with the simpler examples of Warmup tasks only. As recovery progresses, Warmup tasks are "stretched" to greater complexity, and Agenda, then Homework formats are added to the program. The effect is cumulative, not necessarily sequential. At the latter stages of training, the client may practice multiple repetitions of complex Warmup tasks throughout the day, plus manage Agendas and Homework assignments day to day. The paradigm thus expands to incorporate the entire continuum concurrently from narrow, focused, attentional analog tasks to functional survival activities in everyday settings.

Again, the process remains constant, dispensing with much of the confusion that can arise when numerous cognitive skills are practiced according to a schedule of modules, generated from speculation about unobservable, internal "information processing." With Multitasking, the training hierarchy is derived from task analyzing the interaction of the individual with the external environmental contingencies that determine overt behavior. The hierarchy does not derive from task content or type. Visuospatial, language, attentional, and reasoning tasks might all be incorporated concurrently, not in a rigidly prescribed sequence. Difficulty is related to the management of multiple task demands regardless of specific task content. This encourages a simpler training environment, with current performance directly prescribing subsequent task definition.

Evaluation of Multitasking Model

In applying the previously stated criteria for an effective cognitive rehabilitation model, it can be seen that the Multitasking model offers reasons for confidence that it meets the tests. The model derives from a single, coherent, theoretically based conceptual framework. The paradigm integrates evaluation and prescription; the client's performance within the paradigm directly suggests the next training task environment. The model is flexible, enabling different clinicians or caregivers to work within their domain of expertise or interest. The model affords individualization of training by expanding or contracting any or all of the three component operations. The model is easily adapted to generate quantifiable behavioral data.

The final and perhaps most critical criterion, promoting ecological validity, is addressed in numerous ways:

1. Training tasks are selected, to the extent possible, for their direct relevance to the client's expressed goals.
2. Successive approximations of target behaviors are progressively shaped, starting with simple actions, and systematically graduating toward more complex, functional activities.
3. Prompts and cues are faded systematically, both in rate of presentation and specificity, as the client progresses toward the more advanced formats.
4. Reinforcement becomes more intermittent, strengthening the resistance of the learned skills to extinction or forgetting.
5. The number and practical relevance of training settings systematically increases.
6. The target skill remains constant while environmental contingencies are systematically varied.
7. Consistent feedback is provided to focus awareness on performance of the zoom navigation skill, and to enhance self-monitoring.

Each of these factors increases the probability that the executive function skill, zoom navigation, will generalize to those settings most relevant for self-sufficient, autonomous action.

COMPUTER APPLICATIONS

This chapter began with the observation that computer applications in cognitive rehabilitation are being scrutinized with more skepticism than in the past. This is a healthy and appropriate trend that will raise the standards of accountability for those who develop and apply software tools in cognitive rehabilitation. This trend need not, however, obscure the fact that data are ac-

cumulating to demonstrate the positive effect of computer applications.

Overview

The following are examples of recently published empirical studies reporting on the effects of computer-assisted cognitive training:

1. Head-injured persons receiving computer-presented memory training showed lasting and significant gains on an independent memory test. Gains were significantly greater than controls receiving no training (Kerner, 1985).
2. Children with learning disabilities given computer-presented visuospatial training improved their Performance IQ scores on the Wechsler Intelligence Scale for Children–Revised (Wechsler, 1974) by an average of 15 more points than did a control group who received no training (Owen, 1986).
3. Elderly individuals given practice on video games significantly improved their IQ scores (both Performance and Verbal) on the Wechsler Adult Intelligence Scale–Revised (Wechsler, 1981), plus showed gains on other psychometrics. Control subjects showed no gains (Drew & Waters, 1986).
4. Persons with head injury exposed to computer-presented memory training significantly improved their memory test performance. The gains were maintained over time. Controls showed no equivalent gains (Marks, Parenté, & Anderson, 1986)
5. Chronic alcoholics presented with computerized visuospatial training achieved higher post-training scores than did an untrained control group on all of the five visuospatial tests administered (Nicely, 1987).
6. A brain-injured hospital patient showed significantly more effective performance in a cooking task when using computer-generated cuing than she did when the computer "orthotic" was withdrawn (Kirsch, Levine, Fallon-Krueger, & Jaros, 1987).
7. Four persons with brain injury showed attentional skill gains following attention training incorporating computer-presented tasks. Equivalent attentional gains were not demonstrated following visual process training (Sohlberg & Mateer, 1987).

8. Three brain-injured persons with visual neglect improved their reading and other visuospatial abilities following computerized training and verbal mediation strategies (Robertson, Gray, & McKenzie, 1988).

9. Thirty persons with brain injury demonstrated significant improvement on computerized cognitive training tasks, with those most impaired improving to the level of those least impaired. The clients reported significant benefit and preference for the computer-assisted training (Fisher, 1988).

10. Three head-injured persons with attentional problems demonstrated improved attentional performance on untrained measures following training with computerized attentional programs. No improvement was noted during baseline or control periods (Gray & Robertson, 1989).

11. Forty head-injured persons receiving neuropsychological intervention, incorporating computer-assisted cognitive training, demonstrated significant gains on neuropsychological test performance. Performance gains on memory, problem-solving, and attentional measures significantly surpassed those of the control group (Ruff et al., 1989).

12. An individual with Alzheimer's disease showed gains on all measured tasks and increased attention span on therapeutic and real world tasks following computer training in "distraction management" (Nagler, 1989).

The cumulative evidence from the above studies is certainly insufficient to assure that CACR consistently results in improved self-management competence. Indeed, some investigators have found no measurable therapy effect with CACR (Fisk-Price, 1987; Ponsford & Kinsella, 1988). Much further investigation must be undertaken to establish links between specific training paradigms and functional outcomes. Yet, the evidence clearly justifies further research and development toward more effective computer-assisted cognitive rehabilitation methods. Enough successes have surely now been demonstrated to give pause to those who would argue against the potential of CACR.

Further, the above studies demonstrate the diversity of possible approaches to applying CACR. Certainly additional models of application are possible. It might be helpful to classify uses of computers in cognitive rehabilitation as follows:

1. *Computer as "learning laboratory"* This category applies to the use of the hardware or software as a learning environment, apart from specific CACR software applications. For example, a client may receive training in using the disk drive, the mouse, the keyboard, or the printer. A variation on this theme is to learn the commands that allow facility within applications, such as word processors, graphics programs, desktop publishing programs, or spreadsheets. At a more complex level, an individual may receive training by practicing the logic required to maneuver within the operating system or within simple programming languages, such as LOGO (Papert, 1980). In each of these examples, the client practices logic and organizational skills within the practical context of applying computer technology.

2. *Information acquisition* Computer-assisted tutorials provide excellent interactive means of presenting information while affording the learner maximum involvement and control over the pace of instruction. Expert system shells offer the potential to assist those who seek technical expertise when no "expert" is readily available. Such software tools enable experts in particular professional disciplines to create computer-assisted resources that imitate their own decision-making processes and professional judgments.

3. *Computer as orthotic device* Traditional computer applications can be used by therapist or client just as they are used in business, education, or the professions: to simplify otherwise complex tasks. Kreutzer et al. (1989) reported, for example, specific ways in which word processing software assisted in generating memory prompts and checklists. Kirsch et al. (1987) reported on an innovative approach, cited earlier, using a specialized computer programming environment (COGORTH) to prompt and

monitor a cooking task. Chute, Conn, and Di-pasquale (1988) developed "ProthesisWare" for the Macintosh computer line, to provide assistance in managing activities of daily living.

4. *Simulations* This category includes video games, which present artificial environments requiring the user to deduce and apply procedural rules, usually under time pressure. Simulation software provides the opportunity to practice complex tasks (e.g., piloting a jet, running a business, managing a baseball team, driving a race car, administering a city) in a protected, entertaining environment. Such environments are motivating, and provide rich opportunities to observe the learning capacities of the client. They are, however, often too complex and fast-paced for persons with head injury, and tend to allow little control over the many component variables that determine the degree or quality of cognitive challenge.

5. *Drill and practice* This category includes much of the currently applied cognitive rehabilitation software. Unlike video games, very discrete and simple tasks are presented, one at a time, often allowing reasonable control by the therapist over the contingencies of task presentation. These tasks in many ways approximate those traditionally presented on psychometric tests, yet allow significantly more flexibility and interactivity. They also allow component skills to be measured precisely, but typically do not provide the real-world analog that is the strength of simulations.

This overview is clearly not meant as a reference to available software products; such resources are available elsewhere (Kurlychek & Levin, 1987; Lynch, 1986; Story & Sbordone, 1988). The categories are presented to highlight the particular strengths of very different approaches to applying computers. The point has been emphasized that computer applications in cognitive rehabilitation are most appropriately understood as extensions of a particular, theoretically based intervention model. Any or all of these categories of applications may be appropriate for a given individual, depending on how their use is logically derived from particular intervention approaches.

Computer-Assisted Multitasking

None of the categories just mentioned is ideally suited to extend the model developed in this chapter. The Multitasking model, as stated earlier, derives from a behavioral perspective that emphasizes the impact of environmental contingencies on behavior, including cognitive behavior. It is the ability to attend consciously to this environmental impact on one's own behavior (to zoom navigate) that lies at the crux of effective executive function skills, and ultimately, of self-responsibility. In contemplating computer approaches to Multitasking, therefore, the emphasis is directed toward creating ways to help the therapist control environmental contingencies for specific training objectives.

In many respects, this is what is afforded by existing drill-and-practice cognitive rehabilitation software. Different computer-presented tasks provide practice with specific skills, with certain components of stimulus presentation regulated by the therapist. There are reaction-time skills, language skills, visuospatial skills, numerical skills, analogy skills, maze skills, reasoning skills, and so on. It might appear that the quantity of tasks available is the criterion of software quality.

The point is not to disparage the efforts of software innovators who have thus far developed training tools, for much that is currently available is elegant, admirable, and potentially useful. Rather, the point is to return to a premise of this chapter that emphasizes managing integrated task hierarchies according to designated contingencies instead of mastering increasing numbers of unrelated, functionally irrelevant tasks. What is needed is a tool to give us the power to re-combine a few simple components into increasingly complex hierarchies of environmental contingencies. Fortunately, computers provide this power. Unfortunately, most current software tends to focus more on refining the contingencies within any single task rather than on combining multiple, different tasks into a broader working environment.

In theory, software can be written to allow the design and construction of multitask environments. Such software would allow the clinician to replicate the Multitasking paradigm, and would efficiently provide training in "zooming" from task detail to increasingly complex layers of task arrays, agendas, and time schedules. The computer would allow simulation of the Warmup format, simplifying the construction of precise, brief, repetitive task-completion cycles for practicing zoom navigation. In addition, however, the computer could be a link to scheduled behavioral operations, including functional, everyday tasks in the natural environment. It could serve as the check-in point for registering the completion of such tasks, occurring away from the machine. If linked to an optical video disc player (Levin, 1983; Lynch, 1989), the computer could potentially direct the user to an electronic "therapist," captured on video, who instructs the user on the appropriate agenda of activities for the immediate block of time. The video therapist (not to be construed as replacing the direct supervision of the actual clinician), would base each set of instructions on the user's Multitasking performance, as captured by the computer.

Such a computer environment, with or without the interactive video disc component, would combine the strengths of the simulation and drill-and-practice categories. Complex real-world tasks would be presented, and control would be maintained over the specific contingencies of each component task within the Multitasking environment. The result might be a synthesis of a neuropsychometric test battery, a video game, and traditional training in activities of daily living.

A prototype of such a computer environment is currently under development. Existing software, however, can be adapted to be applied within a Multitasking model of intervention. Commercially available business or consumer "memory resident" or "pop-up" programs allow the user to shift from work in one software application (e.g., a spreadsheet) to a different program (e.g., a word processor), at the touch of one or two keys. Simple tasks could be prescribed in each application, with requirements for shifting between them according to con-

tingencies designed to appropriately challenge the client's zoom navigation ability. "Integrated" software products, incorporating word processors, graphics programs, spreadsheets, and database programs, similarly enable rapid shifting across very different cognitive tasks. Additional programs are available for the higher level IBM-compatible computers that provide a graphic interface, similar to the user interface available for the Macintosh computers. Such programs advertise the capability for "multitasking" across applications, allowing the user to dispense with the need to exit one application before beginning work in another. All of these products offer the potential for providing practice in embedding tasks within other tasks, according to environmental contingencies controlled by the therapist.

Since these environments are not designed for the special needs of brain-injured persons or their therapists, they may be too complex for most clients. Another alternative is to use a single software application as one task among several that are presented within a training session. The client must shift among multiple tasks in the clinic, of which a given computer task is only one. For therapists wishing to extend the Multitasking model by using currently available cognitive rehabilitation software, the most relevant programs are those that gradually introduce simultaneous stimuli for monitoring (e.g., Bracy, 1988; Sanford & Browne, 1985). Such programs emphasize the zoom navigation attentional skill, but tend to be limited in the range of attentional shifting they require. In general, they do not present hierarchies of tasks embedded within other, different tasks. They do, however, provide practice in rapid attentional shifting among stimuli, while maintaining simultaneous awareness of the overall context within which the competing stimuli are changing.

These computer applications of the Multitasking model, like the model itself, are preliminary and untested. As stated at the outset, the model and its applications are presented not only as offerings in their own right, but as examples of the importance of applying CACR within the context of a cohesive theoretical model. At present, the field of cognitive rehabilitation is too young to have evolved to a consensus on a given training model. Indeed, many models may emerge for different objectives. At the same time, the field is too advanced to require us to rely on shotgun approaches that are not well grounded in what is known about principles of learning, generalization, and the effects of environmental variables on behavior.

SUMMARY AND CONCLUSIONS

This chapter set as its first objective the presentation of a conceptual foundation for addressing the application of computer technology to the cognitive rehabilitation endeavor. In approaching this objective, the author has presented, as examples, a diagnosis of what is most critically impaired (executive function skills), an explanation of why (impaired zoom navigation skills), and a prescription for how to fix it (Multitasking model). The appropriate use of computer technology becomes apparent only after addressing these prior issues. It is hoped that this discussion will stimulate further progress toward more helpful theories, models of intervention, and computer applications. To the extent that this happens, our opportunities increase for helping individuals with traumatic brain injury to pursue self-sufficiency, and lives of contribution, productivity, and pride.

REFERENCES

Baddeley, A.D. (1982). Domains of recollection. *Psychological Review, 69*, 708–729.

Bayless, J.D., Varney, N.R., & Roberts, R.J. (1989). Tinker Toy Test performance and vocational outcome in patients with closed-head injuries. *Journal of Clinical and Experimental Neuropsychology, 11*(6), 913–917.

Becker, W.C., Engelmann, S., & Thomas, D.R. (1975). *Teaching 2: Cognitive learning and instruction.* Chicago: Science Research Associates.

Ben-Yishay, Y., & Diller, L. (1983). Cognitive remediation. In M. Rosenthal, E.R. Griffith, M.R. Bond, & J.D. Miller (Eds.), *Rehabilitation of the head injured adult* (pp. 367–380). Philadelphia: F.A. Davis.

Boyd, T.M., Sautter, S., Bailey, M.B., Echols, L.D., & Douglas, J.W. (1987, February). *Reliability and validity of a measure of everyday problem solving.* Paper presented at the annual meeting of the International Neuropsychological Society, Washington, DC.

Bracy, O.L. (1986). Cognitive rehabilitation: A process approach. *Cognitive Rehabilitation, 4*(2), 10–17.

Bracy, O.L. (1988). *Foundations II: Simultaneous multiple attention* [computer program]. Indianapolis, IN: Psychological Software Services.

Chute, D., Conn, G., & Dipasquale, M. (1988). ProsthesisWare: A new class of software supporting the activities of daily living. *Neuropsychology, 2*(1), 41–57.

Cicerone, K.D. (1989, December). *Neuropsychological predictors of rehabilitation outcome.* Paper presented at the annual meeting of the National Head Injury Foundation, Chicago.

Cicerone, K.D., & Wood, J.C. (1987). Planning disorder after closed head injury: A case study. *Archives of Physical Medicine and Rehabilitation, 68*, 111–115.

Claxton, G. (1988). How do you tell a good cognitive theory when you see one? In G. Claxton (Ed.), *Growth points in cognition* (pp.1–31). New York: Routledge.

Drew, B., & Waters, J. (1986). Videogames: Utilization of a novel strategy to improve perceptual motor skills and cognitive functioning in the non-institutionalized elderly. *Cognitive Rehabilitation, 4*(2), 26–31.

Engelmann, S., & Carnine, D. (1982). *Theory of instruction: Principles and applications.* New York: Irvington.

Eriksen, C.W., & St. James, J.D. (1986). Visual attention within and around the field of focal attention: A zoom lens model. *Perception & Psychophysics, 40*(4), 225–240.

Fisher, S.N.G. (1988). The use of the computer for rehabilitation of the adult human brain (Doctoral dissertation, University of California–Berkeley, 1987). *Dissertation Abstracts International, 49*(6), 1407A–1408A.

Fisk-Price, T.L. (1987). Comparison of standard treatment and computer enhanced treatment for the remediation of cognitive deficits associated with chronic alcoholism (Doctoral dissertation, University of Kansas, 1986). *Dissertation Abstracts International, 48*(2), 562B.

Gordon, W.A., Hibbard, M.R., & Kreutzer, J.S. (1989). Cognitive remediation: Issues in research and practice. *Journal of Head Trauma Rehabilitation, 4*(3), 76–84.

Gray, J.M., & Robertson, I. (1989). Remediation of attentional difficulties following brain injury: Three experimental single case studies. *Brain Injury, 3*(2), 163–170.

Guilford, J.P. (1973). Theories of intelligence. In B. Wolman (Ed.), *Handbook of general psychology* (pp. 630–643). Englewood Cliffs, NJ: Prentice-Hall.

Kerner, M.J. (1985). Computer delivery of memory retraining with head injured patients (Doctoral dissertation, Pacific Graduate School of Psychology, 1985). *Dissertation Abstracts International, 46*(1), 305B.

Kirsch, N.L., Levine, S.P., Fallon-Krueger, M., & Jaros, L.A. (1987). The microcomputer as an "orthotic" device for patients with cognitive deficits. *Journal of Head Trauma Rehabilitation, 2*(4), 77–86.

Kreutzer, J., Conder, R., Wehman, P., & Morrison, C. (1989). Compensatory strategies for enhancing independent living and vocational outcome following traumatic brain injury. *Cognitive Rehabilitation, 7*(1), 30–35.

Kurlychek, R.T., & Levin, W.L. (1987). Computers in the cognitive rehabilitation of brain injured persons. *Critical Reviews in Medical Informatics, 1*(3), 241–257.

Lawson, M.J., & Rice, D.N. (1989). Effects of training in use of executive strategies on a verbal memory problem resulting from closed head injury. *Journal of Clinical and Experimental Neuropsychology, 11*(6), 842–854.

Levin, W.L. (1983). Interactive video: The state-of-the-art teaching machine. *Computing Teacher, 11*(2), 11–17.

Levin, W.L., Rawlings-Boyd, J., & Clapper, J. (1990, October). *Multitasking: An Interdisciplinary model for training of executive function skills.* Paper presented at the meeting of the Oregon Speech and Hearing Association, Eugene, OR.

Lezak, M.D. (1982). The problem of assessing executive functions. *International Journal of Psychology, 17*, 281–297.

Lezak, M.D. (1987). Relationships between personality disorders, social disturbances, and physical disability following traumatic brain injury. *Journal of Head Trauma Rehabilitation, 2*(1), 57–69.

Luria, A.R. (1979). *The making of mind: A personal account of Soviet psychology* (M. Cole & S. Cole, Eds.). Cambridge, MA: Harvard University Press.

Lynch, W. (1986). An update on software in cognitive rehabilitation. *Cognitive Rehabilitation, 4*(3), 14–18.

Lynch, W. (1989). Microcomputers in cognitive rehabilitation: New directions. *Journal of Head Trauma Rehabilitation, 4*(3), 92–94.

Marks, C., Parenté, F., & Anderson, J. (1986). Retention of gains in outpatient cognitive rehabilitation therapy. *Cognitive Rehabilitation, 4*(3), 20–23.

Mayer, N.H., Keating, D.J., & Rapp, D. (1986). Skills, routines, and activity patterns of daily living: A functional nested approach. In B. Uzell & Y. Gross (Eds.), *Clinical neuropsychology of intervention* (pp. 205–222). Boston: Martinus Nijhoff.

Mesulam, M.M. (1981). A cortical network for directed attention and unilateral neglect. *Annual Review of Neurology, 10*, 309–325.

Nagler, R.A. (1989). "Distraction management" training via microcomputer with a dementia patient: An unexpected outcome [Summary of poster presentation]. *Archives of Physical Medicine and Rehabilitation [Scientific Paper and Poster Abstracts, Annual Meeting Issue], 70*(11), A-80.

Nicely, E.R. (1987). The computer-based remediation of visuospatial deficits in chronic alcoholics (Doctoral dissertation, University of Toledo, 1986). *Dissertation Abstracts International, 47*(10), 3666A.

Norman, D.A. (1980). Twelve issues in cognitive science. *Cognitive Science, 4*, 1–33.

Owen, N.W. (1986). Exploratory study: Effect of computer cognitive rehabilitation on visual-spatial skills of learning-disabled students (Doctoral dissertation, Mississippi State University, 1986). *Dissertation Abstracts International, 47*(4), 1284A.

Papert, S. (1980). *Mindstorms: Children, computers, and powerful ideas.* New York: Basic Books.

Phillips, J.L. (1969). *The origins of intellect: Piaget's theory.* San Francisco: W.H. Freeman.

Ponsford, J.L., & Kinsella, G. (1988). Evaluation of a remedial programme for attentional deficits following closed-head injury. *Journal of Clinical and Experimental Neuropsychology, 10*(6), 693–708.

Posner, M.I. (1990). Structures and functions of selective attention. In T. Boll & B. Bryant (Eds.), *Clinical neuropsychology and brain function: Research, measurement, and practice* (pp. 173–202). Washington, DC: American Psychological Association.

Posner, M.I., & Petersen, S.E. (1990). The attention system of the human brain. *Annual Review of Neuroscience, 13*, 25–42.

Reitan, R.M. (1958). Validity of the Trail Making Test as an indication of organic brain damage. *Perceptual and Motor Skills, 8*, 271–276.

Rizzolatti, G., Gentilucci, M., & Matelli, M. (1985). Selective spatial attention: One center, one circuit or many circuits. In M. I. Posner & O.S.M. Marin (Eds.), *Attention and performance* (vol. XI, pp. 251–265). Hillsdale, NJ: Lawrence Erlbaum Associates.

Robertson, I., Gray, J., & McKenzie, S. (1988). Microcomputer-based cognitive rehabilitation of visual neglect: Three multiple-baseline single-case studies. *Brain Injury, 2*(2) 151–163.

Ruff, R.M., Baser, C.A., Johnston, J.W., Marshall, L.F., Klauber, S.K., Klauber, M.R., & Minteer, M. (1989). Neuropsychological rehabilitation: An experimental study with head-injured patients. *Journal of Head Trauma Rehabilitation, 4*(3), 20–36.

Sanford, J.A., & Browne, R.J. (1985). *Captain's log: Cognitive training system, visual/motor skills module, visual tracking/discrimination* [Computer program]. Richmond, VA: Network Services.

Sidman, M. (1960). *Tactics of scientific research.* New York: Basic Books.

Sohlberg, M.M., & Mateer, C.A. (1987). Effectiveness of an attention-training program. *Brain Injury, 9*(2), 117–130.

Sohlberg, M.M., Mateer, C.A. (1989). *Introduction to cognitive rehabilitation: Theory and practice.* New York: Guilford Press.

Story, T.B., & Sbordone, R.J. (1988). The use of microcomputers in the treatment of cognitive-communicative impairments. *Journal of Head Trauma Rehabilitation, 3*(2), 45–54.

Wechsler, D. (1974). *WISC-R manual, Wechsler Intelligence Scale for Children–Revised.* New York: Psychological Corporation.

Wechsler, D. (1981). *Wechsler Adult Intelligence Scale–Revised.* New York: Psychological Corporation.

CHAPTER 14

Social Skills Training Following Head Injury

CORWIN BOAKE

Therapeutic intervention of social behavior is an important part of head injury rehabilitation because many persons with head injury have difficulty interacting with others. Clients whose social behavior is mildly impaired may show subtle changes in isolated areas, such as difficulty in keeping to the same topic. In clients with more severe impairments, social behavior may be so pervasively altered that family members feel the client has a different personality. Family members rate change in clients' social behavior as the most stressful consequence of head injury, more stressful than changes in cognitive or physical abilities (Brooks & McKinlay, 1983). Clinical experience suggests that social behavior is also a major factor in vocational outcome after head injury.

The goal of this chapter is to review a group of interventions, termed *social skills training,* that have been used to treat behavioral disorders of clients with head injury. The basic model of social skills training is that social behaviors can be learned and used in the same manner as other skills. According to this model, the process of learning a social skill consists of: 1) others' instruction in and modeling of the skill; 2) practicing the skill, with feedback; and 3) shaping the skill until it is used correctly. Most readers are familiar with social skills training as applied to teaching assertiveness. In fact, there is a wide range of applications for social skills training, including its use with persons with mental retardation or cognitive impairments (e.g., Curran & Monti, 1982; L'Abate & Milan, 1985; Liberman, DeRisi, & Mueser, 1989).

The first section of the chapter discusses assessment of the social behavior of persons with head injury. The second section reviews social skills interventions that have been used with head-injured clients, and evaluates evidence of their effectiveness. Finally, the third section discusses issues in the clinical application of social skills training in head injury rehabilitation.

ASSESSMENT OF BEHAVIORAL CHANGE AFTER HEAD INJURY

A major obstacle is that there is no accepted standard procedure for assessing social behavior of persons with head injury. Lezak (1989) summarized the problems that can render traditional self-report questionnaires unsuitable for use with head-injured clients. Research on behavioral change after head injury has increasingly used direct behavioral observation. For example, Godfrey, Knight, Marsh, Moroney, and Bishara (1989) and Milton, Prutting, and Binder (1984) videotaped head-injured clients role playing social interactions and measured their performance in terms of behavioral ratings. Mentis and Prutting (1987) analyzed clients' speech samples in terms of linguistic features.

The Neurobehavioral Rating Scale (Levin et al., 1987) is the only standardized observer rating scale developed for assessment of behavioral symptoms in clients with head injury. Approximately half of the 27 subscales rate deficits in social behavior. Interrater reliability and validity have been demonstrated (Levin et al., 1987). This scale should be considered for use as a screening instrument in most head injury rehabilitation settings, and may also have a role in measuring intervention effects.

Two observer rating scales have been validated for measurement of speech pragmatics skills of clients with head injury. The Pragmatics

Protocol (Prutting & Kirchner, 1983) measures 32 pragmatics skills that are rated in terms of appropriateness. The scale was valid in distinguishing head-injured clients from controls when used to rate brief, role-played interactions (Milton et al., 1984). The Communication Performance Scale (Erlich & Barry, 1989) was adapted from the Pragmatics Protocol and rates six behaviors (Intelligibility, Eye Gaze, Sentence Formulation, Coherence of Narrative, Topic, and Initiation of Communication). Interrater reliability was adequate when the scale was used to rate videotaped role plays of clients with head injury. These two scales should be more widely used in social skills training, but probably need to be supplemented with ratings of emotional behaviors.

Burke (1988) provided a set of observer rating scales that were developed for other client populations, which he recommended based on clinical experience with head-injured clients. There remains, however, a strong need for research on the utility of established social skills assessment instruments with head-injured clients.

SOCIAL SKILLS TRAINING WITH HEAD-INJURED CLIENTS

Social skills training programs that have been used in brain injury rehabilitation can be categorized as follows: videotape feedback, feedback interventions for specific behaviors, pragmatics training, social skills classes, and problem-solving training. The following sections review applications of these programs with head-injured clients, together with evidence of their effectiveness.

Videotape Feedback

The rationale for the use of feedback in training social skills is that clients with head injury may need additional feedback in order to discriminate and monitor their deficits in social behavior. Natural social interaction also produces feedback, but natural feedback may be too subtle or delayed for many head-injured clients. To be effective, feedback may need to be immediate and explicit in terms of discriminating specific behaviors. Videotape feedback may be an effective intervention for many clients because it is objective. Further, as Alexy, Foster, and Baker

(1983) pointed out, observing oneself on videotape may be a rewarding activity for many persons.

A social skills training program using videotape feedback was described by Helffenstein and Wechsler (1982). Their program consisted of individual therapy sessions in which the client and therapist role played and then reviewed one videotaped interaction per session. The interactions were mostly unstructured, as the overall goal was to improve interpersonal and communication skills in general. The major modifications of the original technique were that therapists provided corrective feedback and coached clients to suggest alternative responses as needed.

In the same paper, Helffenstein and Wechsler (1982) reported a study evaluating this program with 16 head-injured clients at Woodrow Wilson Rehabilitation Center, a residential treatment center. Clients were randomly assigned to receive either 20 videotape feedback training sessions or an equal number of individual therapy sessions that did not provide feedback. The results showed that the videotape feedback group improved more than the other group in terms of staff ratings of everyday behavior and observer ratings of two interactions. This study shows that many clients respond to and benefit from videotape feedback, and can generalize improved social skills to outside therapy. The use of random assignment in this study is especially noteworthy and qualifies the study as one of the few true experiments conducted in the field of cognitive rehabilitation.

Alexy et al. (1983) described a social skills training program adapted from Helffenstein and Wechsler (1982) and based on videotape feedback. The program was conducted as a therapy group in an inpatient rehabilitation unit. Alexy et al. emphasized the importance of targeting specific problem behaviors for clients and focusing attention on these goals during training. An interesting feature of their program was that therapists also identified and worked on their own social skills objectives, in order to model how to participate in the exercises and accept feedback.

Brotherton, Thomas, Wisotzek, and Milan (1988) developed a social skills training program that combined videotape feedback with other training techniques. The program was designed for 4 head-injured outpatients who had significant social skills deficits. As a first step, family interviews and client observation were used to identify the most problematic social skills deficits. These were posture; speech dysfluencies; self-manipulative behaviors; and low frequency of responding with personal attention, reinforcing comments, and positive statements. Problem behaviors were addressed in different stages of training according to a multiple baseline design. Clients attended approximately 20 individual training sessions, each consisting of an unstructured interaction, several role-played scenarios, and a training period that used a combination of interventions, including videotape feedback for the target behavior. Clients were also given homework and asked to keep a diary of relevant interactions, and their families were informed of the target behaviors and recommended feedback.

The results showed that 3 out of the 4 clients maintained improvement in at least one behavior at a 1-year follow-up (Brotherton et al., 1988). The most stable improvements were mainly in nonverbal skills such as posture and self-manipulation. Verbal social skills improved in some clients, but the improvements were not maintained at follow-up.

Brotherton et al.'s (1988) study evaluated a combined package of social skills interventions and cannot distinguish the role of any one technique. It is noteworthy, however, because training was planned based on a pretraining assessment, and because tracking of multiple behaviors showed differential effects on the clients' social skills deficits.

Individual Feedback Programs for Specific Behavioral Deficits

A group of social skills training programs have used different forms of feedback in interventions designed for individual clients with specific behavior problems.

Conversational Skills

Gajar, Schloss, Schloss, and Thompson (1984) developed and evaluated a social skills training program to improve conversational skills, using feedback and self-monitoring training in different stages of intervention. Sessions consisted of group discussions and role-played conversations. During the feedback training stage, clients were provided with feedback from lights operated by therapists to indicate whether clients were responding appropriately. Clients were asked to explain the feedback they received and were given written exercises in discriminating appropriate conversation responses. In the self-monitoring training stage, sessions consisted of the same discussions and role plays, with the modification that clients operated their own feedback lights.

This program was evaluated with 2 head-injured outpatients who were selected because of conversational difficulties (Gajar et al., 1984). Training was provided in 12 group sessions. The results showed that appropriate conversational responses increased to within the normal range during both training stages, but fell below normal when training was discontinued. The study can be criticized because the duration of training may have been too brief to test adequately whether training effects would have been maintained over time. However, Gajar et al.'s results indicate that some clients respond to corrective feedback and can learn to self-monitor their social behavior.

Schloss, Thompson, Gajar, and Schloss (1985) developed a training program for male head-injured clients to learn conversational skills for interactions with female peers. The program was developed for 2 head-injured outpatients who had difficulty in heterosexual interactions. The training objectives were to increase their frequency of giving compliments and asking questions, and to decrease their frequency of making inappropriate self-disclosures. Each conversational behavior was addressed in a different stage of training according to a multiple baseline design. Clients participated in 22 training sessions consisting of orientation to the target behavior and training to self-monitor the target behavior during conversations with therapists. The results showed clients were successful in increasing their compliments and questions, but less successful in decreasing their self-disclosures.

Inappropriate Speech

Giles, Fussey, and Burgess (1988) developed a conversational skills training program for a head-injured inpatient who was treated in a psychiatric unit in part because of inappropriate social behavior with severe circumstantiality and tangentiality. The program consisted of training the patient to respond appropriately to three types of interactions: 1) structured interaction requiring the patient to give one-word responses, 2) semistructured interaction requiring specific but brief answers, and 3) unstructured interactions requiring responses of less than 90 seconds. Successful performance was rewarded by attention, praise, and chocolate. Unsuccessful performance was punished by the Time Out On The Spot (TOOTS) procedure, in which the therapist ignored the patient for 20 seconds before resuming therapy.

After 1 month of daily training sessions, the patient's conversational behavior was felt to be satisfactory and the training program was discontinued. Statistical analysis showed significant improvement occurred in all three conversational situations and continued at a 2-month follow-up (Giles et al., 1988). This study is an excellent example of a short-term intensive intervention and is also the only study that used statistical analysis of single-case data. Unfortunately, the patient's improvement may not be wholly attributable to the training program because unit staff used the TOOTS procedure during the same period. This illustrates the practical difficulties in attributing behavioral improvements to different interventions that are being applied simultaneously, as is typical in inpatient or residential settings.

Lewis, Nelson, Nelson, and Reusink (1988) developed and evaluated a training program for an anoxic client with impulsive, disinhibited, and inappropriate social behavior. The intervention was for three staff members at the client's residential treatment center to provide immediate feedback in response to the client's inappropriate speech. Feedback was provided in one of three forms: attention and interest, systematic ignoring, and verbal correction. The program was designed so that each week the staff members rotated between the different forms of feedback. The results showed the client responded best to verbal correction, regardless of the staff member providing it. This study is noteworthy because it demonstrated that social skills training can be conducted in relatively natural settings without formal therapy sessions.

Conclusions

Published individual feedback programs have addressed a limited number of behavioral deficits, including conversational skills and inappropriate speech. There is a need for individual feedback programs to be attempted with a wider range of behaviors such as tangentiality, labile or flat affect, and reduced social initiative.

Pragmatics Training

Pragmatics is the branch of linguistic theory dealing with language use in social communication. Pragmatics can be divided into nonverbal communication, interactional rules of communication between speakers, and propositional rules of message formulation (Hartley & Griffith, 1989). The basic goal of pragmatics training is to train clients to use pragmatic skills appropriately in their social interactions.

Although pragmatics training is widely used in head injury rehabilitation, there are few published descriptions of this type of intervention. One detailed example of a pragmatics training program was described by Erlich and Sipes (1985). The program, which also used videotape feedback, was implemented as a therapy group in a day treatment program for persons with head injury. Sessions followed a curriculum divided into four modules addressing pragmatic skills relevant to head-injured clients. The four modules covered nonverbal communication, conversational interaction, repairing communication failures, and improving cohesion of narrative discourse. Each module began with an orientation to the target skills and a review of a videotaped interaction role played by therapists to demonstrate both appropriate and inappropriate examples of the target skills. In the second stage, clients were asked to role play situations on videotape and their performances were then reviewed by the group.

Erlich and Sipes (1985) reported an uncontrolled study evaluating their training program with a therapy group of 6 head-injured outpatients. Clients showed statistically significant improvement from pre- to post-treatment on a composite rating of pragmatics skills. The results showed pragmatics skills improved differentially, with relatively greater improvement in linguistic skills (e.g., topic maintenance, cohesiveness) and relatively less improvement in nonlinguistic skills (e.g., prosody, facial expression). Although this study can be faulted for obvious methodological limitations, it is important as the first empirical study of pragmatics training; also, the results are supportive of continued development of this intervention.

Sohlberg and Mateer (1990) described a group pragmatics training program that they implemented at the Good Samaritan Hospital Center for Cognitive Rehabilitation, a day treatment center in Puyallup, Washington. Their program is adapted from the Erlich and Sipes (1985) program, with the addition of training components to identify clients' major pragmatics deficits, to improve clients' awareness of these deficits, and to promote generalization beyond the training setting. The first step in their program was to videotape each client in conversation and then to review the videotape during therapy in order to identify the pragmatic skills that should be prioritized for the client. Group training sessions consisted of role-play exercises targeting specific pragmatic skills. Sohlberg and Mateer emphasized the importance of promoting generalization by having clients receive feedback on their pragmatics skills in different situations and from different persons. To accomplish this, they informed the clients' relatives and other therapists about the clients' communication goals, and recommended appropriate feedback.

Sohlberg and Mateer (1990) also described how pragmatics training can be implemented in individual therapy. They stated that the first stage in individual training should be to improve the client's awareness of his or her communication deficits by viewing himself or herself on videotape, while recording target behaviors. Next, therapy sessions can be used to practice dyadic communication exercises with the therapist, focusing on pragmatics goals.

Social Skills Classes

A common approach to social skills training is to develop a curriculum of important social skills and to train clients to perform all the skills correctly. This approach is especially suited for therapy groups of clients with similar rehabilitation goals, such as employment or independent living. Burke (1988) provided a curriculum of social skills that are probably important for most persons with head injury. A similar curriculum was developed for adolescents by Goldstein, Sprafkin, Gershaw, and Klein (1980), who also presented detailed clinical protocols. Dunn, Van Horn, and Herman (1981) developed a social skills curriculum for persons with spinal cord injury that includes problem situations involving bias against persons with disabilities.

Braunling-McMorrow, Lloyd, and Fralish (1986) developed a social skills training program in which clients responded to a series of social situations sampled from six areas: compliments, social interaction, politeness, criticism, social confrontation, and questions/answers. The situations were read to the clients, who responded by suggesting appropriate responses, rather than role playing the responses. The social skills exercise was combined wth a board game in which clients moved their game pieces around the board by making correct responses to the social situations.

This social skills training program was evaluated with 3 clients who were treated as a group for 16 sessions (Braunling-McMorrow et al., 1986). The clients were from the Center for Comprehensive Services, a residential treatment center in Carbondale, Illinois. Results showed that, after training, the clients were able to respond correctly to almost 100% of the problem situations, and also increased their appropriate interactions during mealtime conversations. However, behavioral ratings by residential staff failed to show that any of the 3 improved in their everyday social behavior at the center. This may represent a failure to generalize to some settings.

Problem-Solving Training

The rationale for training problem-solving skills as an intervention for social behavior is that clients' ability to respond appropriately in social situations depends partly on their skills in analyzing situations and determining the optimal responses. Many social situations require clients to choose the correct response from among many alternatives.

Foxx, Marchand-Martella, Martella, Braunling-McMorrow, and McMorrow (1988) developed a problem-solving training program based on a set of 32 problem situations generated from a staff survey at the Center for Comprehensive Services. The situations were divided into four categories, including one category, "Stating One's Rights," which focuses on assertiveness skills. The training program consisted of clients practicing responses to the problem situations. During the first stage of training, clients used cue cards prompting them with questions about the correct solution (e.g., "What should you say?"). Therapists gave corrective feedback and coaching for incorrect responses. During the second stage of training, clients practiced the same problem-solving task without the cue cards.

This training program was evaluated in two studies (Foxx et al., 1988; Foxx, Martella, & Marchand-Martella, 1989) with clients at the residential center. Both studies showed the program was effective in terms of improving clients' solutions to the problem situations. The program was partly revised based on the finding that clients complained of boredom during training sessions. The main modification was that all clients were asked to respond to each problem situation in order to increase their participation. The revised program was published as a package entitled *Thinking It Through* (Foxx & Bittle, 1989), including instructions and forms. This program is noteworthy as one of the few cognitive rehabilitation programs that is empirically developed and fully documented.

CLINICAL ISSUES IN SOCIAL SKILLS TRAINING WITH HEAD-INJURED CLIENTS

Because there is no standardized social skills training program for persons with head injury, clinicians who implement social skills training must deal with a number of practical issues. The following sections are intended to help clinicians address some of these issues.

Selecting Clients for Social Skills Training

The first issue concerns whether social skills training is potentially beneficial for a given cli-

ent. Although research does not provide any firm guidelines, clinicians should consider clients' cognitive abilities and motivation in making this decision. The role of cognitive ability is obvious because social skills training assumes a minimal level of memory, reasoning, and other abilities. For example, clients must have sufficient memory capacity to retain information between sessions. Cognitive requirements may be higher in some forms of social skills training, such as curriculum-based classes, which present more information and rely on clients to generalize their skills. Persons with severe impairments may benefit more from intensive, individual programs.

The role of motivation is equally important because, as Crosson (1987) pointed out, feedback is effective only with clients who are motivated to change behaviors that they recognize as inappropriate. It should not be assumed, however, that all clients with behavior disorders are appropriate for social skills training. Clients can have behavioral deficits despite adequate social skills. They may fail to use appropriate social skills because of emotional distress, incentives for inappropriate behaviors, or other causes. Clients whose behavioral deficits are due to problems with motivation rather than social skills can be considered for other interventions such as psychotherapy or behavior therapy.

Individual versus Group Training

The programs reviewed in this chapter show both group and individual programs can be effective. However, the two have never been directly compared to determine if either approach is more effective for any one clinical problem. Individual programming has been used primarily with clients who have specific, severe behavioral deficits that are different from other clients. On the one hand, the advantage of individual training is that target behaviors can be quickly addressed without exposing other clients to behaviors that may be aversive or disruptive. On the other hand, group programming may be more cost-effective with groups of clients who have similar social skills goals. In addition, some clients may respond better to feedback from other clients rather than from clinicians. A limitation of group training is that individual clients may receive less intensive training in groups.

Social Skills Training versus Pragmatics Training

The choice between these two approaches is to some extent a disciplinary issue because some behaviors targeted by social skills training programs can also be defined in terms of pragmatics skills. The choice between approaches may depend on the clinical problem. Social skills training lends itself to training clients to handle specific problem situations, such as meeting new people and refusing alcoholic drinks. Pragmatics training may be better suited to treat specific problem behaviors that occur in different situations.

Pretraining Assessment

A common finding in the published training programs was that behavioral deficits improved differentially with therapy (e.g., Brotherton et al., 1988; Erlich & Sipes, 1985). This suggests that social skills training improves specific behaviors, perhaps through improved self-monitoring, rather than improving social behavior in general. Therefore, clients should have target behaviors identified before training. The Neurobehavioral Rating Scale (Levin et al., 1987) can be recommended as a screening instrument to identify the most important behavioral deficits of each client. Clients should be directly observed during natural interactions, because indirect reports from family members, friends, and co-workers can be biased by different emotional and cultural expectations (Braunling-McMorrow, 1988). Behaviors should be compared between different situations in order to reveal if problems are due to motivational or situational factors, rather than to social skills deficits per se.

Generalization

An important criticism of cognitive rehabilitation techniques, including social skills training, is that persons with head injury may fail to generalize therapy effects to everyday life. In fact, this problem was directly addressed in most of the programs reviewed in this chapter, many of which included a component to assess or train generalization outside formal training sessions.

Some of the assessment probes that may be clinically practical are unobtrusive observation of natural interactions, global ratings of everyday behavior outside therapy, and staged interactions. These assessment techniques can be used to verify that clients are generalizing improved social skills outside training sessions. It can be strongly recommended that programs should train social skills directly in the community as well as during formal therapy sessions.

Training Awareness of Behavioral Disorders

Finally, it should be noted that persons with head injury are generally less aware of their behavioral deficits than of their cognitive and physical impairments (Hendryx, 1989; McKinlay & Brooks, 1984). This finding suggests that clients may not be aware of the need for social skills training and that they may benefit from interventions to increase their awareness of their behavioral deficits. In addition to the feedback and self-monitoring interventions reviewed in this chapter, clinicians may choose from a variety of group exercises for awareness training that have been described elsewhere (cf., Ben-Yishay & Lakin, 1989; Ben-Yishay et al., 1980; Prigatano, 1986).

SUMMARY

The programs reviewed in this chapter show that different forms of social skills training are effective with some head-injured clients. The fact that the programs were mostly evaluated with single clients does not weaken this conclusion, because the studies used single-case designs to rule out plausible alternative explanations of improvement. In fact, social skills training of head-injured clients is unique among areas of cognitive rehabilitation in having relatively good empirical support.

Clinicians who apply social skills training in head injury rehabilitation centers can adapt several programs shown to be effective with head-injured clients, or they can develop new programs based on these successful models. However, in the absence of standardized programs, clinicians must exercise both care and creativity in developing social skills training programs. Assessment and training of general-ization are areas of special responsibility, in order to ensure that improved social skills translate into improved behavior in everyday life.

REFERENCES

Alexy, W.D., Foster, M., & Baker, A. (1983). Audio-visual feedback: An exercise in self-awareness for the head injured patient. *Cognitive Rehabilitation, 1*(6), 8–11.

Ben-Yishay, Y., & Lakin, P. (1989). Structured group treatment for brain-injury survivors. In D.W. Ellis & A.L. Christensen (Eds.), *Neuropsychological treatment after brain injury* (pp. 271–295). Boston: Kluwer Academic Publishers.

Ben-Yishay, Y., Lakin, P., Ross, B., Rattok, J., Cohen, J., & Diller, L. (1980). Developing a core curriculum of group exercises designed for head trauma patients who are undergoing rehabilitation. In Y. Ben-Yishay (Ed.), *Working approaches to remediation of cognitive deficits in brain damaged persons* (Rehabilitation Monograph No. 61, pp. 175–235). New York: New York University Medical Center, Institute of Rehabilitation Medicine.

Braunling-McMorrow, D. (1988). Behavioral rehabilitation. In P.M. Deutsch & K.B. Fralish (Eds.), *Innovations in head injury rehabilitation* (chap. 8). New York: Matthew Bender.

Braunling-McMorrow, D., Lloyd, K., & Fralish, K. (1986). Teaching social skills to head injured adults. *Journal of Rehabilitation 52*(1), 39–44.

Brooks, D.N., & McKinlay, W. (1983). Personality and behavioural change after severe blunt head injury—a relative's view. *Journal of Neurology, Neurosurgery, and Psychiatry, 46,* 336–344.

Brotherton, F.A., Thomas, L.L., Wisotzek, I.E., & Milan, M.A. (1988). Social skills training in the rehabilitation of patients with traumatic closed head injury. *Archives of Physical Medicine and Rehabilitation, 69,* 827–832.

Burke, W.H. (1988). *Head injury rehabilitation: Developing social skills*. Houston: HDI Publishers.

Crosson, B. (1987). Treatment of interpersonal deficits for head-trauma patients in inpatient rehabilitation settings. *Clinical Neuropsychologist, 1,* 335–352.

Curran, J.P., & Monti, P.M. (1982). *Social skills training: A practical handbook for assessment and treatment*. New York: Guilford Press.

Dunn, M., Van Horn, E., & Herman, S.H. (1981). Social skills and spinal cord injury: Comparison of three training procedures. *Behavior Therapy, 12,* 153–164.

Erlich, J., & Barry, P. (1989). Rating communication behaviours in the head-injured adult. *Brain Injury, 3,* 193–198.

Erlich, J.S., & Sipes, A.L. (1985). Group treatment of communication skills for head trauma patients. *Cognitive Rehabilitation, 3*(1), 32–37.

Foxx, R.M., & Bittle, R. (1989). *Thinking it through: Teaching a problem-solving strategy for community living*. Champaign, IL: Research Press.

Foxx, R.M., Marchand-Martella, N.E., Martella, R.C., Braunling-McMorrow, D., & McMorrow, M.J. (1988). Teaching a problem-solving strategy to closed head-injured adults. *Behavioral Residential Treatment, 3,* 193–210.

Foxx, R.M., Martella, R.C., & Marchand-Martella, N.E. (1989). The acquisition, maintenance, and generalization of problem-solving skills by closed head-injured adults. *Behavior Therapy, 20,* 61–76.

Gajar, A., Schloss, P.J., Schloss, C.N., & Thompson, C.K. (1984). Effects of feedback and self-monitoring on head trauma youths' conversation skills. *Journal of Applied Behavior Analysis, 17,* 353–358.

Giles, G.M., Fussey, I., & Burgess, P. (1988). The behavioural treatment of verbal interaction skills following severe head injury: A single case study. *Brain Injury, 2,* 75–79.

Godfrey, H.P.D., Knight, R.G., Marsh, N.V., Moroney, B., & Bishara, S.N. (1989). Social interaction and speed of information processing following very severe head-injury. *Psychological Medicine, 19,* 175–182.

Goldstein, A.P., Sprafkin, R.P., Gershaw, N.J., & Klein, P. (1980). *Skill-streaming the adolescent: A structured learning approach to teaching prosocial skills*. Champaign, IL: Research Press.

Hartley, L.L., & Griffith, A. (1989). A functional approach to the cognitive-communicative deficits of closed head injured clients. *TEJAS: Texas Journal of Audiology and Speech Pathology, 14*(2), 37–42.

Helffenstein, D.A., & Wechsler, F.S. (1982). The use of Interpersonal Process Recall (IPR) in the remediation of interpersonal and communication skill deficits in the newly brain-injured. *Clinical Neuropsychology, 4,* 139–143.

Hendryx, P.M. (1989). Psychosocial changes perceived by closed-head-injured adults and their families. *Archives of Physical Medicine and Rehabilitation, 70,* 526–530.

L'Abate, L., & Milan, M.A. (1985). *Handbook of social skills training and research*. New York: John Wiley & Sons.

Levin, H.S., High, W.M., Goethe, K.E., Sisson, R.E., Overall, J.E., Rhoades, H.M., Eisenberg, H.M., Kalisky, Z., & Gary, H.E. (1987). The Neurobehavioural Rating Scale: Assessment of the behavioural sequelae of head injury by the clinician. *Journal of Neurology, Neurosurgery, and Psychiatry, 50,* 183–193.

Lewis, F.D., Nelson, J., Nelson, C., & Reusink, P. (1988). Effects of three feedback contingencies on the socially inappropriate talk of a brain-injured adult. *Behavior Therapy, 19,* 203–211.

Lezak, M.D. (1989). Assessment of psychosocial dysfunctions resulting from head trauma. In M.D. Lezak (Ed.), *Assessment of the behavioral consequences of head trauma* (pp. 113–144). New York: Alan R. Liss.

Liberman, R.P., DeRisi, W.J., & Mueser, K.T. (1989). *Social skills training for psychiatric patients.* Elmsford, NY: Pergamon Press.

McKinlay, W.W., & Brooks, D.N. (1984). Methodological problems in assessing psychosocial recovery following severe head injury. *Journal of Clinical Neuropsychology, 6,* 87–99.

Mentis, M., & Prutting, C.A. (1987). Cohesion in the discourse of normal and head-injured adults. *Journal of Speech and Hearing Research, 30,* 88–98.

Milton, S.B., Prutting, C.A., & Binder, G.M. (1984). Appraisal of communicative competence in head injured adults. In *Proceedings from the Clinical Aphasiology Conference* (pp. 114–123). Minneapolis, MN: BRK Publishers.

Prigatano, G.P. (1986). *Neuropsychological rehabilitation after brain injury.* Baltimore: Johns Hopkins University Press.

Prutting, C., & Kirchner, D. (1983). Applied pragmatics. In T. Gallagher & C. Prutting (Eds.), *Pragmatic assessment and intervention issues in language* (pp. 29–64). San Diego: College-Hill Press.

Schloss, P.J., Thompson, C.K., Gajar, A.H., & Schloss, C.N. (1985). Influence of self-monitoring on heterosexual conversational behaviors of head trauma youth. *Applied Research in Mental Retardation, 6,* 269–282.

Sohlberg, M.M., & Mateer, C.A. (1990). Evaluation and treatment of communicative skills. In J.S. Kreutzer & P. Wehman (Eds.), *Community integration following traumatic brain injury* (pp. 67–82). Baltimore: Paul H. Brookes Publishing Co.

CHAPTER 15

Group Interventions for Cognitive Rehabilitation
Increasing the Challenges

ANN V. DEATON

The rubric *cognitive rehabilitation* has been applied to a large number of varied interventions over the last decade or more. By far, the majority of attention has been paid to computer-assisted cognitive rehabilitation (CACR), to the degree that to some family members, insurers, and rehabilitation professionals, cognitive rehabilitation and computers are nearly synonymous. Since the beginning of this specialty area, however, cognitive rehabilitation has included group interventions as well as individual computer- and non-computer-based interventions. This chapter reviews the types of group intervention that have been used to retrain cognitive skills, their inherent advantages and potential problems, and the ways in which their effectiveness can be evaluated.

To review briefly, group interventions in cognitive rehabilitation came into practice in the early 1980s. Perhaps the best known of group interventions are the psychosocial groups in Ben-Yishay's program in New York (Ben-Yishay & Diller, 1981) and the cognitive/psychotherapy groups held at the neuropsychological rehabilitation program at Presbyterian Hospital in Oklahoma City (Prigatano et al., 1986). The developers of these programs were pioneers convinced that group interventions are ideal and essential for addressing the unique cognitive and psychosocial needs of persons with traumatic brain injury. The program at Presbyterian Hospital in particular has been thoroughly documented by Prigatano et al., reviewing the format and the effectiveness of the largely group-oriented intervention program for a small group of clients going through a 6-month rehabilitation program together.

Group interventions occurring separately from an integrated comprehensive treatment program have also been described. Although not labeled cognitive rehabilitation per se, Kagan's (1969) model for Interpersonal Process Recall (IPR) has been adapted by Helffenstein and Wechsler (1982) for use with brain-injured clients to improve their awareness of their social interactions. Similarly, orientation groups for elderly persons in nursing homes have been modified for application to persons with traumatic brain injury (Corregan, Arnett, Houck, & Jackson, 1985). Numerous other group interventions have been described at conferences and in facility brochures for the remediation of deficits in social skills, awareness, memory, and other cognitive areas.

REASONS FOR PROVIDING GROUP INTERVENTIONS

Group interventions should be included in the cognitive rehabilitation of persons with brain injury for several reasons.

1. Cognitive impairments are less likely to be apparent in individual therapy, particularly when the therapist is responsible for structuring the session. In contrast to individual therapy, group therapy provides numerous sources of input as well as multiple distractions and a degree of unpredictability, making it more similar to real life. Subtle cognitive-behavioral impair-

ments (e.g., concentration difficulties, disinhibition) are more likely to emerge under such conditions and, once, apparent, can be effectively
treated.

2.   It is by now well established that a devastating long-term effect of brain injury for many
clients is that of social isolation and loneliness
(Oddy, Coughlan, Typerman, & Jenkins, 1985;
Wagner, Williams, & Long, 1986). It has been
speculated that reasons for this social isolation
include loss of networks at work or school; the
common emotional and behavioral sequelae of
brain injury, which may drive people away; and
the fact that the majority of brain injuries occur
in young people, who have less established
social networks (Wagner & Danse, 1987). Community reintegration programs must, of necessity, include group interventions because persons with traumatic brain injury are returning to
a community of people (Ylvisaker, Szekeres,
Henry, Sullivan, & Wheeler, 1987). It is possible
that early group interventions may reduce social
skills deficits and also decrease social isolation
in the long term by facilitating the relearning of
appropriate interactional skills.

3.   An obvious reason for utilizing group
interventions is that they are cost-effective, in
terms of both personnel and financial resources.
This is an important advantage in a time when:
1) there are still fewer cognitive rehabilitation
therapists available than are needed; and 2) insurers do not always reimburse for cognitive rehabilitation, making a cost-effective means of
cognitive rehabilitation essential for the client
who needs it. Group therapy is less expensive
than individual therapy, *if* it is at least as effective. However, cost-effectiveness is not the only
reason to utilize group interventions and, clinically speaking, it is far from their most important advantage.

4.   Many persons with brain injury manifest symptoms such as apathy, lack of initiative,
and limited motivation. Group interventions
tend to be inherently motivating in that they are
social in nature, may be less threatening than individual sessions, provide peer support, and are
often enjoyable. It may also prove motivating to
be confronted by and encouraged by peers, or

even to feel a sense of competition in the desire
to achieve goals as rapidly as the next person.

5.   Persons with traumatic brain injury often lack awareness or insight into their more subtle cognitive and behavioral impairments. Feedback from peers is often more meaningful and
acceptable than what comes from those in authority positions. Group interventions may therefore function as a means of decreasing denial
and/or increasing awareness. In the long run,
peers will be more important to the head-injured
person than are the professionals he or she
encounters soon after the injury. Due to their
similar experiences, peers may also be more
believable.

6.   In group interventions, the individual
has an opportunity to practice monitoring his or
her own behavior by first carrying out the easier
and less threatening task of monitoring others. It
is frequently simpler to see what someone else is
doing wrong than to recognize one's own errors.

7.   Group interventions provide a variety
of perspectives and feedback as well as a variety
of models for developing compensatory strategies. Having a variety of feedback provides a
number of perspectives to consider and may increase the chance of a client's finding some of
the feedback relevant and understandable. In addition, group interventions provide the opportunity for more ideas than those generated by only
the therapist and client, including models for
how a strategy really works when employed by
someone else who has had a brain injury.

8.   Group interventions are more similar to
real-life social settings than are individual interventions. Because they share many characteristics with nontherapy social settings, skills learned
in group therapy may be more likely to generalize outside the artificial therapy environment.

PLANNING GROUP
INTERVENTIONS FOR PERSONS
WITH TRAUMATIC BRAIN INJURY

Persons with brain injury have variable abilities,
disabilities, and needs; this poses a challenge to
any group intervention (Prigatano et al., 1986;
Sohlberg & Mateer, 1989; Wilson & Moffat,

1984). There are some common characteristics, however. For example, group members: 1) will have compromised intellectual functioning to some extent, frequently in the areas of attention, new learning, and speed and accuracy of information processing; 2) may be in therapy involuntarily, due to their lack of insight into their post-injury sequelae; and 3) may experience difficulties controlling their emotional responses to confrontation, failure, frustration, or increased awareness.

Issues specific to the use of group interventions with brain-injured clients include: criteria for group membership, group format, evaluation of efficacy, and therapist characteristics. These are discussed next.

Criteria for Group Membership

Specific suggestions have been made by others (e.g., Prigatano, et al. 1986; Wilson & Moffat, 1984) regarding the inclusion of brain-injured persons in group interventions: Group members should possess an adequate degree of verbal comprehension and verbal expression, a certain level of intellectual functioning, the ability to control aggressive and disruptive behavior, and a degree of homogeneity. However, these authors were referring specifically to groups appropriate for clients at Level VI and above of the Rancho Los Amigos Scale of Cognitive Function (Hagen & Malkums, 1979); that is, those clients whose behavior is goal directed but who may experience difficulties associated with impairments in memory, judgment, insight, or other cognitive arenas (see also Table 19.1, this volume). Since the current chapter describes group interventions at all levels of cognitive functioning, a different set of guidelines needs to be adopted. Suggestions include the following recommendations regarding group membership:

1. The specific deficit area addressed by the group should be an area of weakness shared by all group members.

2. Should some group members have difficulty controlling their verbal or physical behavior, sufficient therapists or other staff members should be available so that no one in the group is injured and so that the group session can continue after interruptions. It is not recommended that persons be excluded from all groups on the basis of disruptive or aggressive behavior since these are common characteristics of persons with traumatic brain injury and can be dealt with effectively in a social context.

3. Should some group members have difficulty with verbal expression, accommodations should be made such that they can express themselves appropriately, via the use of written communications, sign language, alphabet boards, or augmentative communication devices. Sufficient personnel should be provided to enable efficient communication and to minimize frustration.

Group Format

The format of the group will largely depend upon the level of cognitive functioning of group members and the nature of the setting in which the group intervention occurs. For the most part, group interventions for clients who are early in the recovery process (i.e., at lower levels of cognitive functioning) will include briefer sessions, more frequent meetings, more repetition, a specific routine followed in each session, and a high degree of structure by the therapist(s). Groups for lower level clients are also likely to have a higher staff-to-client ratio than is necessary for groups of individuals later in their recovery.

Whether the group is closed to new members or has new members continually added will depend on the nature of the setting. Long-term inpatient settings, school systems, and outpatient clinics are often able to utilize closed groups, with no addition of new members after the first few sessions. In contrast, acute rehabilitation settings with a shorter length of stay may use exclusively open groups where members join the group or leave the group as they are admitted and discharged. For groups in which skills are being built in a hierarchical fashion (e.g., problem-solving groups), a stable, closed group membership seems to be essential. Even in groups requiring the gradual acquisition of a knowledge base, however, an individual client can sometimes be seen individually initially to provide skills instruction before entering a group of persons who have already learned these basic skills.

Other groups may repeat the same sorts of information on a daily basis (e.g., sensory stimulation and orientation groups) or may cycle through a series of topics repeatedly over a course of weeks or months (e.g., social skills or self-assessment groups). These group formats may allow for the addition of members at any time in the cycle.

Evaluation of Efficacy

Group cognitive rehabilitation often takes place: 1) in the context of a comprehensive rehabilitation program, within which the effects of group therapy per se will be difficult to differentiate from the effects of the intervention program as a whole; and 2) with recently brain-injured persons, in whom spontaneous recovery is likely to play at least as significant a role as any intervention in the reacquisition of cognitive skills. These factors make it difficult to ascertain whether cognitive recovery can be attributed to a group intervention. Nonetheless, failure to evaluate intervention efficacy cannot be excused. The quality of therapy evaluation, even in strictly clinical settings, should be improving as the field develops. For example, some authors (e.g., Sohlberg & Mateer, 1989) have suggested multiple baseline designs as the most reliable way to demonstrate intervention gains. Because these designs involve multiple measures of skills, they are more expensive in terms of time and cost—but they may be worth the expense. In addition, data collection can be readily incorporated into each session, requiring a minimum of additional time as well as facilitating adequate documentation of therapy.

Therapist Characteristics

Persons with brain injury can frequently appear inattentive, unmotivated, disruptive, angry, and easily frustrated. These characteristics certainly affect the therapist directly and have implications for the type of therapist who will work effectively with these individuals. Typically, the therapist must be patient, flexible, knowledgeable regarding the broad range of sequelae from brain injury, and able to remain therapeutic in the face of behaviors that may seem to be deliberate efforts to sabotage rehabilitation. In addi-

tion, as with any therapist, the cognitive rehabilitation group therapist must remain cognizant of his or her own reactions and be willing to model constantly such qualities as effective problem solving and appropriate social skills.

Although little information about burnout in this population of therapists has been published, it seems likely that the burnout rate is high due to the challenging nature of persons with brain injury. In addition, the need to provide frequent repetition can result in burnout as the therapist may not feel he or she is providing anything unique or valuable. One way in which the problem of burnout has been addressed is to rotate therapists among groups or to provide co-therapists for all group interventions so that the therapists can monitor each other as well as "spell" each other when necessary.

CONTINUUM OF GROUP COGNITIVE REHABILITATION INTERVENTIONS

The information provided in this section of the chapter concerns specific "cognitive groups" and their characteristics, and is based on several assumptions:

1.   It is possible to use groups as an intervention for persons functioning throughout the continuum of cognitive functioning. For obvious reasons, the characteristics of the group interventions at each of the levels of functioning may vary, with respect to the length of the group session, the degree of structure provided, the predictability of the session, the degree of repetition, the provision of out-of-group assignments, and so forth.

2.   Many group intervention formats and trials have been carried out, both with brain-injured persons and with other populations of clients. An attempt has been made here to review the significant types of cognitive group interventions that have been implemented; however, some equally worthwhile interventions may have been overlooked.

3.   Some kind of evaluation should be carried out for every type of group intervention. The nature of the evaluative tool may be observational in nature or may be a questionnaire, spe-

cific task performance, or scores on a test. Reliable data are not available on many existing interventions; however, suggestions for evaluative measures are provided here.

4. It should be possible to specify general objectives and client-specific goals for any group intervention and to evaluate whether or not these goals have been achieved at the end of the intervention. Suggested objectives for each of the groups are summarized in Table 15.1. Client-specific goals are developed based on the needs and goals of that individual.

The six groups described include: sensory stimulation, orientation, memory, social skills, problem solving, and self-assessment. All are based on interventions carried out by the author and her colleagues in comprehensive inpatient and outpatient rehabilitation settings. The subtitle of the chapter, "Increasing the Challenges," is reflected in the sequencing of the group presentations: The discussion begins with the lowest level, most structured group and ends with the least structured, most challenging groups.

Sensory Stimulation Group

The first and most controversial of the groups is the sensory stimulation or low-level orientation group. It includes persons at Levels II and III of the Rancho Los Amigos Scale (Hagen & Malkmus, 1979)—those who respond to the environment minimally with generalized or localized responses. Individuals at this level are responding "to some external events without, however, processing much, if any, of the meaning of these events" (Szekeres, Ylvisaker, & Cohen, 1987). To the extent that they do process information, they are likely to find the hospital environment confusing, frustrating, and often frightening. With these persons, disorientation is assumed because there is no obvious way in which they are in contact with and responding to the reality of the world about them. It is also known that as these individuals emerge from this state, they typically act confused and disoriented, suggesting that these are useful targets for intervention and for prevention even while individuals remain unable to respond consistently. Some of the objectives for the sensory stimulation group include providing labels for the sights, smells, sounds, and people in the client's environment; increasing arousal; and reinforcing appropriate responses when they occur (see also Table 15.1).

The group intervention occurs daily on the client's living unit. Each group session lasts 30 minutes and follows a predictable sequence: initial greeting; orienting information regarding the day, date, time, and place; identification of group members; description of the physical environment; presentation of stimuli to various senses; and labeling and reinforcing clients' reactions. During holiday seasons, stimuli may incude traditional songs, pictures, and so forth. Weather variations are also described and clients are told what to expect when they go outside that day.

Data are kept on the stimuli provided and the clients' responses to these stimuli. When consistent responses are occurring and clients are able to discriminate between two stimuli, their involvement in this group is usually ended. They may "graduate" to the orientation group if this appears appropriate.

Orientation Group

At a higher cognitive level, perhaps Levels IV and V on the Rancho Los Amigos Scale (Hagen & Malkmus, 1979), are clients who are obviously confused and disoriented. With repetition, they can frequently learn new information that allows them to begin to make sense of the world around them, and to become more functional and goal directed. They can learn where they are, what happened to bring them to the hospital, and perhaps what month it is. They may begin to make simple connections between the world about them and how they should respond to it. The orientation group intervention occurs on the living unit. Behavioral expectations include staying in the room, taking turns, and participating. Objectives of the group include assessing the clients' ability to use cues, allowing them to experience success, and orienting them. Sessions remain brief (30 minutes) and occur daily. The staff-to-client ratio is about 1:2 due to the level of structure, feedback, and assistance required by the clients. The activities of the group include periods of parallel individual activities as well as involvement of the group as a

Table 15.1.   Sample group objectives

Sensory stimulation group
Therapist strives to:
Provide client with orienting information
Increase client's arousal
Identify client's responses to stimuli in any sensory modality
Encourage client to discriminate between stimuli
Reinforce client's appropriate responses
Provide labels for the sights, smells, sounds, and people in client's environment
Label the client's responses

Orientation group
Therapist strives to:
Decrease client's confusion
Increase client's awareness of environment, both internal and external
Orient client to reality
Reinforce responses and facilitate client's experience of success
Assess client's response to cuing and structure
Structure group participation, modeling, and turn taking

Memory group
Therapist strives to:
Provide client with strategies for improving organization of material for memory
Teach client how to use external aids such as memory journals
Identify the strategies (internal or external) most effective for client in a variety of situations
Facilitate client's recognition of memory impairments

Social skills group
Client learns to:
Recognize nonverbal cues
Match own verbal and nonverbal messages
Initiate interactions
Self-monitor
Inhibit inappropriate remarks
Present himself or herself in an organized manner
Improve word finding
Improve eye contact
Act assertively
Enjoy social interaction
Build self-esteem

Problem-solving group
Client learns to:
Increase cognitive flexibility
Decrease impulsivity
Improve problem-solving effectiveness in daily life
Decrease frustration

Self-assessment group
Client learns to:
Decrease depression and self-deprecating remarks
Decrease denial
Identify ways in which compensatory strategies can reduce effects of the injury
Increase awareness of own strengths and deficits
Increase understanding of brain-behavior relationships
Increase understanding of own injury and its consequences

whole. For example, a typical format includes: initial greetings; a request for group members to identify the day, date, month, and year; placement of this information on a calendar visible to all; a request for group members to identify the weather and put this information (in picture form) on the calendar; group inference about what kind of clothes to wear in this weather; identification of any birthdays, holidays, and special occasions; and individual completion of orientation sheets with staff supervision and cuing as needed.

Data are collected on initiation, interruptions, and performance on the orientation sheet. Clients who are able to demonstrate intact orientation, either through the use of memory or external cues, and who demonstrate adequate basic turn-taking skills are typically ready to graduate from this group and may be appropriate for inclusion in one of the other higher level cognitive groups.

Memory Group

The memory group, as well as the other remaining groups, consists of clients at Levels VI and above on the Rancho Los Amigos Scale (Hagen & Malkmus, 1979). Memory and new learning deficits are identified in a majority of brain-injured individuals. The severity and nature of these deficits vary. Some individuals with traumatic brain injury cannot recall much of anything that occurs from one moment to the next, no matter how important an event may be. Others find that they can remember those events that are especially meaningful to them, such as a weekend home pass or a visit by family members, but cannot remember daily appointments or how to find their way around the hospital. Obviously, objectives for such a group include the development and use of memory strategies (e.g., peg words, clustering, imagery) as well as the use of external aids such as appointment books, journals, and lists. Wilson and Moffat (1984) provided many useful ideas and suggestions for running memory groups. Their groups were typically time limited and closed to new membership. Examples were provided of one group that occurred five times per week and lasted for 3 weeks, and a second group that met

weekly for 15 weeks. The daily group sessions included: memory games, tests, and general stimulation; the use of external aids; and the use of internal strategies. The weekly group, which appears more geared to the generalization of memory skills to a natural setting, included: homework assignments, identification of memory difficulties in everyday life, the teaching of new memory strategies, and a focus on self-assessment of memory performance.

Data on the effectiveness of memory groups often include behavioral observation regarding the use of external cues, and client and family reports on memory failures in everyday life. Neuropsychological measures (e.g., Rey Auditory Verbal Learning Test [Rey, 1964; Taylor, 1959]; Wechsler Memory Scale–Revised [Wechsler, 1987]) can also be used periodically to assess whether effects of memory groups generalize to memory measures.

Social Skills Group

Cognitive deficits frequently interfere with social interactions, as evidenced by the client who sees a therapist 5 days a week but has not learned the therapist's name, the young woman who desperately wants friends but who perseverates on the same topics and statements over and over and over again, or the young man who responds to the concrete content of what is said rather than recognizing the nonverbal cues that change its meaning. All of these situations reflect underlying cognitive deficits that make normal, meaningful social interactions confusing, awkward, and difficult.

Research has demonstrated that psychosocial deficits are frequently those that have the greatest impact on clients' lives. Deficits affecting social skills following brain injury include: reduced capacity for social perceptiveness, an inability to benefit from experience, decreased self-control, decreased initiation, low self-esteem, anxiety, inadequate recall of the rules of social interactions, reduced ability to take alternative perspectives, disorganization, poor self-monitoring, reduced comprehension, disinhibition, and behavioral rigidity (Haarbauer-Krupa, Henry, Szekeres, & Ylvisaker, 1985; Johnson & Newton, 1987; Lezak, 1978). These deficits can be addressed using models such as that of the Advanced Cognitive and Empathic Skills (ACES) group (Cuff & Deaton, 1988), Interpersonal Process Recall (IPR) (Helffenstein & Wechsler, 1982), and various other social skills training formats (e.g., see Chapter 14, this volume). Using the IPR and ACES group formats, the first half of each group session is videotaped and the tape is reviewed during the second half of each session. Tasks may include: introductions, making a request, asking for a date, debates, planning an outing, providing positive feedback, or offering and responding to criticism. Behavioral objectives of the group include: recognition of nonverbal cues, self-monitoring, presenting oneself in an organized manner, and acting assertively.

Evaluation of social skills groups is often based upon ratings of pragmatic skills; that is, those language skills that are "concerned with communicative intentions and interactions" (Erlich & Sipes, 1985, p. 32). Prutting and Kirchner's Pragmatic Protocol (1983) is an example of one such instrument that includes ratings of such diverse aspects of communication as body postures, repair of communication failures, facial expression, initiation, topic maintenance, listening skills, and so forth. Erlich and Sipes, among others, have found communication skills training to be effective in improving turn-taking skills, repair of communication breakdowns, consideration of the listener's needs, cohesiveness of presentation, and topic maintenance. A speech-language pathologist often serves as co-therapist or consultant to a social skills group.

Problem-Solving Group

When problem situations arise, ideally one considers what he or she would like the outcome to be, identifies several possible options for attaining that outcome, chooses the best of the possible solutions, plans and implements a strategy, and later thinks about how it worked out. Most people tend to do this fairly automatically for the minor problems that arise in day-to-day life. The reader may consider the example of a woman who misses the bus in the morning, whose goal may be to get to work on time. She could: 1) wait for the next bus, 2) catch a cab, 3) drive her own car, or 4) have her spouse or a friend drive her. A large number of considerations will affect her

decision in this seemingly minor matter. If parking downtown is difficult, taking her own car may not be quickest. If buses run only every half hour, waiting for another may make her hopelessly late. If there is an empty cab approaching, this may become a more attractive option, and so forth. Eventually the woman chooses and then she may either congratulate herself for getting to work on time and/or curse herself for missing the bus and not getting there. Obviously, this is a complex process—and yet, usually, one does it without even thinking about it.

However, for the person with traumatic brain injury, problem solving can lose its "automatic" quality and become quite difficult. The complexity of considering a large number of relevant variables simultaneously can be impossible for someone with difficulties concentrating or shifting attention from one thing to another. The anger and frustration resulting from missing the bus and being afraid of being late may prevent effective problem solving as the emotional arousal interferes with cognition. Cognitive inflexibility may also prevent the brain-injured person from generating or considering more than one alternative.

Despite these difficulties, however, many brain-injured persons can learn how to problem solve effectively once again. They can do so by making the problem-solving process a conscious and deliberate one, and learning the sequential steps of the process. This is what occurs in problem-solving group interventions, models of which have been developed for other client populations by Kendall and Braswell (1985) and Meichenbaum (1977), and applied to persons with traumatic brain injury by, for example, Allen and Johnson (1987) and others. The initial sessions of the group focus on clients learning the individual steps in the problem-solving process, using problems that are generated by the therapist and are, therefore, perhaps more straightforward and less emotionally laden than those problems actually occurring in the clients' lives at the moment.

Steps are taught through repetition, rehearsal, feedback, and modeling. They include asking the following questions:

What is happening?
What do I want to happen?

How can I make it happen?
How good is each solution?
Did I choose the best one?

Data are collected on acquisition of the steps, ability to apply them appropriately to written and real-life problems, and demonstration of these skills in a group setting. Modifications can include the addition of several individual sessions at the start to teach the steps more quickly and the addition of weekly maintenance sessions to help clients maintain and generalize problem-solving skills after they have met the criteria for graduating from the group. Allen and Johnson (1987) documented that this approach can be implemented effectively with brain-injured persons, although the biggest barrier to success appears to be such clients' impulsivity.

Self-Assessment Group

Coming to terms with a head injury is no easy task. Cognitive deficits interfere significantly with successful accomplishment of this task. For example, cognitive flexibility is often impaired as a result of frontal lobe injuries. This can make it difficult for head-injured persons to see themselves in a new light, to reconsider future plans, or to identify new possibilities for themselves. New learning and memory are often impaired; head-injured persons may have difficulty recalling what has happened to them and why they are so different now from the way they were. Or there may be denial, a sometimes organically based and sometimes functionally based tendency not even to acknowledge that anything has changed.

The self-assessment group intervention was developed for the highest functioning clients to address some of these issues. This group is the most variable of all the groups with respect to content and structure: The clients have the most responsibility for structuring the group for themselves and providing feedback regarding the rules of the group to others. In addition, this

group is probably most similar to a traditional psychotherapy group and, as such, is typically run by a psychologist or social worker, often with a cognitive rehabilitation therapist as co-leader. Groups occur two to four times weekly. Sessions may have a specific topic chosen by therapist or client or may be based on a concern arising in the group. Groups require leaders who are themselves flexible enough to track what is happening in the group and respond appropriately.

Efforts to evaluate the efficacy of self-assessment or self-awareness groups have involved the use of questionnaires for determining the clients' awareness of their strengths and impairments. Other means of evaluation may include the use of self-esteem scales, comparison of family and client ratings of skills, and quantification of staff observations. Several studies have demonstrated this kind of group to be effective in increasing awareness of both assets and impairments as well as decreasing emotional distress (e.g., Deaton, 1986; Prigatano et al., 1986). Because such groups typically occur in the context of comprehensive intervention programs, these changes may not be group specific.

SUMMARY AND CONCLUSIONS

Group interventions are an important method for cognitive rehabilitation, both in terms of their efficacy and their cost-effectiveness. The present chapter reviewed some of the unique aspects of doing group cognitive rehabilitation with brain-injured clients, and described the nature of the six most popular types of groups.

At present, the most glaring gaps in the use of group interventions have to do not with the availability of various models and formats, but rather with the documentation of group effectiveness in improving cognitive skills—in particular, as these skills generalize to other social environments. This remains the most significant issue needing to be addressed in future work in this area.

REFERENCES

Allen, D., & Johnson, A. (1987). *Retraining the head-injured adolescent: A model for improving problem solving skills.* Unpublished manuscript, Cumberland Hospital, New Kent, VA.

Ben-Yishay, Y., & Diller, L. (1981). Rehabilitation of cognitive and perceptual deficits in people with traumatic brain damage. *International Journal of Rehabilitation Research, 4,* 208–210.

Corregan, J.D., Arnett, J.A., Houck, L., & Jackson, R.D. (1985). Reality orientation for brain injured patients: Group treatment and monitoring of recovery. *Archives of Physical Medicine and Rehabilitation, 66,* 626–630.

Cuff, M., & Deaton, A.V. (1988, March). *Retraining social skills: A Continuum of group interventions for the brain injured adolescent.* Presentation at the Houston Neurotrauma Conference, Houston.

Deaton, A.V. (1986, August) *Self assessment group: An intervention strategy for head injured adolescents.* Presentation at the American Psychological Association Annual Convention, Washington, DC.

Erlich, J.S., & Sipes, A.L. (1985). Group treatment of communication skills for head trauma patients. *Cognitive Rehabilitation, 3*(1), 32–37.

Haarbauer-Krupa, J., Henry, K., Szekeres, S.F., & Ylvisaker, M. (1985). Cognitive rehabilitation therapy: Late stages of recovery. In M. Ylvisaker (Ed.), *Head injury rehabilitation: Children and adolescents* (pp. 311–343). San Diego: College-Hill Press.

Hagen, C., & Malkmus, D. (1979, November). *Intervention strategies for language disorders secondary to head trauma.* Paper presented at the American Speech-Language-Hearing Association Convention, Atlanta.

Helffenstein, D., & Wechsler, F. (1982). The use of interpersonal process recall in the remediation of interpersonal and communication skill deficits in the newly brain injured. *Clinical Neuropsychology, 4,* 139–143.

Johnson, D.A., & Newton, A. (1987). HIPSIG: A basis for social adjustment after head injury. *British Journal of Occupational Therapy, 50*(2), 47–52.

Kagan, N. (1969). Interpersonal process recall. *Journal of Nervous and Mental Disease, 148,* 365–374.

Kendall, P.C., & Braswell, L. (1985). *Cognitive-behavioral therapy for impulsive children.* New York: Guilford Press.

Lezak, M.D. (1978). Living with the characterologically altered brain injured patient. *Journal of Clinical Psychiatry, 39,* 592–598.

Meichenbaum, D. (1977). *Cognitive behavior modification: An integrative approach:* New York: Plenum.

Oddy, M., Coughlan, T., Typerman, A., & Jenkins, D. (1985). Social adjustment after closed head injury: A further follow-up seven years after injury.

Journal of Neurology, Neurosurgery, and Psychiatry, 48, 564–568.

Prigatano, G.P., Fordyce, D.J., Zeiner, H.K., & Roueche, J.R., Pepping, M., & Wood, B.C. (Eds.). (1986). *Neuropsychological rehabilitation after brain injury.* Baltimore: Johns Hopkins University Press.

Prutting, C.A., & Kirchner, D.M. (1983). Applied pragmatics. In T.M. Gallagher & C.A. Prutting (Eds.), *Pragmatic assessment and intervention issues in language* (pp. 29–64). San Diego: College-Hill Press.

Rey, A. (1964). *L'examen clinique en psychologie* [The clinical examination in psychology]. Paris: Presses Universitaires de France.

Sohlberg, M.M., & Mateer, C.A. (1989). *Introduction to cognitive rehabilitation.* New York: Guilford Press.

Szekeres, S.F., Ylvisaker, M., & Cohen, S.B. (1987). A framework for cognitive rehabilitation therapy. In M. Ylvisaker & E.M.R. Gobble (Eds.), *Community re-entry for head injured adults* (pp. 87–136). San Diego: College-Hill Press.

Taylor, E.M. (1959). *The appraisal of children with cerebral deficits.* Cambridge, MA: Harvard University Press.

Wagner, M.T., & Danse, M.B. (1987). Cognitive rehabilitation: Psychosocial issues. In J.M. Williams & C.J. Long (Eds.), *The rehabilitation of cognitive disabilities* (pp. 139–148). New York: Plenum.

Wagner, M.T., Williams, J.M., & Long, C.J. (1986). The influence of social support on the recovery from head injury. *Journal of Clinical and Experimental Neuropsychology, 8,* 142.

Wechsler, D. (1987). *Wechsler Memory Scale–Revised.* New York: Psychological Corporation.

Wilson, B., & Moffat, N. (1984). Running a memory group. In B.A. Wilson & N. Moffat (Eds.), *Clinical management of memory problems* (pp. 171–198). Rockville, MD: Aspen.

Ylvisaker, M., Szekeres, S.F., Henry, K., Sullivan, D.M., & Wheeler, P. (1987). Topics in cognitive rehabilitation therapy. In M. Ylvisaker & E.M.R. Gobble (Eds.), *Community reentry for head injured adults* (pp. 137–220). San Diego: College-Hill Press.

CHAPTER 16

Rehabilitating Cognitive Impairments Through the Use of Games

ANN V. DEATON

The fact that available treatment tools, including computers, are used to treat noncognitive as well as cognitive impairments makes it misleading to identify cognitive rehabilitation with any one technique. (Kreutzer & Boake, 1987, p. 200)

While it should come as no surprise to the reader that games serve a wide variety of social, cognitive, and leisure functions, it has come as a bit of a revelation to the field of cognitive rehabilitation that popular tabletop games can be valuable tools for cognitive rehabilitation. Many individuals in the field have used computer tasks and computer games in assessing and remediating cognitive skills. However, if the literature and conference syllabi are any indication, few have focused on demonstrating the value of popular games to address these same cognitive deficits. Games have long been recognized as teaching tools: ways to teach cooperation and competition, rule following, new information, and the mastery of specific skills (Boehm, 1989). As teaching tools, they lend themselves admirably to the task of cognitive rehabilitation.

In cognitive rehabilitation (and other rehabilitative therapies), the quality and effectiveness of the therapy depends as much or more on the knowledge and skills of the therapist as on the nature of the tools they use. This chapter focuses specifically on assisting therapists in developing an understanding of how they can incorporate games into their repertoire of tools for cognitive rehabilitation. Topics covered will include how the principles of cognitive rehabilitation apply to games; what the unique advantages of games are; specific ways in which games can be used for cognitive rehabilitation, including modifications that enable a single game to be used to address a variety of cognitive deficits in clients at varying levels of functioning; and, finally, how game performance can be quantified to measure and demonstrate improvement in skills. Although the focus of the chapter is on commercially available, tabletop games, readers may readily generalize some of the concepts involved to more active games (e.g., Simon Says; Duck Duck Goose) that may be particularly appropriate with children.

The author has chosen not to provide a thorough review of the problem of acquired brain injury in this chapter, due to space limitations and the fact that this is available elsewhere (Levin, Benton, & Grossman, 1982; Rosenthal, Griffith, Bond, & Miller, 1983). Suffice it to say that over 400,000 traumatic brain injuries occur in the United States annually (Kalsbeek, McLaurin, Harris, & Miller, 1980), along with an approximately equal number of nonfatal strokes (Wolf, Kannel, & Verter, 1984). These brain insults result in a host of cognitive, physical, and psychosocial difficulties that require remediation. Rehabilitation professionals must use every tool at their disposal to address these difficulties. Games can be one of those tools.

This chapter is an extension and substantial revision of a presentation by Ann V. Deaton and Debra Allan at the first annual Cognitive Retraining Conference, Williamsburg, VA, September 11–13, 1987.

PRINCIPLES OF COGNITIVE REHABILITATION AS APPLIED TO GAMES

Cognitive rehabilitation using games involves the same principles as cognitive rehabilitation via other therapy modalities (e.g., Craine & Gudeman, 1981). Game selection and progression in therapy are based on a recognition of the hierarchy of cognitive abilities, such that attentional skills are typically addressed before memory; sequencing skills are addressed before planning and organizational skills; and memory is addressed before problem solving.

Identifying Cognitive Components of Games

Recognition of the components of a game facilitates its use as a tool for cognitive remediation. It is necessary to identify the requisite cognitive skills for a game and ensure that the more basic cognitive skills are intact or deficits compensated for before higher level cognitive abilities are required. Task analysis, the process of examining a task in detail for the steps or the cognitive processes that are required for its completion, can be useful in this regard. When applied to games, task analysis involves identifying all the cognitive (and other) abilities that will be required to play the game. Even the simplest of games is complex in the sense that a large number of cognitive skills (e.g., attention, visual discrimination, sequencing, memory, planning) are typically necessary for engaging in the game. For example, checkers requires, at a minimum, vigilance, visual scanning, color discrimination, sequencing, and planning. This list of underlying requirements can then be used to select a game that will be especially challenging to a client or to rule out a game for which he or she has few of the necessary abilities.

Another strategy for identifying component skills is that of reducing a game to a hierarchically organized list of activities rather than cognitive skills per se. Such a list might include such activities as choosing the game, reading the rules, setting up the game materials, and so forth (Savage & Wolcott, 1988). Any reasonable and systematic strategy for breaking down a game into its component skills is likely to enable the

task or game to be effectively used for cognitive rehabilitation.

Beginning at the Client's Level

A second principle of cognitive rehabilitation is that of beginning at the client's level. This is as important in using games as in using any other rehabilitative intervention. Choosing a game that is too difficult results in excessive frustration for the client and does not allow him or her to enjoy the game or to practice the appropriate cognitive skills. At the same time, beginning at too low a level does not challenge the client to attempt to utilize skills in which he or she may need work. Therapists should structure therapeutic play activities so that the cognitive, physical, and emotional demands can be systematically increased (Haarbauer-Krupa, Moser, Smith, Sullivan, & Szekeres, 1985).

The difficulty level of games can be determined via task analysis, identifying the component cognitive skills required for game playing, and by taking into account the guidelines provided on the game box regarding the ages for which the game was designed. Games can also be adapted to increase or decrease their difficulty level. For example, games can be adapted by modifying the materials used, by providing supplementary materials (e.g., paper and pencil), by omitting or modifying some of the rules, by altering the client's approach to the game, by organizing as teams, and so forth. Adapting a game to a client's level ensures that it is not frustrating (i.e., that it remains enjoyable to the client), facilitates focusing on the specific cognitive deficits on which the client is working, and allows fairness in competitive games.

Providing Repetition and Practice

Repetition is a prime requirement of cognitive rehabilitation, allowing learning to take place with repeated trials. This is essential for most individuals with acquired brain injury. Games lend themselves to repetition because they are enjoyable. They provide social interaction as well as cognitive remediation. Moreover, they are somewhat different every time they are played and therefore remain fun and challenging, perhaps resulting in increased frequency of practice outside of scheduled therapy sessions. The repetition involved, while not identical each time, allows for practice and acquisition of identified cognitive skills.

Providing Feedback

Feedback is also a necessary characteristic of effective cognitive rehabilitation interventions. Feedback can be concrete and immediate, as in the feedback a player receives in a checkers game when he or she moves a piece and his or her opponent makes a triple jump, or as in a game of Concentration when a player turns over two cards that match. Such feedback tells a player immediately whether he or she made a right or a wrong move. Feedback can also be delayed, as in the feedback received upon winning or losing the entire game. Delayed feedback is directed not to any single move made, but rather to a player's overall approach to the game.

Ensuring Relevance

Games are also useful in cognitive rehabilitation because they are meaningful to the client and, therefore, motivating. While games may not be "real life" in the sense that holding a job is, many people, both with and without brain injury, view games as pleasant ways to spend leisure time and to interact with others. They do not mind learning and practicing cognitive skills when it does not feel like a "therapy task." Games may also feel more "normal" to clients than many of the other tools that can be used for cognitive rehabilitation. Moreover, they can be a comfortable and enjoyable means of families and friends interacting with the brain-injured person in a therapeutic way.

Varying Level of Difficulty

Finally, games can be a useful tool for cognitive rehabilitation because they vary in their difficulty levels. The same game can be played in a number of different ways to change its difficulty level—for example, a game of Concentration can be played with 12 cards (six pairs), or with 52. Moreover, the circumstances in which the game is played can be varied to make it more difficult (e.g., by turning on the radio during a game, by playing the game with several other people, by providing a more skilled opponent). Characteristics that can be varied range from the rules of the game to its materials, its familiarity, and the environment in which it is played. The appendix at the end of this chapter includes suggestions for modifying the difficulty level of specific games. The individual therapist will likely come up with many others.

Planning for Generalization

In addition to using games to facilitate acquisition and maintenance of cognitive skills, it is also essential to plan for generalization to occur. Opportunities for generalization within a therapy setting can be provided by altering the circumstances, materials, or rules of a game as well as by substituting other games requiring the same or similar cognitive skills. In addition, the effective therapist should identify situations in everyday life where the client might be required to use these same skills, and should then work with the client to anticipate how to do so effectively. Games are useful because they provide a nonthreatening way to focus initially on skill development. Generalization of game skills will thus extend beyond their use in a specific therapy setting.

ADVANTAGES OF GAMES

Given that games can be used for cognitive rehabilitation, one still wonders why they should be used. That is, what advantages do they have over already available workbooks, computer software, and so forth?

The advantages of games are many. Among them are the following.

1. *Games are inexpensive* Most popularly available games cost less than $25. A deck of playing cards for Concentration, slapjack, and so forth can be had for about 50¢, considerably less than most of the other tools available for cognitive rehabilitation. Their minimal cost ensures that a variety of games can be purchased by therapists, facilities, or families.

2. *Games are readily available* The games discussed in this chapter are commonly available in most toy stores, as well as many drug and department stores. At least some of

these games are probably already available in most hospitals and rehabilitation centers, homes, and classrooms. Thus, games are accessible to nearly any client, family, or therapist as a tool for retraining lost or impaired cognitive skills.

3. *Games are inherently rewarding and motivating* If an intervention proves effective in improving cognitive skills but is not particularly motivating, it is less likely to be used, and ultimately less effective. The rewards inherent in games also enable the brain-injured client to get through frustrating moments when deficit areas are most apparent and most difficult to overcome.

4. *Specific games may be familiar to the client* The majority of persons with brain injury experience memory problems. Using familiar games may allow the client to rely on remote memory for the rules of the game and/or previously learned strategies in order to play the game well. Familiar games may also help to decrease a client's denial as he or she becomes aware that a game previously played well now presents challenges he or she had not anticipated. Providing such "guided failures" may enhance the client's motivation for learning compensatory strategies as well as relearning specific skills or strategies (cf. Chapter 11, this volume).

5. *Games have the advantage of being different each time* Different settings, different opponents or teammates, and different sequences of the actual game moves as a result of chance (the roll of the dice or the luck of the draw) all occur. This variability provides opportunities for generalizing acquired skills to slightly different circumstances and increases the chances of generalization to other settings.

6. *Games are enjoyable and typically nonthreatening to the brain-injured person if they are selected appropriately and if necessary adaptations are made* Many recently brain-injured persons complain that the worst thing about having a brain injury is that life becomes "all rehab and no fun." Long after the injury, many note that one of the long-term effects is that of isolation and loneliness. Including games as a cognitive rehabilitation tool is a way of facilitating clients' having fun again as well as having a skill they can use in interacting comfortably with family and friends. Thus, games allow for

remediation of some of the psychosocial difficulties as well as the cognitive difficulties secondary to brain injury (e.g., Wagner & Danse, 1987).

GAMES AND COGNITIVE DEFICITS ADDRESSED

Given that games lend themselves to being tools for cognitive rehabilitation, what are some of the specific games that can be used and what are the cognitive areas that they address? The appendix at the end of this chapter presents a summary of several games, including the cognitive abilities they target. The appendix can be used as a guideline in selecting games to address specific skills deficits and modifying these games to an appropriate difficulty level.

Attention deficits are present to some extent in most brain-injured persons, whether in the form of limited attention span; distractibility; or deficits in selective attention, vigilance, or attention to detail. Although nearly all games require attention, a few games have attention as a primary focus. These may include such games as slapjack and Uno. Slapjack, played with an ordinary deck of cards, requires vigilance to the cards so that the next jack that comes up is responded to quickly with a slap of the hand. The goal of the game is to acquire the most cards. Being the first person to slap a jack results in being awarded all the cards under the jack. The goal of Uno is to use up all one's cards before anyone else does. Similar to Crazy 8s, this requires that cards be played that are either the same number or the same color as the top card in the discard pile. To increase the challenge, when a player is on the verge of winning, rules of this game require that the player say "Uno" to warn the other players that he or she has only one card left. The failure of a player to recognize that he or she has only one card remaining and to say "Uno" results in his or her having to put additional cards in his or her hand—but only if one of the other players notices the error. Thus, this game rewards vigilance (to the number of cards in one's own and others' hands), attention to detail (color and number), and shifting attention among two salient dimensions—color and number—and the number of cards held by oneself and the other players.

Perceptual skills are also addressed in most games directly or indirectly. Perceptual skills required may include discrimination, matching, and scanning. Candyland, for example, is a game of chance rather than skills. However, it requires the player to move pieces by perceiving a color card accurately, scanning the board for the next space of that color, and then moving the marker to that colored space. Checkers requires discriminating red from black checkers and scanning the board to identify potential moves. In Gridlock, the player must place pieces in a grid so that all the pieces fit, requiring that salient aspects of the pieces be accurately discriminated.

Sequencing is required in a basic sense for most games in that turn taking occurs and moves take place in a specified sequence. Scrabble, solitaire, Simon, Numbers Up, and Boggle are all games that involve sequencing as a central requirement of the game. Each of these games requires players either to follow a specified sequence or to generate a sequence of their own.

Memory skills are tapped by such games as Concentration, Memory, Numbers Up, and Enchanted Forest. These games can facilitate the acquisition and use of strategies such as rehearsal or association. They also lend themselves to teaching the use of external memory aids such as lists, as it will quickly become apparent to the client that his or her performance on the game improves dramatically when this additional tool is available to aid in recall. Memory is also rewarded by many games in that strategies are developed over time by players with intact memory so that one gradually becomes a more skilled player. Remote memory or fund of information is tapped by all familiar games to some degree, but in particular by games such as Whatzit?; Trivial Pursuit; and Win, Lose, or Draw—in which players with the ability to retrieve information from long-term memory have an advantage.

Problem-solving and planning skills are involved in most of the "strategy" games that are popular with adults as well as with children and adolescents. Connect Four is a relatively simple game dependent upon good planning skills and reflective problem solving. The goal of this game is for a player to get four colored pieces in a row (row, column, or diagonal) before his or her opponent does so. In addition to good planning and problem-solving abilities, Connect Four requires a number of other underlying skills such as: visual scanning, visualization of the result of one's move, simultaneous attention to one's own moves (desire to win) and one's opponent's moves (prevention of his or her winning), and problem-solving or reasoning skills. When played repeatedly, performance on Connect Four is also enhanced by learning and memory, since certain strategies result in greater likelihood of winning this game. Who Dun It? and Clue rely on problem-solving and reasoning abilities as well, particularly those involved in divergent and convergent reasoning.

While not every game can be described in detail here, it is important to recognize that nearly any cognitive impairment can be addressed by one or more popular games if the therapist is knowledgeable about the client's cognitive strengths, deficits, and interests, and the games that are available. The therapist's ability to think flexibly and to modify games as needed is also essential in utilizing popular games, since they are not as likely as computer software to include varying difficulty levels (although some game instructions do provide suggestions for varying the difficulty; e.g., Outburst, Scattergories).

QUANTIFYING GAME PERFORMANCE AND REVISING GOALS

Cognitive rehabilitation is still in its infancy and, as such, research on its effectiveness is a necessary component of good clinical practice. There are practical as well as theoretical reasons for wanting to quantify the gains attributable to cognitive rehabilitation. Cognitive deficits are not as readily observable as are physical impairments. Third-party payers are sometimes reluctant to pay for cognitive rehabilitation if it does not obviously contribute to an individual's recovery. This can be further complicated in that the use of popular games is not as impressive or face valid as computer-assisted cognitive rehabilitation. Given the lack of obvious validity as an intervention, it becomes increasingly important to document change and cognitive gains associated with this intervention modality.

A second concern is that of the attitudes of the client and family. Many families have been told that there is a critical period for cognitive recovery. Their reactions to hearing that their loved one is spending precious hours in cognitive rehabilitation therapy playing games may be negative unless they understand clearly the goals of this intervention and are able to see documented changes. Similarly, the client who wants to facilitate his or her own recovery will be frustrated if he or she does not understand how therapeutic activities contribute to recovery.

Each of these issues—documentation of clinical efficacy, reimbursement for services, and consumer satisfaction—makes it essential that what is done with a client be quantifiable and that its effectiveness be demonstrable to the client, third-party payers, and the family.

Quantification

Tabletop games do not lend themselves as readily to quantification as do computerized tasks and games. However, it is possible to quantify performance and measure improvement. Data sheets for recording performance can be developed, as demonstrated by the example in Figure 16.1 for one specific game: Connect Four. While this figure includes several specific behaviors, not all of them will be relevant to each client. Thus, first it is important to identify the performance variables relevant to a given client. Data collection of some formalized type is essential. Figure 16.1 works well in that it is relatively quick to complete during the game itself and allows review of a number of different aspects of game-playing performance. This may be especially useful in a multiple baseline design when the therapist expects to affect only one or two specific abilities and anticipates that other dimensions of performance will remain essentially unchanged until they are specifically addressed.

Second, criteria for success need to be established. An initial criterion may be not to lose the game in fewer than six moves; later, the criterion may increase in number of moves, or

change to winning the game a certain percentage of the time.

Third, setting new goals involves the previous step of setting criteria for success. The objectives should be revised periodically to reflect increasing skills. This may involve increasing the expectations for success (e.g., no omission errors in playing slapjack) or increasing the game's difficulty level while retaining the same criteria for success (e.g., playing the game in a distracting environment). When a goal has been achieved, it may be possible to move on to another cognitive skill area, building on previously learned skills. Examples of some goals that may be addressed through the use of specific games are provided in the appendix at the end of this chapter.

Fourth, frequency of reassessment should be established. This may occur frequently during therapy sessions or, if the games are part of a home- or unit-based program, may occur on a periodic basis. Ideally, periodic reassessment should include cognitive tasks/games with which the client is familiar. Also included should be unfamiliar tasks/tests requiring the same underlying cognitive abilities in order to assess generalization or transfer of skills.

Documentation

In addition to identifying goals and quantifying game performance, documentation is required by third-party payers for payment and by most rehabilitation facilities for the purposes of program evaluation and utilization review. Documentation includes the listing of specific goals and whether or not they are achieved as well as regular notations regarding progress. Figure 16.2 provides an example of a client's documentation in the form of goal, method, progress notes, and intervention summary.

A specific suggestion regarding documentation is that "cognitive task" rather than "game" be used to ensure that it is understood that the game is being used as a therapeutic task rather than a leisure activity. This is helpful not only to those reading the documentation but also to the therapist involved, as it ensures that the therapist focuses on the cognitive nature of the task and

Data sheet for: Connect Four
Name of client: A. Jones
Date initiated: 1-3-89
Intervention goal: Client will be able to attend to two aspects of a cognitive task simultaneously (i.e., his own moves and those of his opponent).

Criteria for discontinuation: 30% wins; no losses in fewer than eight moves

Date	#Blocks	#Cues	#Useless	#Moves	Outcome	Conditions
1–3	0	5	0	5	lost	office; T

Therapist began game; client put each of his markers on top of hers. Did not respond to cues, did not attempt to block.

1–4	1	6	0	6	lost	office; T

Client began game; blocked one horizontal sequence but failed to block therapist building vertically. Appeared not to understand that win could occur with sequence of four vertically, diagonally, or horizontally.

(data collected during seven intervening sessions with gradual improvement)

2–14	0	2	0	8	won	office; T
	2	1	0	12	won	office; T

Client won both games; requiring fewer prompts. Will make task more difficult by providing competitive peer.

2–17	2	0	0	8	lost	office; P

Peer began game. Client lost but handled his frustration well. Client noted that he can beat his opponent and knows how he will do so.

2–18	3	0	0	14	won	office; P

Client has not required any prompts for past two sessions. Has mastered the art of attending to his own and opponent's moves simultaneously. Is also able to alter strategy following his opponent blocking a move. Will advance to more complex game and new goals due to client's meeting criteria of 30% wins (75% this week) and no losses in fewer than eight moves.

#Blocks = making a blocking move when one exists.
#Cues = verbal prompts by therapist.
#Useless = # moves that have no value for either blocking opponent or winning game.
#Moves = markers played by client.
Outcome = win or loss.
Conditions = place; competition: T = with therapist, P = peer.

Figure 16.1.   Sample data collection sheet for Connect Four.

his or her specific cognitive goals rather than the content of the game itself.

SUMMARY AND CONCLUSIONS

Although many individual therapists utilize popular games as a tool for cognitive rehabilitation, little has been written on the subject. This chap-ter described how games can be incorporated as cognitive rehabilitation interventions, utilizing many of the same principles that apply to the use of other therapy modalities.

It is hoped that this chapter will assist thera-pists in their use of games, both with respect to appropriate clinical usage and with respect to documentation of therapeutic gains. It is unlikely

Goal: Client will decrease time needed for decision making without decreasing the quality of his decisions.
Tool: Poker, using regular playing cards.
Quantification: Number of hands played during a 30-minute therapy session; quality of decisions as assessed by therapist; percentage of hands won by client.

Sample progress note

Week of: 1-12-90
Skill areas: Decision making; cognitive flexibility
Method: Poker
Subjective: "I still can't do this as well as I could before. I get so confused."

Objective: Client continues to work on cognitive task requiring complex decision making involving probability assessment. Client's decision making is typically of good quality but remains slow. Client was able to complete the task an average of four times in a therapy session as compared to one time per session during first week with no decrease in the quality of his decisions.

Assessment: Client shows improvement in speed of information processing and decision making without sacrifice in accuracy/quality.

Plan: Utilize timer to increase time constraints and difficulty level of task. Discuss with therapeutic recreation personnel and with client's family how to incorporate poker into leisure activities to enhance generalization as well as providing client with additional practice.

Sample Therapy Summary

Client participated in cognitive rehabilitation therapy sessions five times per week from December 1, 1989, through February 15, 1990, for a total of 44 sessions. Goals addressed included the following:

- Client will demonstrate the ability to make decisions, utilizing available information as well as anticipation of the consequences of his decisions.
- Client will decrease time needed for decision making without decreasing the quality of his decisions.
- Client will identify how decision-making skills learned in a therapeutic setting can be applied to problem situations in his daily life.
- Client will demonstrate the ability to make decisions effectively outside of a therapy setting.

These goals were initially addressed via the use of cognitive tasks and games in a quiet, supportive setting. The client initially demonstrated very slow decision making and numerous errors in considering the options available to him in decision-making situations. Once the client had learned how to consider the multiple options available to him, the focus changed to speed of decision making. As the client demonstrated the ability to make decisions effectively in a structured therapy session, therapy's focus moved to transferring these decision-making skills to problem situations outside of therapy.

The client was able to identify situations in which his poor or slow decision making led to difficulties (e.g., trying to decide what kind of cigarettes to buy while a long line of people waited behind him; trying to decide what movie to see when a friend asked him; being unable to decide on which route to drive, in the midst of rush-hour traffic). The client was able to learn strategies for deciding more quickly in situations such as these and then to evaluate the adequacy of his decision making afterward when no time constraints existed.

At discharge, the client was able to demonstrate quick and thoughtful decision making consistently in a therapy setting, even with time constraints. He continued to experience some difficulty in making quick decisions in everyday situations due to his fear that he might make a wrong decision or overlook some important aspect of the situation.

The client and his family were encouraged to continue to evaluate decisions made after the fact in order to further improve the quality of the client's decisions. It was also recommended that the client engage in enjoyable and meaningful activities involving decision making such as planning outings or parties or participating in popular games such as Scruples or Scattergories that involve taking into consideration multiple factors while making decisions.

Figure 16.2.   Example of documentation of the use of games for cognitive rehabilitation.

and probably undesirable that games be the sole method used for the cognitive rehabilitation of any client. However, as the field of cognitive rehabilitation continues to evolve, therapeutic tools accrue in the cognitive rehabilitation therapist's repertoire. Popular games can be one such tool.

REFERENCES

Boehm, H. (1989, September). Toys and games to learn by. *Psychology Today,* pp. 62–64.

Craine, J.F., & Gudeman, H.E. (1981). *The rehabilitation of brain functions, principles, procedures, and techniques of neurotraining.* Springfield, IL: Charles C Thomas.

Haarbauer-Krupa, J., Moser, L., Smith, G., Sullivan, D.M., & Szekeres, S.F. (1985). Cognitive rehabilitation therapy: Middle stages of recovery. In M. Ylvisaker (Ed.), *Head injury rehabilitation: Children and adolescents* (pp. 287–310). San Diego: College-Hill Press.

Kalsbeek, W.D., McLaurin, R.L., Harris, B.S.H., III, & Miller, J.D. (1980). The National Head and Spinal Injury Survey: Major findings. *Journal of Neurosurgery, 53*(Suppl.), 19–31.

Kreutzer, J.S., & Boake, C. (1987). Addressing disciplinary issues in cognitive rehabilitation: Definition, training, and organization. *Brain Injury, 1*(2), 199–202.

Levin, H.H., Benton, A.L., & Grossman, R.G. (1982). *Neurobehavioral consequences of closed head injury.* New York: Oxford University Press.

Rosenthal, M., Griffith, E.R., Bond, M.R., & Miller, J.D. (Eds.). (1983). *Rehabilitation of the head injured adult.* Philadelphia: F.A. Davis.

Savage, R., & Wolcott, G. (Eds.). (1988). *An educator's manual: What educators need to know about students with traumatic brain injury.* Southborough, MA: National Head Injury Foundation Task Force on Special Education.

Wagner, M.T., & Danse, M.L.B. (1987). Cognitive rehabilitation: Psychosocial issues. In J.M. Williams & C.J. Long (Eds.), *The rehabilitation of cognitive disabilities* (pp. 139–148). New York: Plenum.

Wolf, P.A., Kannel, W.B., & Verter, J. (1984). Cerebrovascular diseases in the elderly: Epidemiology. In M.L. Albert (Ed.), *Clinical neurology of aging.* New York: Oxford University Press.

Game title (maker)	Targeted deficits	Modifications	Quantification	Observations	Sample goals
Battleship (Milton Bradley)	Visual discrimination Planning Response to feedback	Work in teams Provide verbal cuing	# moves taken to sink opponent's ships # opponent's ships sunk	Development of strategies Ability to keep track of hits and misses	Client will demonstrate ability to shift his or her attention between two aspects of a cognitive task Client will demonstrate ability to learn a strategy and to apply it in later trials of the same task Client will demonstrate ability to use available information efficiently to solve a problem
Boggle (Parker Bros.)	Visual scanning Sequencing Speed of information processing Word retrieval Cognitive flexibility	Allow two- and three-letter words Eliminate time limit	# words # of different initial letters # letters in longest word	Flexibility in approach Frustration tolerance Response to time limits	Client will increase speed of task performance in response to time limits Client will sequence letters correctly in order to form words
Checkers (various)	Visual scanning Attention Planning Cognitive flexibility	Eliminate "kinging" rule	Amount of time game played # missed jumps # jumps # multiple jumps	Client's ability to attend to opponent's moves while planning his or her own Consideration of variety of possible moves before deciding	Client will demonstrate ability to attend to an enjoyable cognitive task for 20 minutes Client will demonstrate ability to consider several options before making a decision Client will accurately predict or anticipate the results of a chosen course of action
Concentration (various)	Attention Spatial organization Memory	Decrease number of pairs Provide cues for rehearsal and association	# pairs in time period # moves to get certain # of pairs # recall errors	Strategies used for recall Impulsive versus reflective approach	Client will learn strategies to facilitate his or her organization and recall of visual information Client will utilize reflective rather than trial-and-error approach to a difficult task
Connect Four (Milton Bradley)	Visual scanning Planning Cognitive flexibility	Omit diagonal series	# opponent's moves blocked # moves before game won/lost	Ability to attend to own and opponent's pieces simultaneously Impulsivity	Client will demonstrate ability to anticipate/predict the consequences of a course of action Client will demonstrate ability to attend to two aspects of a cognitive task (e.g., winning, preventing opponent's win)

Game	Cognitive skills	Grading/Modifications	Measurement	Behaviors observed	Sample goals
(Ideal)	discrimination Spatial organization Planning Cognitive flexibility Error recognition	...ut several key pieces in place Verbal cues regarding stimulus aspects	Time taken to complete task # prompts required	Frustration tolerance Perseveration	Client will be able to modify his or her approach to a visual organizational task as needed to complete task Client will persist at a frustrating task, requesting help as needed
Guess Who? (Milton Bradley)	Visual discrimination Categorization Visual scanning Low-level reasoning Initiation	Provide list of appropriate questions Increase difficulty by choosing two targets and asking "and/or" questions	# questions required to guess target # targets eliminated with one question # incorrect guesses	Ability to generate questions Appropriate use of information Perseveration on same question Efficiency of strategy	Client will identify salient characteristics of a visual stimulus Client will be able to generate questions to get needed information Client will demonstrate ability to develop a time-efficient strategy for solving a problem Client will improve his or her efficiency over repeated trials
Jenga (Milton Bradley)	Visual discrimination Perceptual-motor coordination Cognitive flexibility Response to tactile feedback Error correction	Decrease # levels Provide verbal prompts (e.g., "Take your time")	# levels achieved Time taken to complete move	Impulsivity Ability to respond to feedback	Client will demonstrate ability to use tactile and visual feedback to alter his or her course of action Client will demonstrate ability to evaluate the quality of his or her response and modify it as needed
Poker (various)	Visual discrimination Decision making Cognitive flexibility Categorization Sequencing	Provide written explanation of scoring Provide reminders regarding factors to consider when planning hand	# hands played in given time period Won/lost record	Quality of decisions made Ability to consider and use different scoring options (e.g., flush)	Client will increase the speed with which he or she makes decisions Client will demonstrate ability to consider several different options before making decision Client will be able to use external aids (list of scores) to maximize his or her performance
Scattergories (Milton Bradley)	Word retrieval Organization Perspective taking Cognitive flexibility Categorization	Delete time limit Delete multiple credits rule Omit limitation on repeated use of same word Provide dictionary to refer to when generating words	Score on several trials Time taken to generate responses	Consideration of quality of his or her own response Catastrophic reaction Getting stuck on one response	Client will identify options that are in keeping with set criteria (e.g., initial letter, category) Client will demonstrate ability to complete as much of a task as possible despite difficulty on some parts Client will learn self-cuing strategies Client will decrease time taken to complete cognitive task by 30%

(continued)

Game title (maker)	Targeted deficits	Modifications	Quantification	Observations	Sample goals
Scrabble (Selchow & Righter)	Sequencing Visual scanning Word retrieval Math calculation (scoring) Cognitive flexibility	Provide dictionary as external aid Eliminate double and triple scoring Add time limit to increase difficulty	# letters in longest word Score # turns in which more than one word was generated	Visual inattention Flexibility in making response	Client will demonstrate ability to consider complex information before making a response Client will utilize more sophisticated strategies with repeated trials Client will accurately perform sequential math calculations
Scrabble Sentence Cubes (Selchow & Righter)	Sequencing Reading Planning Cognitive flexibility Turn taking	Omit bonus points Have client play against self	# cubes used Score	Trial-and-error approach	Client will complete complex sequencing task within set time limit Client will be able to tolerate brief waiting periods Client will identify and self-correct errors
Scruples (Milton Bradley)	Decision making Perspective taking Abstract thinking Awareness of others	Omit challenges to responses Play with familiar others Use questions without the predictions in more of a social interaction format	# cards remaining in hand at end	Social appropriateness Improved accuracy of predictions Confidence Verbal fluency	Client will respond appropriately to hypothetical questions Client will use available information about others to predict their responses Client will improve in confidence in own performance in ambiguous situations
Simon (Milton Bradley)	Attention Sequencing Memory	Rehearse before responding Work as teams	Length of longest sequence	Attention Perseverance Improvement across trials	Client will demonstrate ability to attend to and replicate a sequence of visual stimuli
Slapjack (various)	Attention/vigilance Impulse control Speed of information processing Perceptual-motor coordination Visual discrimination	Use any face card as target Hold hand on lap to reduce impulsive responding Verbalize name of card displayed Increase difficulty by changing target stimulus each game	# response errors # seconds to respond # nonresponse errors	Kinds of errors made Response to errors Impulsivity	Client will decrease response (or nonresponse) errors by 20% Client will demonstrate ability to shift attention to a new target stimulus

Game	Areas assessed	Modifications	Quantitative measures	Qualitative measures	Goals
Trivial Pursuit (Horn Abbott Ltd.)	Fund of information, Remote memory, Reading, Verbal fluency	Form teams, Provide clues, Award a "pie" for any correct answer	# "pies" received, # correct answers	Recognition of own knowledge strengths, Use of self-cuing strategies	Client will demonstrate ability to tolerate perceived failures; Client will use strategies to cue recall of previously learned information
Uno (International Games)	Attention/vigilance, Divided attention, Visual discrimination, Low-level decision making	Omit "Uno" rule, Omit wild cards, Focus on color alone before adding number, Verbal prompts, Play as teams	Won/lost record, Time taken to respond, # incorrect plays	Failure to recognize playable card, Ability to attend to own and others' hands, Anger control	Client will demonstrate ability to attend to multiple aspects of a cognitive task; Client will show appropriate control of emotions in competitive situation; Client will demonstrate ability to match colors and numbers
Whatzit? (Milton Bradley)	Fund of information, Abstract reasoning, Cognitive flexibility	Select simpler cards for play, Provide list of possible relationships between words	# guesses per card, % cards guessed	Response to frustration, Use of strategies	Client will attempt to solve problems by using a variety of strategies
Who Dun It? (Selchow & Righter)	Reasoning, Cognitive flexibility, Memory, Attention, Use of external aids	Provide additional forms for recording information, Work in teams	% items correctly eliminated, # errors in summarizing information, % items correctly guessed	Quality of questions asked, Ability to make inferences	Client will identify when he or she has gathered sufficient information to solve a problem; Client will develop strategies for more effective problem solving
Win, Lose, or Draw (Milton Bradley)	Word retrieval, Response to feedback, Perceptual-motor coordination, Cognitive flexibility	Delete time limit, Verbal prompts to change approach, Choose easiest items	Time taken to guess, % items correctly guessed	Ability to vary strategy, Quality of drawings, Consistency of guesses with known information	Client will respond to feedback by altering his or her strategy as needed; Client will generate more than one option for communicating information; Client will demonstrate ability to translate words into visual images

CHAPTER 17

Functional Cognitive-Communicative Impairments in Children and Adolescents
Assessment and Intervention

ROBERTA DEPOMPEI AND JEAN L. BLOSSER

Traumatic brain injury is particularly devastating when it involves a growing child or adolescent. In most cases, this child/adolescent was developing into a contributing member of society and could be expected to participate with responsibility in activities of home, school, and community. Traumatic brain injury alters the individual's potential to be involved with peers, family, and teachers at the same level as prior to the injury. This alteration in potential causes difficulty for professionals who treat children or adolescents, and for parents, relatives, and friends who live, learn, and play with them.

Because children and adolescents are not "little adults," there are a variety of different factors that must be considered when providing assessment and intervention. These factors are all related to the inescapable truth that children and adolescents are in ongoing developmental stages—physical, cognitive-communicative, and psychosocial. While the brain injury may have affected that development, creation of assessment and intervention procedures to determine its affect on performance must also be guided by these normal developmental issues.

Bruce (1978) reported that, generally, children/adolescents have a better functional prognosis than adults with similar injuries. However, Blosser and DePompei (1989a), Lehr (1990), Lehr and Savage (1990), and Ylvisaker et al. (1990), indicated that there are major residual impairments in children and adolescents that will require individualized assessment and intervention over long periods of time. These impairments may be subtle or obvious, depending on the extent of injury. Because the impairments can exist in unique and unusual combinations, assessment and intervention must be functional and appropriate to the individual needs of the child/adolescent.

Ylvisaker et al. (1990) and DePompei and Blosser (1989) indicated that while many problems exist with this population, the cognitive-communicative impairments that can be experienced appear to be the main deterrents to successful reintegration into home, school, and community. These cognitive-communicative impairments must be understood by all individuals who design and execute programs in the hospital, rehabilitation facility, school, and home so that the best progress can be achieved. The ultimate goal of professionals at hospitals and rehabilitation facilities is to return the child/adolescent to home, friends, and "workplace"—the school. The functional cognitive-communicative skills that are stimulated by therapists, parents, teachers, and friends are critical to the successful implementation of the return. It is, therefore, essential for professionals to develop assessment and intervention strategies that include input and participation by immediate family, other relatives, and peers wherever possible.

While formal assessments and intervention are frequently indicated and provide much needed structure, they often ignore individual differences of the child/adolescent that are critical to acceptance by family and friends. For the most complete return possible, functional aspects of cognitive communication within school and home that foster "normal" communication among family and friends are extremely significant to the overall progress of the child or adolescent. To that end, the purposes of this chapter are to:

1. Define functional cognitive-communicative impairments in children and adolescents
2. Discuss the impact of impaired cognitive-communicative skills on families and peers, and its relationship to learning in children and adolescents
3. Outline some issues that affect cognitive-communicative assessment and intervention
4. Suggest methods for functionally assessing cognitive-communicative impairments
5. Recommend intervention strategies for therapists, parents, teachers, and peers that are based in stimulating cognitive-communicative behaviors in home, school, and community

DEFINITION OF COGNITIVE-COMMUNICATIVE IMPAIRMENTS

The American Speech-Language-Hearing Association (ASHA, 1987) defined cognitive-communicative impairments as "those communicative disorders that result from deficits in linguistic and non-linguistic cognitive processes" (p. 4). ASHA further stated there are many cognitive processes that underlie language development. When these cognitive processes are impaired, deficits in language will be the outward manifestation that indicates the underlying problems. These cognitive processes include:

Impaired attention, perception, and/or memory
Inflexibility, impulsivity, disorganized thinking
Difficulty processing complex information
Problems learning new information
Inefficient retrieval of stored information
Ineffective problem solving or judgment
Inappropriate social behavior (pragmatics)
Impaired executive functioning

The result of impairments in cognitive-communicative abilities for children and adoles-

cents is ineffective learning in school and poor social interaction. Both conditions may ultimately interfere with acceptance by family and peers. These cognitive-communicative impairments can be subtle in some children/adolescents and obvious in others. For example, a child/adolescent who has anomia (word-finding problems) may exhibit inconsistent difficulty with vocabulary exercises at school and be able to circomlocute the definition with lengthy responses that are somewhat related; another child/adolescent will demonstrate an inability to name, and be unable to locate any related words that would carry through the attempt at naming. The child/adolescent who spoke at length about the word may be seen by the teacher as performing adequately in the exercise, while the child/adolescent who simply did not respond may be seen as severely delayed. In truth, both may have equal word-finding problems.

It is often the behavior, rather than the underlying deficit causing the behavior, upon which teachers, family, and peers focus. It is also often the behavior, instead of the underlying deficit, upon which the therapist focuses attention in intervention. In functional cognitive-communicative assessment and intervention, it is important to recognize both aspects and incorporate them into a remediation program. It is essential to begin with underlying deficit areas and to develop as much ability to compensate as possible. It is also important to recognize that if family, teachers, and peers are to be involved in communication with the child/adolescent with traumatic brain injury, the outward behaviors of both the child/adolescent and the communicator must be understood and modified.

IMPACT OF IMPAIRMENTS ON FAMILIES AND PEERS

Cognitive communication is an essential component of adequate reintegration into home, school, and community. As time spent at home, at school, and with friends in the community constitute the entire daily experience of the child or adolescent with traumatic brain injury, it is important to understand how each environment is affected by cognitive-communicative impairments.

Home

Communication in the home is based on a variety of factors, including how the family is organized around operational aspects such as roles, rules, and structure (DePompei & Zarski, 1989). Other authors (DePompei, Zarski, & Hall, 1987; Waaland, 1990; Williams & Kay, 1991; Zarski, DePompei & Hall, 1987) have dealt with the multiple concerns of the family and it is recognized that the family is a complex unit with many possible reasons for poor interactions. However, a major factor in the success of reinvolving the child/adolescent with traumatic brain injury at home will be his or her ability to communicate with the family and vice versa. Difficulties reported by the family may include the inability to resume home routines, the disruption of family schedules, or the ignoring of rules and traditions.

It is especially difficult for siblings to deal with the inappropriate social interactions of their brother or sister. They find their sibling's behaviors embarrassing. Their lack of understanding about how the cognitive-communicative deficits will have an impact on behaviors will interfere with their ability to develop positive interactions. Families often believe that the return home signals a return to "normalcy," and when problems emerge, they become frustrated.

There are many communication behaviors that families may require of the child/adolescent. These include:

Following family rules
Responding to questions
Participating in conversations in a give-and-take manner
Using appropriate language
Respecting others
Showing interest in family activities (baseball, chess, running, poetry, music)
Expressing or withholding expression of feelings
Completing household chores
Comprehending written notes on the refrigerator door about who is where or what is to be done at home
Controlling behavioral outbursts

By determining what is important within the family, the therapist is able to plan intervention that is meaningful to the child/adolescent with traumatic brain injury, as well as to the family. By understanding the cognitive-communicative strengths and weaknesses of the child/adolescent and matching those to the functional needs within the family, useful skills can be developed.

For example, Susan, a 12-year-old who sustained a traumatic brain injury, came from a family where the three children had specific jobs in the household. Susan was responsible for garbage collection and for unloading the dishwasher. When she returned home, it was anticipated that she would resume these responsibilities. Fatigue, poor organization, and memory difficulties were impairments that interfered with completion of her jobs. This resulted in numerous family arguments as other siblings assumed that she was taking advantage of her recent injury to get out of her responsibilities. Therapy was focused on several aspects. First, explanations about the deficits and how they could affect Susan's behavior in the home were described for the family. Second, specific techniques were introduced to Susan to help her remember her jobs. Third, family members were included in a problem-solving session with Susan to devise reminders that would trigger her recall and help her complete her jobs. Fourth, Susan was encouraged to state clearly when she was tired so that jobs could be delayed until after a rest period or scheduled at a different time.

Therapists in rehabilitation centers or hospitals can focus on family communication needs such as Susan's in order to prepare the child or adolescent to participate as much as possible within the home communication setting. The family often can provide information that will guide the selection of situations in which to practice valuable communication skills.

School

School is a language-based environment and learning is a language-based activity (Berlin, Blank, & Rose, 1980; Blosser & Secord, 1989; Silliman, 1984; Wiig & Semel, 1980). The success of reintegrating the child/adolescent with traumatic brain injury into home and school will depend heavily on his or her ability to communicate effectively with others and perform adequately to meet classroom requirements and situations (Blosser & DePompei, 1989b). Difficulties may be reflected in the student's expression and understanding of language within the context of the school setting.

There are many communication behaviors needed to meet objectives and daily classroom requirements (Blosser, 1990). These include:

Using appropriate phonology, syntax, semantics, and pragmatics to meet verbal and written expression requirements

Responding appropriately when asked a question

Understanding the meaning of vocabulary and concepts unique to subject areas

Interacting socially

Formulating and asking questions to obtain information

Following written and spoken instructions

Organizing thoughts

Understanding word relationships

Using listening skills to learn from both classroom discussion as well as informal verbal interactions with peers in the classroom

Comprehending large amounts of information presented in a specified time period

By knowing the curricular demands, analyzing the cognitive-communicative skills needed for successful performance, and comparing this information to what is known about the student's strengths and weaknesses, one can determine where problems might arise in the classroom. For example, in reading, the student must be able to read a lengthy passage and answer the teacher's queries, recall facts and details, organize segments into appropriate sequences, and/or predict outcome based on portions of stories. Success in math requires an understanding of vocabulary and concepts, the ability to detect hidden questions and implied meanings, and knowledge of symbolic representation. In a class such as social studies, the ability to understand figurative language, spatial and temporal concepts, and language related to chronology is necessary. Similar examples could be generated for each subject area.

The student with traumatic brain injury who attempts to return to school with deficits in these areas can be expected to experience some level of difficulty, especially with performance in the academic subjects and relating to others (fellow students as well as teachers). These difficulties must be recognized and understood by teachers and clinicians who are responsible for working with the student. Cognitive-communicative rehabilitation in the hospital or rehabilitation center, outpatient treatment programs, home tutoring programs, or school setting needs to focus efforts in these areas in order to prepare students for reintegration. In addition, assessment prior to school reentry should evaluate these skills and capabilities so that educational plans can be developed to maximize areas of strength and target areas of need.

Community

A third factor in successful reintegration for the child or adolescent with traumatic brain injury is participation with siblings and/or peers within the community. Many young people are involved with activities such as scouting, YMCA/YWCA, gymnastics, athletics, music, art, dances, theater, or shopping in malls. Becoming reinvolved in these activities with friends is a crucial element to reintegration. It is often this area of maintaining friends and social activities that is neglected in therapy. Yet, it is one of the most important facets in total rehabilitation.

Abilities in cognitive communication that may affect the individual's ability to perform and communicate effectively with friends and within the community include the following:

Using age-appropriate vocabulary (including slang expressions)

Responding within adequate time (processing time is not so delayed as to "turn off" peers)

Understanding puns, humor, sarcasm

Participating equally in a conversation rather than monopolizing it

Controlling anger, frustration

Using "social space" appropriately (not standing too close or too far away)

Controlling disinhibited speaking out

Following the rules of a game or activity correctly

Generalizing from one social situation to the next

Formulating questions to obtain necessary information

Therapists, teachers, and family members are encouraged to consider functional situations where these valuable social skills might be rehearsed (cf. Chapter 14, this volume). By anticipating where the communication breakdowns may occur and providing strategies for handling them, valuable information is provided for the child/adolescent when he or she attempts to return to these activities. Peers also learn valuable lessons about how to aid their friend successfully in these situations.

ASSESSMENT AND INTERVENTION ISSUES

There are several issues that must be considered when planning assessment and intervention for the cognitive-communicative problems of children/adolescents with traumatic brain injury. These include developmental, educational, medical, family, and psychosocial areas.

Developmental Issues

Developmental issues must be considered in planning assessment or intervention for children or adolescents with cognitive-communicative impairments. If we are to put faith in the words and works of Piaget (Furth, 1970; Gruber & Vonech, 1977), then we must acknowledge that the developing child moves through a series of cognitive stages that influence what cognitive skills would be expected to be present at various ages. For example, a teenager who is unable to rationalize waiting for a reward, such as a movie at the end of the week for good behavior, may be viewed as delayed, while a preschooler may be seen as behaving normally for his or her age. Intervention could be devised for the teenager to restimulate abilities that were present previously; however, intervention to develop the ability to wait may be inappropriate for the preschooler.

According to Gans, Mann, and Ylvisaker (1990), some normal developmental cognitive patterns might include:

Centration to decentration: moving from self-centeredness to considering others' perspectives

Concrete to abstract: moving from trial and error to hypothetical problem solving

Growth of knowledge base: addition of factual information that aids learning new information

Increased capacity: developing speed of processing and flexibility of the retrieval system

Improved situational behavior: moving from indiscriminant behavior to appropriate behavior based on the specific situation.

Savage (1991) pointed out that an elementary-age child who sustains a traumatic brain injury may "look fine" during the first year or two after returning to school. It is when the additional cognitive skills of deductive reasoning, organization, and reliance on verbal rather than written directions are introduced at junior high levels that the same child, now an adolescent, falls apart. He indicated that it is necessary, whenever possible, to follow the development of brain-injured children/adolescents over extended periods of time. It is also important for therapists, teachers, and parents to understand that problems may emerge later that can be attributed to the traumatic brain injury.

The development of cognitive-communicative abilities is dependent on ability, progress, and basic inherent skill levels. When determining where to begin in assessment and intervention for children/adolescents, there are several questions that should be asked:

1. What was the developmental level of the child/adolescent prior to injury?
2. Was the child/adolescent developing normally prior to the accident?
3. Are the developmental delays that are noted now different from what was occurring previously? (This is especially difficult to describe in preschool populations where extremely wide gaps in what is considered normal development are possible.)
4. What cognitive levels are appropriate for the child/adolescent to have achieved?

Educational Levels

Preinjury educational levels of the child/adolescent should be noted. The abilities of the child/adolescent to participate in educational settings will not be better than they were prior to the injury. Several questions that may be asked include:

1. What were the academic abilities of the child/adolescent prior to the traumatic brain injury?
2. Were any special class placements or academic services provided previously? (For example, if the child could not read prior to the injury, inability to read now is not necessarily related to the injury.)
3. Who at the school can provide information about the child/adolescent as a student and as a social member of the class?
4. How did the child/adolescent learn best prior to the injury?
5. What rewards previously worked best in motivating the child/adolescent in the classroom?

Medical Information

The severity of the injury should be determined by obtaining accurate information from medical personnel. There are not particularly good data to indicate that the more severe the injury, the worse the cognitive-communicative impairment. However, Ylvisaker et al. (1990) reported that there is a significant chance that cognitive-communicative impairments will be the residuals that interfere with return to home and school for children/adolescents. Therefore, it is important to document the extent of the injury and the concomitant communication problems. Several questions to be asked include:

1. What is the extent of the brain injury?
2. Are there motor control problems that affect speech-and-language production?
3. What is the Rancho Los Amigos Scale of Cognitive Function (Hagen & Malkmus, 1979) level at the time of discharge of the child/adolescent from the rehabilitation facility (see Table 19.1, this volume, for description of levels)?
4. What is the ability of the child/adolescent to understand what is said or written to him or her?
5. What is the expressive level of the child/adolescent?

Family Issues

Family involvement and support are critical to the returning child or adolescent. Families who are responsive and dealing from a point of information and strength as a unit will provide a better framework for a return to home and community. They offer the child/adolescent a better opportunity to reintegrate successfully. DePompei and Blosser (1989), Fay (1990), and Williams and Kay (1991) indicated that family and peers may be one of the most significant factors in a well-defined and successful school and home return.

Ethnic and cultural issues may also have an affect on the brain-injured child/adolescent and his or her family. Blosser and DePompei (1990), DePompei and Zarski (1991), and Williams and Savage (1991) indicated that cultural and ethnic backgrounds of families have major importance to how the family communicates and cooperates with professionals. It is essential that professionals consider family backgrounds and account for differences when understanding the functional communication patterns within the family. These differences can indicate how useful means of teaching family members about language development can best be accomplished. It is often the professional who must adapt his or her approach to educating and working with the family and peers of the child or adolescent with traumatic brain injury. Obtaining information about the family by asking the following questions will assist in that adaptation:

1. What is the family structure?
2. Who lives in the home?
3. What is the cooperation level of the family?
4. What ethnic or cultural factors exist?
5. What other stress factors (e.g., financial, relationships, illnesses) may be operating in the family?
6. What does the family know about the injury and its impact on their communication abilities?

Psychosocial Development

The psychosocial development of the child/adolescent prior to the injury may also be a factor in determining the direction of intervention and assessment. A child/adolescent may have been aggressive, maladjusted, disorganized, abusive, lacking in social abilities, or nonconforming prior to the injury. If so, some behaviors that are present postinjury may not be related directly to the injury itself. Some questions that may be asked include:

1. Was the child/adolescent shy or outgoing prior to the injury?
2. Were there incidents of aggressive behavior?
3. Were there incidents of any type of abuse in the family or with the child/adolescent?
4. Were there incidents with juvenile court or the law involving the child/adolescent?

FUNCTIONAL ASSESSMENT

Determining the most appropriate intervention for a child or adolescent with cognitive-communicative impairments following traumatic brain injury is a complex process that requires considerable thought and planning (Lovaas & Favell, 1987). It is, therefore, important when determining intervention selection to understand the variables that contribute to the behavior that needs to be stimulated or altered. Standardized tests certainly contribute to the understanding of that process (Begali, 1987; Telzrow, 1991). However, at the present time no standardized test has been normed for use with children and adolescents with traumatic brain injury. While information that is obtained from standardized tests is necessary for placement decisions and for baseline information about a particular child, generalization beyond that would be dangerous.

Functional assessments would appear to offer more flexibility to the practitioner who is hoping to effect changes in the cognitive-communicative behaviors of the child/adolescent with traumatic brain injury. Functional assessment denotes the observation and documentation of antecedent and consequent events that contribute to cognitive-communicative behaviors with both positive and negative results. Determining pertinent situations that hold significance for the teacher, family, or friends, and aiding the child or adolescent to function adequately in those situations would be the goal of functional assessment and intervention.

Carr and Durand (1985) and Day, Rea, Schlusser, Larson, and Johnson (1988) indicated that there is some validity for basing intervention procedures directly on functional assessment of the behaviors. Durand and Carr (1987) also called for prior functional assessment when devising procedures to reduce problem behaviors. Lennox and Miltenberger (1990) suggested that not completing a functional assessment prior to initiating therapy may present risks because: 1) the client may be exposed to an ineffective intervention regimen that is counterproductive; 2) effective procedures may be delayed; and 3) the intervention selected may have aversive results, as it was not appropriate to the needs or goals of the client.

In addition, Andrews and Andrews (1986), DePompei and Blosser (1989), and Ylvisaker and Goebbel (1987) suggested that inclusion of the family in assessment gives the best overview of the child/adolescent and allows professionals a window to past behaviors and personality. Information from the family is often the most useful in determining appropriate intervention goals.

There are several types of functional assessment that may be helpful. These include interviews and surveys, direct observation, and experimental manipulation of variables believed to be related to the behavior in question (including classroom simulations).

Interviews and Surveys

Interviews and surveys are often a main source of obtaining information about cognitive-communicative behaviors. However, they are probably the most effective when combined with direct observations, self-monitoring, and rating scales (Cone, 1987; O'Leary & Wilson, 1986). Interviews can be conducted with parents, peers, relatives, teachers, and rehabilitation therapists to determine the child/adolescent's pre- and post-injury cognitive-communicative behaviors.

In order to obtain the most useful information, it would be helpful to devise a checklist of pertinent information that can be applied to home, school, or community, according to specific needs at the time. This information can then form the basis for intervention sessions. Figure 17.1 is a model of one questionnaire/checklist that the authors have found useful. It is based on information that is deemed necessary for development of home or school cognitive-communicative skills that would be important for acceptance by peers or family.

It is important that we understand the activities in which your child participated. This information will help us design intervention that is meaningful to your child and you. Please fill in all information as completely as possible.

1. List the names, ages, and relationship of everyone living in your home.

2. Are there other children, relatives, or individuals who previously lived in your home? Please list names, ages, and where they are now.

3. What special hobbies or interests does your child have?

4. What kind of food does your family like to eat?

5. What holidays does your family enjoy celebrating?

6. Are there any special traditions that you have when celebrating holidays or birthdays?

7. Indicate who in your family routinely completes the following tasks. Place a star on those items for which your child has been or could be responsible.

Task	Father	Mother	Child	Comments
Setting table				
Cooking meals				
Clearing table				
Washing dishes				
Grocery shopping				
Unpacking groceries				
Laundry				
Ironing				
Putting clothes away				
Sewing/mending				
Cleaning house				
Care of pet				
Emptying garbage				
Yard cleanup				
Mowing grass				
Repairs around house				
Car maintenance				
Homework				
Attendance at school activities				
Attendance at school conferences				
Other				

8. If discipline were necessary for your child, how would this be done and who would do it?

9. When there is a major family decision to be made, who makes it?

10. List activities you enjoy as a family.

(continued)

11. List names and ages of your child's friends, and activities they enjoy.

    Name   Age   Activities

12. What school activities has your child enjoyed in the past?

13. Would you classify your child as outgoing or shy?

14. List any community activities in which your child participates (scouts, swimming lessons, art classes, library hour, etc.).

15. Write any additional information about your child that you think we should know.

Figure 17.1.   Family informational sheet.

Self-monitoring questionnaires can also be very helpful in developing executive functioning skills in the older child or adolescent. Use of this type of survey would be dependent on the cognitive-communicative abilities of the client as well as the ability to self-assess and determine personal strengths and weaknesses. Figure 17.2 is a self-monitoring questionnaire developed for Paul, an adolescent who functioned at Level VIII (Rancho Los Amigos Scale; Hagen & Malkmus, 1979) and had returned to school. Paul was having specific difficulty with restraining himself from "humorous" outbursts in the classroom. While the teacher reported that some of his speaking out was appropriate and humorous, she indicated that he had no ability to know when to stop or when he was offending her or his classmates. This self-monitoring questionnaire was based on work completed by Blackwood (1973). It was employed to help Paul assess his behavior. It then formed a basis for modification as he used the information obtained from the first evaluation as a baseline against which behaviors on subsequent days were measured. One peer in the class as well as the teacher also answered similar questionnaires so that Paul had additional input about his achievements in altering his behavior.

Lennox and Miltenberger (1990) suggested that there are several formalized scales that evaluate problem behaviors. While these scales were devised to look at problem behaviors of individuals with severe developmental disabilities, it appears that some application might be possible with brain-injured children and adolescents. The Motivation Assessment Scale (Durand & Crim-mins, 1988), which looks at how a behavioral problem is reinforced, is one instrument that could prove useful. Donnellan, Mirenda, Mesaros, and Fassbender (1984) devised a formalized instrument to determine the communicative function of problem behaviors. Different ways a behavior may be reinforced by actions of another is provided for professionals to evaluate. Also, adaptation of any of these formalized scales can provide another means of confirming the patterns of behavior and how they appear to others who are communicating with a child or adolescent with traumatic brain injury.

Direct Observation

Direct observation of the child or adolescent with cognitive-communicative problems is often the most useful means of understanding what is happening within a classroom or family. Many assessment and intervention sessions take place in a one-to-one, optimal performance situation. Behaviors that appear to be appropriate in a one-to-one situation often are not so in the larger classroom. For example, a child/adolescent may be able to maintain adequate attention to task in a quiet environment but unable to transfer that behavior to the classroom where many distractions in the form of bells, movement in the class, and classmates' conversations interfere with maintenance of attention to the assigned task.

Because behaviors may be very different in the classroom or home, the best means of determining the factors that may account for lack of performance is to spend time observing in the classroom or with family and friends and the

Date: _____

1. Mark the number of times you interrupted Mrs. McCann's class today.

    1 2 3 4 5 6 7 8 9 10   more than 10

2. How did Mrs. McCann respond to your interruptions?

Response	Number of times
____ She smiled and laughed	_____
____ She didn't laugh	_____
____ She ignored me	_____
____ She talked while I was talking	_____
____ She interrupted me	_____
____ She told me to stop	_____

3. How did the kids in the class respond?

Response	Number of times
____ Laughed	_____
____ Were quiet	_____
____ Looked at me funny	_____
____ Told me to stop	_____
____ Didn't care	_____

4. What did you do wrong in Mrs. McCann's class?

5. What happens that you do not like when you speak out in Mrs. McCann's class?

6. What should you have been doing?

7. What happens that you like when you raise your hand and speak only when called on by Mrs. McCann?

Figure 17.2.   Classroom monitoring form designed for Paul, an adolescent with traumatic brain injury who had returned to school.

child/adolescent with traumatic brain injury. It is also possible to observe behavior patterns among families and friends when they visit a rehabilitation facility. Ylvisaker et al. (1990) suggested a variety of probes for exploring cognitive-communicative behaviors in children/adolescents. Figure 17.3 is an adaptation (Duerk, 1990) of these behaviors that might appropriately be used on a checklist while completing direct observations.

Experimental Manipulation of Variables

When a particular behavior is of concern, experimental manipulation of controlling variables may be helpful in completing a functional assessment. Durand and Carr (1987) completed an assessment of variables hypothesized to be associated with problem behaviors in a classroom. They systematically exposed the student to sequential phases of easy or difficult tasks and low or high attention. The authors were able to identify the variables that controlled the behavior by examining the differential rates of the behavior under each condition. While most professionals who work with children and adolescents with traumatic brain injury may not have the time to develop such extensive procedures to evaluate behaviors, the procedures present a viable option for examining problem behaviors and suggesting alternatives for modification of the behavior. The time expended may be worth the effort if undesirable behaviors can be modified by understanding the controlling variables and employing modifying controls.

FUNCTIONAL INTERVENTION SUGGESTIONS FOR COMMUNICATION PARTNERS OF CHILDREN AND ADOLESCENTS WITH COGNITIVE-COMMUNICATIVE IMPAIRMENTS

The child or adolescent with traumatic brain injury will return to family and friends in the home, school, and community settings. In order to be functional, intervention should be ongoing throughout the day and implemented by individuals in these environments. Formal as well as informal communicative interactions and teaching activities can offer unique opportunities for facilitating functional skill practice and developing important cognitive-communicative skills. The remainder of this chapter provides suggestions of strategies and techniques families, teachers, and peers can use to aid in the development of appropriate and functional cognitive-communicative behaviors.

The child/adolescent's family, teachers, and peers will need to understand the nature of traumatic brain injury and those aspects of the individual's inappropriate behavior that can be directly attributed to the effects of the injury. In cases of mild head injury, this is not always apparent; people often feel the child/adolescent has undergone a personality change due to the circumstances of the injury, puberty, drugs or alcohol, or a variety of other reasons. Rehabilitation professionals should plan to teach the family, teachers, and peers workable strategies so they can respond more appropriately to the child/adolescent and gain the skill and confidence necessary to provide effective interaction and therapy. Family members and friends who are very close to the child/adolescent, as well as teachers and other relatives, can provide needed stimulation and support if they are made aware of specific nonverbal and verbal response techniques and learn how and when to implement them.

The following sections describe general strategies and techniques that can be applied by all.

Interactive Cognitive-Communicative Strategies and Techniques

The interactive cognitive-communicative strategies and techniques discussed in this section have been found to be helpful with children and adolescents who exhibit cognitive-communicative impairments as a result of traumatic brain injury. Not all strategies are appropriate for all children/adolescents. Not all should be implemented simultaneously. They should be matched and adjusted to meet the individual's needs based on the presenting behaviors and characteristics. Decisions regarding which strategy to implement and when to implement it should be made in consultation with professionals who understand cognitive-communicative impairments; the individual's capabilities and needs; and the home, school, and community situation. When selecting a strategy, several factors should be considered:

Level of severity
Combination of impairments
Remaining strengths and needs
Skills identified as strengths that can be used as avenues for success
Skills targeted for improvement or strengthening
Relationship of the "helper" to the child/adolescent
Helper's abilities to understand and provide meaningful assistance
Circumstances of the interactions

Figure 17.4 provides an outline of cognitive-communicative strategies that can be used while interacting with and teaching children/adolescents with traumatic brain injury. Following formal and informal assessment procedures, communication partners should place a checkmark next to those cognitive-communicative skills that are impaired and those strategies to be implemented and/or modified. It is recommended that communication partners select a few to try at a time. This will enable them to develop an understanding of how to implement the procedures, when to implement them, and to decide which ones are effective or not.

Monitoring Quality of Conversations

Due to slowed processing time and impaired comprehension skills, the speaker's rate and quality of speech will be an important factor for consideration. Length, complexity, and rate should be altered to accommodate needs. Important information should be presented with shorter, less complex sentences, and at a slower rate. Key points can be emphasized by varying voice and intonation patterns.

Student name _____   Date of birth _____
School _____   Diagnosis _____
Classroom _____   Date _____

		Y	N
ATTENTIONAL PROCESSES	1. Can be aroused		
	2. Can maintain attention		
	# minutes during testing		
	# minutes during therapy		
	# minutes during favorite acitivity		
	3. Attention span increase:		
	when distractions are reduced		
	when task is familiar		
	when reward is offered		
	when instructed to pay attention		
	4. Can shift attention from one activity to another		
	Maintains topic appropriately		
	Shifts topic appropriately		
	Perseverates		
	Can maintain conversation while performing a motor task		
PERCEPTUAL PROCESSES	1. Eyes focus on people		
	Eyes focus on objects		
	2. Eyes track moving objects/people		
	Cross midline		
	3. Can identify familiar objects in a picture		
	Can complete a puzzle		
	Can sort objects		
	4. Matches pictures		
	Identifies object that is different		
	Completes math problems		
	5. Can find a specific item among many		
	Can find an object in a picture		
MEMORY/ LEARNING PROCESSES	1. Able to recall: events from day to day		
	locations around the building		
	2. Can answer yes/no questions: about a story told to them		
	about a story they read		

(continued)

		Y	N
	3. Can retell a story: with props		
	without props		
	with distractions		
	without distractions		
	with incentive		
	without incentive		
	4. Can list words in a category		
	5. Shows use of rehearsal strategy		
	6. Asks for repetition/clarification		
ORGANIZING PROCESSES	1. Can describe: how to play a game		
	a familiar object		
	2. Can select materials to complete a project		
	3. Can sequence events of the day: with cues		
	without cues		
	4. Can construct things with building blocks		
	5. Can answer main-idea questions		
REASONING/ PROBLEM-SOLVING PROCESSES	1. Can sort according to a rule		
	2. Can predict outcomes		
	Prevents negative outcomes		
	3. Can complete if-then statements		
	4. Completes word analogies		
	5. Explains proverbs		
	6. Provides several possible solutions		
	7. Asks for help		
	8. Keeps working		
	9. Gives up		

Figure 17.3.   Cognitive communication observational checklist. (From Duerk, B. [1990]. *Informal assessment considerations of cognitive-communicative disorders.* Unpublished manuscript, University of Akron, Akron, OH; used with permission.)

Giving Instructions and Directions
Quality and style of instruction delivery will greatly affect a child's/adolescent's ability to perform required tasks. Instructions should be repeated more than once and delivered through a variety of modes (auditory, visual, kinesthetic). The greater the level of severity, the higher need there will be for assistance from the speaker. Visual clues such as pictures, modeling, combined written and spoken instructions, listing the instructions in 1-2-3 order, and prompting will enable greater understanding of instructions.

Explaining New Concepts and Vocabulary
Learning new information poses significant problems for many individuals with traumatic brain injury. As new concepts and vocabulary are presented, words should be defined and explained and visual representations should be provided

Below is an outline of cognitive-communicative strategies that can be used while interacting with and teaching children/adolescents with traumatic brain injury. Following formal and informal assessment procedures, check those cognitive-communicative strategies to be implemented and or modified when interacting with or teaching the child/adolescent.

For example, under MONITORING QUALITY OF CONVERSATIONS, if assessment revealed that the child/adolescent has difficulty understanding long, complex sentences, the communication partners should make attempts to modify their communication styles by using short, simple sentences.

MONITORING QUALITY OF CONVERSATIONS
____ Reduce length of utterances
____ Reduce complexity of utterances
____ Reduce rate of speech
____ Vary voice patterns
____ Vary intonation patterns to emphasize key words

GIVING INSTRUCTIONS AND DIRECTIONS
____ Reduce length of instructions
____ Reduce complexity of instructions
____ Reduce rate of delivery
____ Repeat instructions more than once
____ Alter mode of instruction delivery
____ Give prompts and assistance

EXPLAINING NEW CONCEPTS AND VOCABULARY
____ Give definitions for terms
____ Show visual representations of concepts and vocabulary
____ Present only a restricted number of new concepts at a time
____ Ask questions to be sure of understanding

MONITORING SPEECH SELECTION
____ Avoid sarcasm
____ Avoid idiomatic expressions
____ Limit humor
____ Avoid puns

ORGANIZING AND SEQUENCING INFORMATION
____ Present information in clusters and groups
____ Introduce information with attention-getting words

ATTENDING TO THE CHILD'S/ADOLESCENT'S BEHAVIORS, QUERIES, AND COMMENTS
____ Redirect behaviors
____ Reinforce queries and appropriate behaviors and comment
____ Select material appropriate for skill, age, interest

SUPPORTING VERBAL COMMUNICATION
____ Use or reduce gestures dependent on student response
____ Use visual clues
____ Incorporate imagery to increase understanding

PERMITTING ADEQUATE RESPONSE TIME
____ Provide ample time for responses

ANNOUNCING AND CLARIFYING TOPIC OF CONVERSATION
____ Introduce topic to be discussed
____ Restate topic of discussion

MAKING THE CHILD/ADOLESCENT AWARE OF OTHERS' RESPONSES
____ Inform child/adolescent of verbal signs and their meaning
____ Inform child/adolescent of nonverbal signs and their meaning

READING TO THE CHILD/ADOLESCENT
____ Reduce rate
____ Reduce length
____ Reduce complexity
____ Determine comprehension through questioning
____ Redirect child's/adolescent's attention to important details and facts

(continued)

COMMUNICATING THROUGH WRITING
____ Evaluate quality
____ Provide ample time for task completion
____ Evaluate accuracy
____ Assist with organizational structure
____ Guide changes in legibility and structure

REINFORCING THE CHILD'S/ADOLESCENT'S COMMUNICATION ATTEMPTS
____ Redirect so responses are pragmatically appropriate
____ Inform child/adolescent if message is not understandable
____ Model correct productions
____ Correct error productions

REQUIRING AND EXPECTING COMMUNICATION
____ Provide communication opportunities

ENCOURAGING RESPONSIVENESS
____ Have child/adolescent reread instructions and materials
____ Ask child/adolescent to repeat instructions and information to ensure understanding
____ Guide child/adolescent through proofreading work
____ Assist child/adolescent in evaluating quality of work and accomplishments

FOSTERING COMMUNICATION THROUGH ANY MEANS POSSIBLE
____ Introduce alternative/augmentative communication systems

ARRANGING PHYSICAL ENVIRONMENT FOR COMMUNICATION
____ Reduce distractions
____ Eliminate physical barriers
____ Guide child/adolescent in understanding appropriate proximity

STRUCTURING COMMUNICATION ACTIVITIES
____ Provide opportunities for group interactions
____ Vary group size
____ Vary composition of group
____ Vary formality of interaction opportunities

DEVELOPING MEMORY SKILLS
____ Encourage child/adolescent to categorize information
____ Encourage child/adolescent to make associations
____ Provide opportunities for rehearsing information
____ Assist child/adolescent in visualizing information
____ Encourage child/adolescent to chunk information

PRACTICING HIGHER LEVEL THINKING AND COMMUNICATING
____ Provide opportunities for problem solving
____ Provide opportunities for decision making
____ Provide opportunities for making judgments
____ Ask questions to elicit solutions, judgments, and decisions

WELCOMING DISCUSSION OF FRUSTRATIONS, CONCERNS, AND PROBLEMS
____ Invite open discussion

Figure 17.4.   Checklist for planning interactive cognitive-communicative strategies.

where possible. The number of concepts introduced at a given time should be limited. Multiple opportunities for hearing, using, or understanding the new concept or vocabulary should be provided. The child/adolescent should be stimulated to elicit recall of important facts, concepts, and vocabulary.

Monitoring Speech Selection Some children/adolescents will have difficulty understanding sarcasm, idioms, puns, and humor. While use of these types of speech are common in social communication situations, they may lead to difficulties when used in the classroom or as a means of trying to convey important information at home. Therefore, their use should be avoided in instructional situations. During informal communication interactions, these forms of speech can be used if followed by an explanation of their meaning. This will facilitate learning the meanings of this type of speech.

Organizing and Sequencing Information

Because children/adolescents may have difficulty understanding information presented out of context and in a random manner, it is suggested that important information be presented in a clear, organized, sequential format. This means stating important information in clusters and small groups, and perhaps initiating utterances with attention-getting words such as "first," "next," and so forth.

Attending to the Child's/Adolescent's Behaviors, Queries, and Comments

The speaker must often compensate for the weaknesses presented by the child/adolescent with traumatic brain injury. This means observing and interpreting each behavior and responding accordingly. If the child's/adolescent's response is one of confusion or misunderstanding, changes should be made in mode or format of presentation or additional support and cues should be given. If the child/adolescent is distracted or disengaged, steps should be taken to redirect attention. For example, a system of nonverbal signals to cue the child/adolescent to alter his or her behavior can be prearranged and implemented (calling the child's/adolescent's name, touching him or her on the shoulder, using a hand signal). In addition, reinforcement techniques or high-interest materials can be introduced.

Supporting Verbal Communication

Incorporating gestures, visual cues, and imagery into conversations can often enhance what is said verbally. When using these supportive communication techniques, care must be taken because they will become distracting for some children/adolescents. Often verbal messages will be understood better if the communication partner points to an object or accompanies explanations with notes or pictures.

Permitting Adequate Response Time

Conversations and classroom discussions generally move very rapidly from one speaker to the next. This interaction style can prove very frustrating for the child/adolescent with traumatic brain injury. By the time thoughts are organized and responses are formulated, it is likely the conversation will have moved in another direction.

Communication partners should be made aware of these difficulties and purposefully slow down the pace of the discussion to account for the child's/adolescent's processing time needs.

Announcing and Clarifying Topic of Conversation

Individuals stand a better chance of succeeding in an interaction if they are aware of what is being discussed. Because of attention or memory problems often displayed by persons with traumatic brain injury, the topic may be lost. Introducing the topic, restating it frequently throughout the discussion, and assessing the child's/adolescent's awareness of the topic will be beneficial practices.

Making the Child/Adolesent Aware of Others' Responses

As long as the child/adolescent is oblivious to the way others are responding to inappropriate behaviors, he or she can make no attempt to change them. Therefore, attention should be directed to verbal and nonverbal signs indicating lack of interest or desire to interject a comment. This should be done cautiously and in a situation that will not result in embarrassment. Showing and discussing videotapes of communication interactions may provide some insights and understanding.

Reading to the Child/Adolescent

As in speaking, reading rate, length, and complexity should be monitored and reduced according to the child's/adolescent's response. It may be difficult to maintain attention during reading activities, so frequent questioning and redirecting may be necessary.

Communicating through Writing

Classroom work is often relayed through written communication. Quality, speed, accuracy, organization, legibility, and space planning all might be affected. Therefore, it is important that written communication activities be suited to the individual's performance capabilities in terms of structure and complexity. Efforts to develop written capabilities can be fostered by exercises that include giving dictation, providing written questions to answer, and helping develop simple scripts and essays.

Reinforcing the Child's/Adolescent's Communication Attempts

Providing the child/adolescent with feedback regarding the accuracy and quality of his or her communication attempts is important. The individual should be made aware of whether his or her communication attempts are pragmatically appropriate for the situation, fully understood, or produced correctly. In this way, assistance and guidance for improving communication skills can be given. All persons working with the child/adolescent should be aware of what can realistically be expected and how to correct inappropriate behaviors and communication errors tactfully. Explaining and modeling the correct behavior may be helpful as long as explanations remain simplistic. Confrontation and lengthy attempts at reasoning with the child/adolescent should be avoided. These will only foster a sense of failure on the part of both parties.

Requiring and Expecting Communication   Often persons in the child's/adolescent's environment will behave in ways that will actually give the child/adolescent the message that they do not want him or her to communicate. This may be because communication is a laborious process or because the resulting communication is embarrassing for family, friends, and teachers to witness. Regardless of the reason, communication at whatever level possible and through whatever means possible should be encouraged. It is through the channels of communication that change and improvement can occur. It is important that the requirements, expectations, and demands placed upon the child/adolescent are commensurate with actual capabilities.

Encouraging   Responsiveness   The child/adolescent with traumatic brain injury can also be encouraged to use several strategies to increase the potential for more accurate performance in the learning and communication interaction situation. These include rereading written directions, repeating verbal instructions verbatim and with paraphrasing, proofreading written work, evaluating the success and quality of communicative attempts, and asking questions when confusion is noticed. Some children/adolescents with traumatic brain injury have difficulty responding to direct questioning. Therefore, caution should be used when asking questions of the child/adolescent. If presented in association with a specific context such as a story, *wh* questions (who, what, where, why, when, how) can help facilitate development of organized communication skills. Directing the context, amount, and type of responses the child/adolescent gives can be accomplished by using directive instructions such as "Tell me more" and "How many did you see?" In addition, asking leading questions designed to help the child/adolescent identify a problem and plan out a solution will be helpful.

Fostering Communication through Any Means Possible   Some children/adolescents are left with such severe communication disabilities that they cannot communicate through verbal means. In these cases, alternative or augmentative methods of communication may be necessary. The decision to introduce alternative means of communication should be made as early as possible so that the child/adolescent does not become frustrated by his or her inability to communicate, and so that the doors of interaction and learning will be opened. Waiting for "normal" speech to emerge could waste valuable time. Significant persons in the child's/adolescent's environment should learn to use the alternative method of communication so that it will be considered an acceptable and functional mode. This suggestion also extends to the use of tape recorders, calculators, and computers for making accomplishment of classroom tasks more efficient.

Arranging Physical Environment for Communication   Distractions, physical barriers, and person-to-person proximity can all interfere with the communication process. These factors should be taken into consideration and barriers that prohibit interactive communication removed. Sometimes this means blocking out visual and auditory distractions, rearranging furniture, or reducing the number of persons engaged in a discussion.

Structuring Communication Opportunities   Because of the complex and extensive nature of the recovery process, children/adolescents with traumatic brain injury are often removed from informal communication opportunities. This situation, in combination with weakened skills, can prove devastating when it is time to resume social interactions. Throughout the recovery and reintegration process, group interactions ranging from very informal to formal should be provided so that opportunities for communication can be developed. The size, composition, and formality of the group should be increased as skills increase (see Chapter 15, this volume). At first, a few intimate family members and close friends should be encouraged to talk with the child/adolescent. Over time, experience with more friends and larger groups should be provided. Once the child/adolescent is reintegrated back into the school and community settings, extracurricular activities should be regularly planned and scheduled. When following this recommendation, it will be very important for all group participants to understand the child's/adolescent's cognitive-communicative problems and behaviors and how they should respond to them.

Developing Memory Skills The inability to remember assignments and previous communications will prove extremely frustrating for the child/adolescent and others with whom he or she is communicating. Teaching techniques such as categorizing, associating, rehearsing, visualizing, and chunking information should prove of assistance in developing memory skills. (The reader is referred to Chapter 12, this volume, for further discussion of memory training.)

Practicing Higher Level Thinking and Communicating Often day-to-day basic communication is not affected by the head injury, while complex thinking and communicating is. It will be important to provide the child/adolescent with opportunities to explain how he or she would solve problems, make decisions, and make judgments. Assisting with development of these skills will necessarily be dictated by ability levels. In general, however, the child/adolescent should be confronted with simple situations related to his or her own experiences at first. The difficulty level and relationship to other more far-removed situations should be gradually increased as improvement is observed. Through directive questioning, the child/adolescent should be asked to explain answers and provide rationale and reasons for beliefs. This can be practiced especially well during excursions

throughout the community when unexpected circumstances arise.

Welcoming Discussion of Frustrations, Concerns, and Problems Children/adolescents with traumatic brain injury will suffer great frustrations. As painful as it may be, open discussion about feelings and experiences should be encouraged so that problems can be properly handled.

Opportunities for Implementing Cognitive-Communicative Strategies

Home, school, and community environments each present unique opportunities for targeting cognitive-communicative skills and implementing the suggested techniques. Home and family members offer opportunities for assimilating the child/adolescent back into routines, familiar surroundings, and informal interactions. In the home setting, informal relearning of routines and informal interactions can best be reinforced during grooming and meal activities. In addition, family relaxation activities such as sports, watching TV programs together, reading books or magazines, or playing board games will offer opportunities for improving direction-following skills, pragmatic language skills, memory skills, and vocabulary development. Care should be taken to ensure that the assistance does not become the major focus of each verbal exchange. Rather, it would be more effective to select several key time periods during each day for implementation of one or two strategies. Implementation of strategies in the home setting should be monitored and guided by a professional who can help the family develop confidence and success in using the strategies.

School serves as a site for play and work where interactions can occur with teachers and schoolmates. There, relearning and new learning can take place. Throughout the school day, the student will be confronted with structured as well as unstructured situations that demand formal "academically oriented" communication or informal communication interactions. These variations and changing demands can pose high levels of stress on the student's cognitive-communicative abilities. Because there are so many different people in the school world, care should be taken when selecting communication partners and opportunities for practice. The communication demands and requirements should be monitored and modified frequently if necessary. Observations during classroom activities can be made to determine appropriate times and situations for implementing cognitive-communicative strategies. Performance requirements during discussion-type subjects such as reading and language arts should be closely analyzed. Those tasks that result in a high degree of teacher-to-student interaction will afford opportunities for the teacher to implement strategies. Informal small-group activities such as circle activities, science projects, relaxation time, and socialization activities (art, music, gym) will offer opportunities for student-to-student interactions. School affords development of all aspects of cognitive communication, but especially for direction following, concept and vocabulary development, organizing and sequencing information, pragmatic skills, memory, and communicating through writing. Classrooms that stimulate and reinforce communication attempts and are designed to require some form of communication will most benefit the child/adolescent.

Reintegration into community activities offers opportunities for socialization and functioning in unexpected and unstructured circumstances with relatives and friends as well as strangers. Situations such as purchasing food in a restaurant, buying tickets to a movie, attending church, or visiting a local amusement park all require the use of a different vocabulary and communication exchanges. Activities such as these offer unique opportunities to help the child/adolescent organize thoughts, problem solve, understand written language, ask questions, follow instructions, observe subtle verbal and nonverbal behaviors, and hear different types of speech. Communication partners familiar with techniques for assisting the child/adolescent should accompany him or her on these excursions.

CONCLUSIONS

Parents, friends, and teachers can all provide great support to children and adolescents with traumatic brain injury who are ready to be reintegrated back into home, school, and community. Their contributions will be much more effective if they are armed with strategies for helping and the confidence to implement the help when needed. After conducting assessment appropriate to the child/adolescent, rehabilitation professionals can promote and develop that confidence by providing information and guidance.

REFERENCES

American Speech-Language-Hearing Association, Task Force on Cognitive-Communicative Impairments. (1987). *Working draft of the role of speech-language pathologists in the habilitation and rehabilitation of cognitively impaired individuals.* Unpublished manuscript.

Andrews, J.R., & Andrews, M.A. (1986). A family-based systemic model for speech-language services. *Seminars in Speech and Language, 7*(4), 359–365.

Begali, V. (1987). *Head injury in children and adolescents: A resource and review for schools and allied professionals.* Brandon, VT: Clinical Psychology Publishing.

Berlin, L.J., Blank, M., & Rose, J.A. (1980). The language of instruction: The hidden complexities. *Topics in Language Disorders, 1*(1), 47–58.

Blackwood, R. (1973). *Operant control of behavior: Elimination of misbehavior and motivation of children.* Akron, OH: Exordium Press.

Blosser, J.L. (1990). *Making your speech-language pathology program relevant to educational needs.* Scranton, PA: Luzerne County Schools Speech-Language Pathologists.

Blosser, J.L., & DePompei, R. (Eds.). (1989a). Cognitive-communicative impairments following head injury. *Topics in Language Disorders, 9*(2).

Blosser, J.L., & DePompei, R. (Eds.). (1989b). The head injured student returns to school: Recognizing and treating deficits. *Topics in Language Disorders, 9*(2), 67–77.

Blosser, J.L., & DePompei, R. (1990, April). *Family and friends of the re-entering head injured student: Too often forgotten; always important.* Paper presented at Council for Exceptional Children International Conference, Toronto, Canada.

Blosser, J.L., & Secord, W. (1989, March). *Curriculum referenced language assessment.* Miniseminar, the Ohio Speech and Hearing Association Annual Convention, Dayton.

Bruce, D.A. (1978). Outcome following severe head injuries in children. *Journal of Neurosurgery, 48,* 679.

Carr, E.G., & Durand, V.M. (1985). Reducing behavior problems through functional communication training. *Journal of Applied Behavior Analysis, 18,* 111–126.

Cone, J.D. (1987). Behavioral assessment with children and adolescents. In M. Hersen & V.B. Van Hasslet (Eds.), *Behavior therapy with children and adolescents: A clinical approach* (pp. 29–49). New York: John Wiley & Sons.

Day, R.M., Rea, J., Schlusser, N.G., Larson, S.G., & Johnson, W.L. (1988). A functionally based approach to the treatment of self-injurious behavior. *Behavior Modification, 12,* 565–589.

DePompei, R., & Blosser, J. (1989, November). *The path less traveled: Counseling family and friends of TBI survivors.* Short course presented at the American Speech-Language-Hearing Association National Convention, St. Louis, MO.

DePompei, R., & Zarski, J.J. (1989). Families, head injury, and cognitive-communicative impairments: Implications for family counseling. *Topics in Language Disorders, 9*(2), 78–89.

DePompei, R., & Zarski, J.J. (1991). Assessment of the family. In J. Williams & T. Kay (Eds.), *Head injury: A family matter* (pp. 101–120). Baltimore: Paul H. Brookes Publishing Co.

DePompei, R., Zarski, J.J., & Hall, D.E. (1987). A systems approach to understanding CHI family functioning. *Cognitive Rehabilitation, 5*(2), 6–10.

Donnellan, A.M., Mirenda, P.L., Mesaros, R.A., & Fassbender, L.L. (1984). Analyzing the communicative functions of aberrant behavior. *Journal of The Association for Persons with Severe Handicaps, 9,* 201–212.

Duerk, B. (1990). *Informal assessment considerations of cognitive-communicative disorders.* Unpublished manuscript, University of Akron, Akron, OH.

Durand, V.M., & Carr, E.G. (1987). Social influences on self-stimulatory behavior: Analysis and treatment application. *Journal of Applied Behavioral Analysis, 20,* 119–132.

Durand, V.M., & Crimmins, D.B. (1988). Identifying the variables maintaining self-injurious behavior. *Journal of Autism and Developmental Disorders, 18,* 99–117.

Fay, G. (1990, March). *Neuropsychological consequences of closed head injury.* Paper presented at the Iowa State Conference on Innovative Practices in Special Education, Cedar Rapids.

Furth, H. (1970). *Piaget for teachers.* Englewood Cliffs, NJ: Prentice-Hall.

Gans, B.M., Mann, N.R., & Ylvisaker, M. (1990).

Rehabilitation management approaches. In M. Rosenthal, E. Griffith, M. Bond, & J.D. Miller (Eds.), *Rehabilitation of the adult and child with traumatic brain injury* (2nd ed., pp. 593–614). Philadelphia: F.A. Davis.

Gruber, H., & Vonech, J.J. (1977). *The essential Piaget.* New York: Basic Books.

Hagen, C., & Malkmus, D. (1979, November). *Intervention strategies for language disorders secondary to head trauma.* Paper presented at the American Speech-Language-Hearing Association Convention, Atlanta.

Lehr, E. (1990). *Psychological management of traumatic brain injuries in children and adolescents.* Rockville, MD: Aspen.

Lehr, E., & Savage, R.C. (1990). Community and school integration from a developmental perspective. In J.S. Kreutzer & P. Wehman (Eds.), *Community integration following traumatic brain injury* (pp. 301–310). Baltimore: Paul H. Brookes Publishing Co.

Lennox, D.B., & Miltenberger, R.G. (1990). Conducting a functional assessment of problem behaviors in applied settings. *Journal of The Association for Persons with Severe Handicaps, 14*(4), 304–311.

Lovaas, O.I., & Favell, J.E. (1987). Protection for clients undergoing aversive/restrictive interventions. *Education and Treatment of Children, 10,* 311–325.

O'Leary, K.D., & Wilson, G.T. (1986). *Behavior therapy: Application and outcome.* Englewood Cliffs, NJ: Prentice-Hall.

Savage, R. (1991). Identification, classification, and placement issues for students with traumatic brain injuries. *Journal of Head Trauma Rehabilitation, 6*(1), 1–9.

Silliman, E.R. (1984). Interactional competencies in the instructional context: The role of teaching discourse in learning. In G.P. Wallach & K.G. Butler (Eds.), *Language learning disabilities in school age children* (pp. 228–317). Baltimore: Williams & Wilkins.

Telzrow, C. (1991). The school psychologist's perspective on testing students with traumatic head injury. *Journal of Head Trauma Rehabilitation, 6*(1), 23–35.

Waaland, P.K. (1990). Family response to childhood traumatic brain injury. In J.S. Kreutzer & P. Wehman (Eds.), *Community integration following traumatic brain injury* (pp. 225–247). Baltimore: Paul H. Brookes Publishing Co.

Wiig, E.H., & Semel, E.M. (1980). *Language assessment and intervention for the learning disabled.* Columbus, OH: Charles E. Merrill.

Williams, J., & Kay, T. (Eds.). (1991). *Head injury: A family matter.* Baltimore: Paul H. Brookes Publishing Co.

Williams, J., & Savage, R. (1991). Family culture and child development. In J. Williams & T. Kay (Eds.),

Head injury: A family matter (pp. 219–238). Baltimore: Paul H. Brookes Publishing Co.

Ylvisaker, M., Chorazy, A., Cohen, S., Mastrill, J., Molitor, C., Nelson, J., Szekeres, S., Valko, A., & Jaffe, K. (1990). Rehabilitative assessment following head injury in children. In M. Rosenthal, E. Griffith, M. Bond, & J.D. Miller (Eds.), *Rehabilitation of the adult and child with traumatic brain injury* (2nd ed., pp. 558–584). Philadelphia: F.A. Davis.

Ylvisaker, M., & Goebbel, E.M. (1987). *Community re-entry for head injured adults*. Boston: Little-Brown.

Zarski, J.J., DePompei, R., & Hall, D.E. (1987). Closed head injury patients: A family therapy approach to the rehabilitation process. *American Journal of Family Therapy, 15*(1), 62–68.

REHABILITATION IN COMMUNITY SETTINGS

T raditionally, rehabilitation has been carried out in medical environments. To some extent, family members have also participated in the rehabilitation process by learning about therapy from professionals and applying therapeutic procedures in the home environment. Many family members have relied on common sense to implement their own version of cognitive rehabilitation. Frequently reported techniques include structuring environments, developing schedules and routines, and conducting living skills training.

Recently, concerns have been expressed regarding the generalization of therapy gains demonstrated in center-based rehabilitation programs. There is little evidence to support the notion that success in traditional rehabilitation settings assures success in real-world environments. These concerns have arisen partly from research indicating that many persons with brain injury have long-standing, severe memory problems. The failure of most persons with brain injury to gain and maintain employment also casts doubt on the efficacy of traditional center-based programs.

Within the last several years, creative clinicians have endeavored to develop intervention programs in home and work environments. Therapy intended to enhance daily living and vocational activities is provided by professionals who travel to the client's home or job. Family members, friends, and employers are exposed to cognitive rehabilitation techniques intended to directly benefit skills required for daily living. Professionals return to visit the client, reinforce learned skills, and teach new skills. Because the techniques are taught in the environment in which the skills will be used, few, if any, assumptions about generalization are required.

Reports about the benefits of cognitive rehabilitation efforts in the home and workplace have been promising. Within this section, a variety of real-world cognitive rehabilitation techniques are described and techniques for their application are discussed.

CHAPTER 18

Cognitive Remediation within the Context of a Community Reentry Program

SALLY KNEIPP

At the point of referral to community reentry programs, many persons with traumatic brain injury admit to being "therapied out"—a kind of burnout resulting from the physical and mental energies already expended in comprehensive rehabilitation therapies. Having been discharged from hospital-based therapies, they and their family members often underestimate the need for additional intervention to promote successful reintegration into the community. Since the focus of clients and their families during inpatient rehabilitation has primarily been on physical recovery, their understanding of the importance of cognitive remediation is frequently limited. In particular, the relationship between cognitive impairments and psychosocial behavior may not be appreciated.

In addition to the individuals who have been recently discharged from hospital-based therapies and feel therapied out, there are other individuals, some many years postinjury, who have not had recent therapy and who are only now being referred for community reentry programs. The growing number of community reentry programs has led to greater awareness on the part of rehabilitation specialists/case managers of their suitability for persons with traumatic brain injury who have been residing in the community but who are not integrated within it. These individuals may have adapted to their circumstances and may not understand the rationale for a referral to a community reentry program. The challenge for therapists in a community reentry program becomes how to motivate persons with traumatic brain injury to continue to work on improving their cognitive abilities, so that optimal functional outcomes are achieved.

This chapter addresses salient issues related to cognitive remediation within the context of a community reentry program. These issues include the rationale for and definition of cognitive remediation, conceptual considerations for cognitive remediation, and measurement of outcomes. A model for nonresidential community reentry programs is also presented, which includes descriptions of individual and group intervention approaches.

RATIONALE

The periodical literature in the field of traumatic brain injury rehabilitation is consistent with clinical observations that persistent cognitive impairments affect one's ability to reintegrate successfully into the community. Fryer and Haffey (1987) reported that, for many of the clients with traumatic brain injury in rehabilitation programs during the past decade, "persistent cognitive deficits were the primary barrier to successful community readaptation" (p. 51). Cervelli (1990) reported that "the long-term nature of deficits and disability following mild, moderate and severe brain injury may be grouped into five patient performance areas: health, physical function, cognitive function, behavior, and role resumption" (p. 465). Cervelli included, as elements of cognitive function, "concentration, memory, complex ideational skills, cognitive perceptual-motor skills, verbal and written expression, conceptual organization, reception, [and] self-regulatory skills" (p. 465).

Levels of independent living and employability have been used as measures of community integration. Among the reasons for failure to

239

achieve gainful employment, Ben-Yishay, Silver, Piasetsky, and Rattok (1987) identified cognitive impairments (e.g., deficits in attention, persistence, memory, and executive skills), impaired interpersonal skills, social isolation, unrealistic vocational goals, lack of awareness of the implications of the injury, and a failure to apply compensatory strategies. The interactive relationship between cognitive impairments and ineffective psychosocial behavior has been described by Prigatano (1986) and is increasingly being addressed by other clinicians and researchers. Prigatano proposed a four-step process to improve interpersonal skills: 1) improvement of attentional skills to reduce generalized cognitive confusion, 2) awareness of strengths and deficits through group and individual counseling, 3) recognition of the need for compensatory behaviors, and 4) understanding of the impact of cognitive deficits on interpersonal skills.

Clinical observations and descriptive reports certainly provide a rationale for cognitive remediation during the community reentry process. In addition to the improved quality of life for the individual with traumatic brain injury, greater independence in community living should result in a reduction in costs for services to the individual over his or her lifetime. While reports of the cost benefits of cognitive remediation during the community reentry process are generally not yet available, outcomes to date would yield positive conclusions.

DEFINITION

Various definitions of cognitive rehabilitation/remediation have been proposed, and usually they reflect the emphasis at a particular phase of intervention. For example, the definition of cognitive remediation used by clinicians working with individuals with traumatic brain injury soon after injury may reflect an emphasis on restitution of cognitive function, whereas the definition used by therapists in the postacute phase may reflect an emphasis on amelioration rather than restoration. Dougherty and Radomski (1987) discussed the value of approaches stressing amelioration in the postacute phase of trau-

matic brain injury rehabilitation. They cited three theoretical assumptions:

> 1. The brain-injured adult requires repetition and over-learning in order to master new skills and learn to utilize compensatory strategies. . . .
> 2. Self-monitoring is fundamental to the client's ability to accept feedback, modify performance, and ultimately set realistic goals. . . .
> 3. It is possible for brain-injured adults to relearn domain-specific skills and specific work behaviors. . . . (p. 3)

For purposes of this chapter, the definitions proposed by Ben-Yishay and Prigatano (1990) and Fryer and Fralish (1989) are the most relevant. Ben-Yishay and Prigatano defined "the aim of cognitive rehabilitation following a traumatic head injury as being the amelioration of deficits in problem-solving abilities in order to improve functional competence in everyday life situations" (p. 235). Fryer and Fralish defined cognitive rehabilitation as "the attempt to restore functional goal-directed activity . . . to remove the barriers impeding a person's ability to meet the cognitive and social challenges being presented by his or her environment" (p. 7-3). Both of these definitions stress the ability to function in the individual's natural environment.

CONCEPTUAL CONSIDERATIONS

As more day treatment and community reentry programs have been established, reports of approaches to cognitive remediation have appeared in the neuropsychological and rehabilitation literature. Fryer and Fralish (1989) classified the modes of cognitive rehabilitation into the instrumental skills approach, the hierarchical task approach, and the functional activities approach. The functional activities approach incorporates the instrumental skills and hierarchical task approaches so that structured training is provided.

Like Ben-Yishay and Prigatano (1990) and Fryer and Fralish (1989), Sohlberg and Mateer (1989) also emphasized improving the ability to function in everyday life, and stated that the success of the process-specific approach to cognitive rehabilitation "must be improvements in level of vocational ability and independent living" (p. 22). Sohlberg and Mateer advocated the process-specific approach from among the three approaches they determined were usually used in the United States and Canada: 1) general stimulation approach, 2) functional adaptation approach, and 3) process-specific approach. The process-specific approach emphasizes remediation of targeted cognitive areas and is considered a restorative model, although compensatory methods may be used if restoration to a functional level is not achieved. Tasks are organized in a hierarchy and repetition of specific tasks takes place until criterion is reached.

A significant concern in relation to the process-specific approach is the amount of time that may be required to achieve functional levels sufficient for or during community reentry. At the point of community reentry, many, if not most, persons with traumatic brain injury are well aware of the amount of time they have been out of the mainstream. It is anxiety producing, for example, for adolescents to know that their injury has prevented them from graduating with their class or for adults to know that they have missed opportunities for career advancement. These facts frequently contribute to low self-esteem. The greater the delay in reentering the community, the harder the transition. The amount of gain that could be made by continuing to work on restoration of a specific cognitive function must be compared with the amount of psychological damage that may result from a delay in becoming involved in the community on at least some functional level. To prevent additional psychosocial problems, cognitive remediation approaches must facilitate reentry into the community at the earliest possible time (i.e., when some degree of success can be assured based on level of functioning).

Specific factors to be considered in providing cognitive remediation within the context of a community reentry program for persons with traumatic brain injury follow.

Viability of Any Activity for Cognitive Remediation

Since cognitive abilities are used in planning, organizing, and carrying out all human activities, virtually any activity can be used for purposes of cognitive remediation. If the activity is to be considered a basis for cognitive remediation, however, it must be clear how the activity will improve one or more cognitive functions. The objective of the activity, the specific tasks, and the means of evaluating performance must be agreed upon.

Fryer and Haffey (1987) studied outcomes of an outpatient cognitive retraining model and a residential community reentry model. They concluded:

> For some patients, the minimum mastery levels needed to support relatively independent community living and role restitution outcomes can be achieved by training routines directed at reestablishing cognitive skills that previously supported performance in residential and occupational activities. For other patients direct training on functional behaviors in which minimum mastery levels are supported through reliance on alternative, compensatory strategies based on residual cognitive capacities as contrasted with pre-injury cognitive process can be effective. Direct training does not imply mere practice of functional behaviors. Competency is dependent on individually tailored cognitive orthoses. (p. 62)

Increased Motivation through Participation in High-Interest Activities

Since motivation is a primary variable in one's level of functional attainment, personally relevant, high-interest activities are recommended to serve as a context for cognitive remediation of individuals with brain injury. For example, rather than working with an adolescent on initiating and planning a hypothetical activity, cognitive tasks to address these needs could be structured in relation to an actual rock concert of his or her choosing.

Interaction of Cognitive Abilities

As stated by Fryer and Fralish (1989), traumatic brain injury may result in multiple cognitive impairments. Therapists must be aware of the processes involved in each cognitive ability and must keep in mind "that no single function stands alone; all rely upon one another, interact in an integrative manner and function in unity" (Fryer & Fralish, 1989, p. 7-9).

Cognitive remediation approaches must address not only the interactive effects of cognitive functions but also the integration of activities into a meaningful activity pattern or routine.

Application of Cognitive Abilities to Naturalistic Settings

There is growing consensus that, as Sohlberg and Mateer (1989) stated, "experience has shown that greater functional gains can be achieved when mechanisms to apply improved cognitive abilities to naturalistic settings are pursued" (p. 21). However, even naturalistic settings may not be sufficient. Because persons with brain injury frequently have difficulty generalizing their skills across settings (and often across behaviors as well) or carrying over problem-solving strategies to other situations, cognitive remediation should take place in the setting where the skills are to be applied. The best outcomes are likely if activities are carried out in the client's home and community, not in the locale of a community reentry program's office or facility, or even in a naturalistic setting that has no personal significance for the individual.

The focus on therapy in the setting where skills are to be applied is not intended to suggest that all efforts to restore function or promote generalization in other settings should be abandoned. However, at this late point in the recovery process, the emphasis should be on helping the individual with brain injury to achieve success in functional activities as quickly as possible. Competence in community activities is necessary, as mentioned earlier in this chapter, to prevent the potentially destructive effects of repeated or frequent failures. Success will also go a long way toward motivating the individual to continue to improve.

Need for Opportunities to Integrate Information and Skills

At the point of readiness for community reentry (during the process of recovery from traumatic brain injury), an integrative approach is indicated. Up to this point, discipline-specific intervention rendered by a multidisciplinary or interdisciplinary therapy team has generally been provided. What is often needed by the individual at the point of community reentry is guidance in *integrating* the information and skills acquired during earlier phases of rehabilitation. Learning

to "pull it all together" is a primary goal at this point. In many therapy settings prior to community reentry, therapists encourage their clients to assume responsibility for planning their therapy sessions, but these generally last not more than an hour or two. It is a far more complex undertaking to learn how to integrate disparate skills and abilities as required in day-to-day living, or to plan the many activities that make up a typical day (e.g., household chores and errands, meal preparation, work and/or school, recreation, leisure).

In discussing the need for a holistic approach, Ben-Yishay and Prigatano (1990) explained:

1. Rehabilitation programs for traumatically head injured individuals must consist of well-integrated interventions that exceed in scope, as well as in kind, those highly specific and circumscribed interventions that are usually subsumed under the term "cognitive remediation."
2. An adequate, effective program of neuropsychological rehabilitation must, of necessity, be organized and operated along holistic lines.
3. . . . cognitive remediation must be completely embedded in the totality of the rehabilitation endeavor, wherein its expected outcomes, the specific techniques it employs, and the process of . . . application must be subservient to the wider goals of the rehabilitation endeavor.
4. Cognitive rehabilitation programs in which the "treatment" is primarily focused on computer-assisted cognitive retraining are unlikely to achieve successful treatment outcomes. This may be a consequence of the lack of generalization of treatment effects, narrowness of the "computer" approach, and failure to consider the context in which cognitive and interpersonal deficits occur. (p. 400)

Need for Ongoing Assessment

Ongoing assessment of the individual's cognitive abilities, particularly as they are manifest in various real-life contexts, is essential during community reentry. In addition to measuring performance, ongoing assessment is needed to assure that cognitive remediation tasks are suitable for the individual and lend themselves to progression through a hierarchy of tasks constituting a functional activity. Situational assessment must address one's ability to complete a task, an activity, and a series of coordinated activities. While neuropysychological assessments are unquestionably valuable in their delineation of cognitive strengths and weaknesses, they are not sufficient to measure or predict one's functional capabilities as required in day-to-day living.

Concept of Social Role Valorization

Social role valorization (Wolfensberger, 1983) is an important component of cognitive remediation during community reentry. Condelucci and Gretz-Lasky (1987) emphasized the importance of contributing value to the social role of persons with disabilities in the community by providing culturally normative, age-appropriate activities and training methods in real community settings. They also stressed the importance of working to change societal perceptions and attitudes about the abilities of persons with brain injury.

Impact on the Family

Traumatic brain injury not only affects the individual who sustains it but also his or her family members. While Deutsch (1989) and Jennett (1990) advocated for family members to become the disability managers or therapy providers, respectively, for their family member with brain injury, it must be recognized that some family members are not good candidates to assume these roles and/or would not choose to assume them. Nonetheless, they may play a vital role in decision making about the kind and scope of services, as well as who is to provide them and where. Their opinions can and should be sought; whether or not they themselves can take on the responsibility for care or case management is a very personal decision. During community reentry, the ability of family members to help design, structure, or reinforce performance of cognitive tasks must be assessed. Even if they choose not to be actually involved in cognitive remediation efforts, they must understand the objectives/purposes of the cognitive remediation activities and how they can support and encourage progress.

MODEL FOR COGNITIVE REMEDIATION IN A COMMUNITY REENTRY PROGRAM

The foregoing conceptual considerations have been presented to relate the following model to the research results now available and to theoretical positions that have been espoused by others in the field. The model was designed in response to clinical problems identified at the point of community reentry—problems faced by individuals with traumatic brain injury, their family members, and professionals. Professionals reported feeling frustrated by the failure of most of their clients to proceed smoothly from hospital-based care to community living. Even those individuals who made excellent progress within the hospital environment frequently encountered problems in returning to their home (or the home of their family of origin), to work or school, or to the community at large. A functional, integrative, holistic model was generated. The model has the following elements:

1. Individualized, personalized program plan
2. Variable scheduling
3. Combination of individual and group intervention
4. Transdisciplinary, extended one-to-one approach
5. Systematic reduction of therapy and staff support
6. Ongoing functional observations

Individualized, Personalized Program Plan

An individualized, personalized program plan is designed, based on the individual's high-interest activities, and is carried out in the individual's own community. The goals and methods for working on cognitive problems within the context of the high-interest activities are decided upon and are specified in a written, individualized program plan. The individual with brain injury and his or her family members, as appropriate, are involved in the development of goals, selection of activities related to them, establishment of compensatory strategies, and so forth.

Variable Scheduling

Therapy schedules vary from client to client and are established in response to the individual's needs and those of his or her family members. For example, the therapy schedule may coincide with a single parent's work schedule of 3:00–11:00 P.M., making it unnecessary for the parent to make arrangements for the client's supervision at that time. Therapy is also scheduled at times to take advantage of high-interest activities (e.g., a tennis class, which could address right-left discrimination, decision making, and planning skills while also offering opportunities to work on physical conditioning and psychosocial behavior).

Therapy schedules may be part time or full time, based on need. Part-time schedules (e.g., 2 or 3 days per week) may be implemented while an individual is still receiving traditional outpatient therapies or day programming at a clinic or facility 2 or 3 days per week. Coordination of schedules to provide a full complement of therapeutic activities for the individual may enable family members to adhere to their usual routines. Moreover, the introduction of community-based therapy while still receiving facility-based therapy provides opportunities to assess the individual's ability to carry over into his or her community those skills being addressed or learned in a clinic or facility. Communication between therapists increases the relevance of the therapy in both settings.

Cognitive skills acquired during earlier phases of rehabilitation are reinforced and monitored for their effectiveness in real-life activities during community reentry. Staff routinely meet with the hospital-based treatment team making the referral, prior to the individual's enrollment in the community reentry program. Meeting together prevents "reinventing the wheel" or the introduction of new strategies or techniques that could be confusing to the client. The purpose is to assist the client to carry over skills acquired into community living.

Combination of Individual and Group Intervention

Individual intervention focused on a client's specific cognitive impairments constitutes the majority of therapy time. This is due to the need to assist the client to master the cognitive skills needed for integration in his or her own community. However, because of the interactive effects of cognitive functioning and psychosocial behavior, therapeutic group activities are also needed.

Group activities are established in locations convenient to a small group of individuals in the community reentry program. In other words, wherever there is a small group of persons living in reasonable proximity to one another (e.g., within an hour's drive), group activities are offered and become part of their intervention plan. If the program's offices are not centrally located, community organizations may have available space to accommodate a group at low cost (e.g., Knights of Columbus Hall). Clients' homes may also be used. (Specific cognitive remediation activities within a group context are described in more detail later in this chapter.)

Transdisciplinary, Extended One-to-One Approach

Working together over an extended therapy period (usually 5 hours per day initially), the therapist-client dyad is able to focus on higher level skills involved in the planning, organization, and implementation of therapeutic activities throughout the day. Several variables are taken into account in matching the therapist with the client. The variables include the therapist's skills in relation to the primary clinical problems; areas of common interest, since the cognitive remediation will revolve around the interests of the client; geographical proximity between the client's and the therapist's homes, to assure familiarity with the client's community; and so forth. This "matching" of therapist and client offers consistency and continuity that may be difficult to achieve using a multidisciplinary team approach. (It is important to keep in mind, however, that the single therapist-to-client approach is recommended *only* at this postacute, community reentry phase of therapy because it is believed the focus needs to be on integration.) Also, families often prefer to have one community reentry therapist, rather than several, because the presence of therapists in the home may, among other things, interfere with a family's privacy.

The extended amount of therapy time and the one-to-one approach also provide more opportunities to involve the individual actively in the therapeutic process. Unfortunately, when faced with extreme time pressures, therapists have sometimes resorted to making decisions *for* their clients rather than *with* them. As emphasized by Fryer and Fralish (1989),

> persons with brain injuries must be involved in the process as their level of functioning permits, with a primary goal of rehabilitation being to empower the person with a brain injury through increased skills, so that he or she is able to become a completely active participant in negotiating goals and outcomes. The purpose of cognitive rehabilitation is to restore the individual's ability to function effectively in his or her world and to maintain his or her individuality while participating in social activity.
>
> Effectively assuming responsibility for setting goals is the key to this restoration. (p. 7-17)

The extended one-to-one approach also provides, on a routine basis, the opportunity to review, discuss, evaluate, and interpret the activities during the day. Feedback is given and the client is encouraged to use a metacognitive approach to increase self-monitoring and self-regulation.

An additional advantage of this extended therapy approach is that cognitive remediation tasks can focus on structuring activities or tasks to be carried out by the individual with brain injury on nontherapy days. During the next therapy session, the degree of success in performing the tasks or activities can be evaluated.

Systematic Reduction of Therapy and Staff Support

As gains in cognitive abilities occur and competence in functional activities is exhibited, therapy and staff support is systematically reduced. In particular, reductions in therapy occur when the individual with brain injury demonstrates improved executive functions as evidenced by an ability to plan, organize, and carry out specific tasks or a series of tasks consistently throughout the day. Learning the cognitive skills required in utilizing the resources of the community may include, for example, relearning how to read a bus schedule and accessing public transportation to go to a local health spa or YMCA, where the client carries out an exercise program tailored to his or her needs and uses a checklist to adhere to the exercise program as well as to chart progress. Once this activity can be completed independently, therapy time can be reduced (or directed to other cognitive remediation goals, if necessary). The overall goal is to reduce therapy gradually and systematically to the point of minimal, critical support (i.e., to the point of least support and greatest independence while assuring sustained outcomes).

Ongoing Functional Observations

Neuropsychological test results, progress notes, and discharge summaries are frequently included with the material received at referral. This information, coupled with input from the individual with brain injury and his or her family members, assists the community reentry therapist to target the cognitive impairments needing remediation. There is not always a strong correlation, however, between performance on neuropsychological tests and actual performance on tasks of community living. Observation of the individual is needed while he or she carries out real-life, age-appropriate tasks in the community. Moreover, while it is important for the therapist to document observations, the documentation must be done in a way that does not detract from the naturalness of the activity. In particular, the extended therapy time provides opportunities to observe the client's ability to plan and sequence activities throughout the day in a time-efficient manner. It should be noted that problems with time awareness are major deterrents to effective psychosocial and vocational behavior.

Not only must assessment be ongoing, but also performance must be evaluated in relation to the standards of the family and community in which the client resides. Moreover, compensatory strategies that work for the client are best not changed, even if a "better" way seems obvious to the therapist. For example, one of the author's clients with head injury simply could not make brief notations in his datebook; he insisted on writing in complete sentences, such as, next to 7:00 A.M., "Sally will pick me up to go to breakfast," (rather than "Sally—breakfast" as might be sufficient for someone else). His system worked for him and suggested the need for a datebook with enough space to write his sentences, instead of the need to learn to use simple cue words (the prospect of which was so frustrating to him that temper outbursts would result).

In another case, it became important to search for a datebook that would stay in the shallow pockets in the style of pants preferred by a client; he was not about to choose a different style of pants even though the kind of datebook he had been given as an inpatient kept falling out of his pocket.

EXAMPLES OF INTERVENTION APPROACHES

As emphasized previously, the efficacy of cognitive remediation will be increased if it has a high degree of relevance and meaning for the individual with brain injury. The individualized program plan must be realistic for that individual—that is, it must make sense in relation to the individual's cultural or subcultural environment and family functioning. Creativity in programming is encouraged to enhance the appeal of the intervention. Enhancing the appeal is especially important in designing cognitive remediation tasks for persons with limited awareness of the need for remediation. Also, because of the rebellion that is characteristic during adolescence, teenagers usually respond much better to tasks that incorporate ideas that are "big" at that time. Two examples (of one adult and one adolescent) of one-to-one cognitive remediation within the context of community reentry programming follow. Also, an example of group intervention is provided.

One-to-One Intervention for an Adult

D.R., a 33-year-old male, separated from his spouse at the time of his head injury, had been living alone in his own home. After his injury, he lived with family members, but was not satisfied with that arrangement. Cognitive remediation efforts were directed toward helping him acquire the skills necessary to move back into his own home.

D.R. could not live alone in his own home due to cognitive, perceptual, and sensory impairments; obvious safety issues; and financial reasons. Home health aides or a live-in elderly person were suggested as possible solutions, but there were negative aspects to each of these solutions: 1) The home health aides might assume a custodial role, and compromise D.R.'s potential for more independent functioning; and 2) D.R. stated emphatically that he did not believe he could relate to an elderly person, *and* he desired some social interaction. Problem solving resulted in a decision to try to find two tenants/roommates (two would be needed for financial reasons, and for adequate supervision).

Tasks related to the goal of assisting D.R. to return to his home were addressed through one-to-one cognitive remediation. Some of the tasks in this process, which required various cognitive abilities, were:

1. Placing an advertisement for roommates
   a. Deciding where to place the advertisement (e.g., newspapers, bulletin boards, university housing offices)
   b. Making a list of information to be included in the advertisement (e.g., description of housing, location, amount of rent, when the room would be available, telephone number for responses)
2. Writing the advertisement on cards for placement in areas selected (e.g., university housing office), and for reference when placing the ad in the newspaper
3. Calculating the amount of money available to spend on newspaper advertisements
4. Placing the telephone call(s) to the classified advertisement department of the newspaper and placing the advertisement
5. Deciding what information needed to be obtained when receiving telephone calls in response to the advertisement, and deciding who would be interviewed
6. Developing a list of questions for interviewing prospective roommates (e.g., reliable source of income), and developing a rental agreement
7. Scheduling interviews
8. Inspecting the home and deciding what needed to be done before anyone could move in, since it had been unoccupied for more than a year (e.g., repairs, repainting, turning on utilities)
9. Identifying structural equipment/modifications needed to compensate for D.R.'s sensory deficits (e.g., because of deficits

in recognizing odors, an alarm that would signal escaping natural gas was needed)

10. Establishing strategies to compensate for D.R.'s memory deficits (e.g., association strategies for turning off the lights and the stove, and systems for labeling perishable items in the refrigerator with the date of purchase and when the item should be discarded)

11. Practicing laundry skills (e.g., doing light and dark clothes separately rather than separating by items—socks, underwear, shirts)

12. Learning public transportation routes (previously, D.R. had a car) to grocery stores, and so forth

13. Understanding the role and responsibilities of a landlord (i.e., the "roommates" were, in reality, tenants)

14. Making written lists of procedures for emergencies (e.g., no electricity or water)

The cognitive demands in carrying out the aforementioned tasks were numerous and took a substantial amount of time; thus, therapy was scheduled 5 days per week, 5 hours per day. Additional activities were incorporated into these 5 days of therapy to address other needs, such as the need for some recreation, leisure, and social-ization (and later, job search for competitive employment).

To promote recall of routine activities and tasks, a weekly schedule was developed that remained consistent from week to week (until addition of a new activity dictated a revision in the schedule). Figure 18.1 illustrates D.R.'s therapy schedule while working toward his return home.

One-to-One Intervention for an Adolescent

B.F., 8 years old at the time of his brain injury, attended special classes in a public school and, at age 13, was referred to the community reentry program for one-to-one therapy intended to supplement his educational program and to improve his ability to function in the community. B.F. had significant speech and gait impairments, cognitive deficits, and some psychosocial difficulties. In interaction, all of these problems contributed to B.F.'s poor consumer skills. In stores, he had difficulty identifying the location of items, planning effectively to search systematically for items, and asking appropriately for assistance when needed. To work on his consumer skills in a way that would be enjoyable for B.F. and that would address each of his areas of difficulty, a shopping mall scavenger hunt was designed by his therapist.

Time	Monday	Tuesday	Wednesday	Thursday	Friday
10–11	Review of plans for the day	Review of plans for the day	Review of plans for the day	Review of plans for the day	Group activities
11–12	Tasks related to finding tenants	Tasks related to finding tenants	Tasks related to finding tenants	Tasks related to finding tenants	Group activities
	Activities at his home, in preparation for return (e.g., repairs)	Lunch (out in community)	Activities at his home, in preparation for return (e.g., repairs)	Lunch (out in community)	Group activities
1–2	Preparation/lunch at home	Noncredit class at local university—"Achieving Self-Dignity"	Preparation/lunch at home	Noncredit class at local unviersity—"Achieving Self-Dignity"	Group activities
2–3	Review of tasks completed; planning for tomorrow	Review of tasks completed; planning for tomorrow	Review of tasks completed; planning for tomorrow	Review of tasks completed; planning for tomorrow	Group activities

Figure 18.1. Therapy schedule designed for D.R., a 33-year-old man with traumatic brain injury, to facilitate his return home.

The activity is simple to do and can actually be made relevant to adolescents or older persons. It can be carried out on an individual or group basis. In advance of going to the mall, a list of items found in a mall should be developed, keeping the age level and interests of the participants in mind (see Figure 18.2). Next to the item should be a place to record the location where the item was found (e.g., name of the store) and the price. Each individual should be given a copy of the list, a clipboard, and a pencil or pen.

Upon arriving at the mall, the individuals should be guided in consulting the directory and planning the way they will go. As items are located, their location and price are recorded. (No real purchasing is done.) This can be done as a contest, with time limits set for finding the items. If a group of people are involved, they can be divided into teams, with the winner being the team that completes its list first. A certain store or other landmark (e.g., fountain) can be set as a "finish line." Rules can also be added to make it more difficult, such as "No two items can be located in the same store." It also can be done as a real activity, complete with purchasing, if a list is made with that in mind (e.g., items needed for a party).

Item	Location	Price
1. Record album		
2. Baseball glove		
3. Sweatshirt		
4. 10-speed bicycle		
5. Sneakers		
6. Birthday cards		
7. Model kit (car or airplane)		
8. Photograph album		
9. Sony Walkman		
10. Blue jeans		
11. Skateboard		
12. Hot dogs		

Have Fun!

Figure 18.2. Sample list for shopping mall scavenger hunt designed for B.F., a 13-year-old boy with traumatic brain injury.

The trick to the enjoyment of this activity is including high-interest items on the list, and positively reinforcing the individual(s) for completion of the activity, with a reward also available at the mall. Reward suggestions include a movie (if the mall has a theatre), ice cream, or a small gift.

Group Intervention

Group intervention is intended to promote continued improvement in cognitive abilities, especially as they affect psychosocial, communication, and consumer skills. Higher level skills of decision making, planning, and organizing are emphasized through an extended group day in which the same therapist-client dyads (who work together one to one) participate. The group meets 1 day per week from 9:30 A.M. to 3:00 P.M. The therapist-client dyads take turns leading the day's activities, with the therapist providing only as much assistance as needed. The individual with brain injury assumes increasingly greater responsibility for the planning and leading of the activities.

One group decided on a format that includes some routine agenda items and some time for activities selected by the coleaders. The coleaders are responsible for arriving 30 minutes before the group starts in order to write the agenda for the day on the flip chart and take care of any other advance preparations. The basic format for the day is shown in Figure 18.3.

MEASUREMENT OF OUTCOMES

The problem of how to define and measure the outcomes of cognitive remediation is complex, particularly since intervention is so individualized at the point of community reentry. Intervention outcomes may be affected by such variables as the severity of neuropsychological impairments, emotional disturbances, age at onset, educational level, amount of time postinjury, economic resources, substance abuse, previous access to therapy, family dynamics, and so forth. One way to measure outcomes is simply to look at whether, following cognitive remediation, an individual has met his or her personal goals. However, the major drawback to this

9:30 A.M.–10:00 A.M.	Socialization
10:00 A.M.–11:00 A.M.	Personal sharing
11:00 A.M.–11:15 A.M.	Break
11:15 A.M.– 2:40 P.M.	Activity varies*
2:40 P.M.– 3:00 P.M.	Cleanup and review

Figure 18.3. Basic schedule for group intervention agenda. (*Activities may include trips to museums, movies, a local park for whiffleball, bowling, lunch out, board games, videotaping and playback—whatever.) (*Note:* Including the therapist-client dyads in the group rather than having one group leader offers the opportunity to follow up, within a supportive peer group, issues that surface during one-to-one therapy, and vice versa. It also provides sufficient staff for trips in the community to assist persons with mobility impairments and impaired safety awareness, and to provide transportation as needed.)

method is that there are insufficient standardized data from which to draw conclusions about the efficacy of cognitive remediation for individuals with brain injury in general. In a study of community readaptation outcomes, Fryer and Haffey (1987, p. 56) defined the following as desired outcomes: 1) reduction of the brain-injured individual's need for supervision in the residential setting, and 2) role restitution (i.e., return to vocational or educational activities, even if this required a job change or a reduction in the number of hours each week the person with brain injury engaged in such activities).

These outcome criteria seem logical, especially since they provide a means of estimating the amount of case dollars saved (e.g., the costs of supervision provided through home health aides, which may be reduced or unnecessary following therapy, can be extrapolated over the individual's lifetime to estimate the long-term benefits). However, more specificity may be desired as a means of evaluating intervention approaches and determining where to put more emphasis (e.g., a measure of job retention at various levels of employment—part- or full-time volunteer, sheltered, supported, or competitive employment without a supportive approach). Research related to outcomes of cognitive remediation

during community reentry of persons with traumatic brain injury is needed.

SUMMARY

Impairments in cognitive functioning diminish the efforts of individuals with brain injury to function successfully in the community. In particular, cognitive impairments compromise psychosocial and family functioning and limit one's potential for independent living and employment.

As the number of community reentry programs has increased, there has been greater awareness among rehabilitation specialists and case managers of the need to provide cognitive remediation for effective community living. Various cognitive remediation approaches have been described in the literature, but few approaches for use during community reentry have been discussed.

Cognitive remediation approaches must facilitate reentry into the community at the earliest possible time (i.e., as soon as some degree of success can be assured based on level of functioning). Since cognitive abilities are used in organizing and executing all purposeful activities, virtually any activity can be utilized for purposes of cognitive remediation. If the activity is to be a basis for cognitive remediation, however, the objective(s) of the activity, the specific tasks, and means of evaluation must be clearly specified.

Functional gains are most easily achieved when cognitive remediation is carried out in the client's home and community and involves activities that have high interest to the individual. This approach to cognitive remediation is advocated. The model presented in this chapter emphasizes the individual's needs, variable scheduling to coincide with the needs of the individual and his or her family, a combination of individual and group intervention, transdisciplinary therapy rendered on an extended one-to-one basis, a systematic reduction of therapy, and ongoing functional evaluations.

REFERENCES

Ben-Yishay, Y., & Prigatano, G. (1990). Cognitive remediation. In M. Rosenthal, E.R. Griffith, M.R. Bond, & J.D. Miller (Eds.), *Rehabilitation of the adult and child with traumatic brain injury* (pp. 393–409). Philadelphia: F.A. Davis.

Ben-Yishay, Y., Silver, S.M., Piasetsky, E., & Rattok, J. (1987). Relationship between employability and vocational outcome after intensive holistic cognitive rehabilitation. *Journal of Head Trauma Rehabilitation, 2*(1), 35–48.

Cervelli, L. (1990). Re-entry into the community and systems of posthospital care. In M. Rosenthal, E.R. Griffith, M.R. Bond, & J.D. Miller (Eds.), *Rehabilitation of the adult and child with traumatic brain injury* (pp. 463–475). Philadelphia: F.A. Davis.

Condelucci, A., & Gretz-Lasky, S. (1987). The concept of social role valorization in community-based programming. *Journal of Head Trauma Rehabilitation, 2*(1), 49–56.

Deutsch, P.M. (1989). Family-centered rehabilitation. In P.M. Deutsch & K.B. Fralish (Eds.), *Innovations in head injury rehabilitation* (pp. 2-1–2-10). Albany, NY: Matthew Bender.

Dougherty, R.M., & Radomski, M.V. (1987). *The cognitive rehabilitation workbook: A systematic approach to improving independent living skills in brain-injured adults*. Rockville, MD: Aspen.

Fryer, J., & Fralish, K. (1989). Cognitive rehabilitation. In P.M. Deutsch & K.B. Fralish (Eds.), *Innovations in head injury rehabilitation* (pp. 7-1–7-35). Albany, NY: Matthew Bender.

Fryer, L.J., & Haffey, W.J. (1987). Cognitive rehabilitation and community readaptation: Outcomes from two program models. *Journal of Head Trauma Rehabilitation, 2*(3), 51–63.

Jennett, B. (1990). Scale and scope of the problem. In M. Rosenthal, E.R. Griffith, M.R. Bond, & J.D. Miller (Eds.), *Rehabilitation of the adult and child with traumatic brain injury* (pp. 3–8). Philadelphia: F.A. Davis.

Prigatano, G. (1986). *Neuropsychological rehabilitation after brain injury*. Baltimore: Johns Hopkins University Press.

Sohlberg, M.M., & Mateer, C.A. (1989). *Introduction to cognitive rehabilitation theory and practice*. New York: Guilford Press.

Wolfensberger, W. (1983). Social role valorization: A proposed new term for the principle of normalization. *Journal of Mental Retardation, 21*, 234–239.

CHAPTER 19

Cognitive Rehabilitation Services in Home and Community Settings

TAMARA B. STORY

Traditionally, rehabilitation efforts have focused on the period immediately following incidence of brain injury, trauma, or stroke (Condelucci, Cooperman, & Seif, 1987). This is due partly to services being provided in the hospital setting with insurers' reimbursement requirements influencing treatment guidelines. There was some consensus that after spontaneous recovery there would be little or no progress. Evidence is now emerging that this is not necessarily true for persons with traumatic brain injury (Bigler, 1990). It appears that recovery of function continues for up to 10 years postinjury (Sbordone, 1989). Recent technological advances keep more head-injured persons alive and also reduce the effects of the injury (Wehman & Goodall, 1990). Spin-offs from the technological explosion of the space age provide prosthetic devices and adaptive environments that facilitate greater participation in the community, at work, and in the home. In sum, there are more persons who survive the injury, longer periods of recovery, and greater potential recovery. Unfortunately, this is linked to spiraling costs due to lengthy hospitalizations, use of expensive technology, and rising health care costs. An alternative to the traditional medical model must be explored (Zola, 1986).

Providing services for persons with brain injury in their homes and communities is an alternative. The optimal time for initiating home/community services varies with each client. Depending on the complexity and severity of the injury, the appropriate time can range from emergency room discharge to several years postinjury. There are indications that providing long-term services for traumatically brain-injured persons in isolated settings, using a medical model, is of questionable validity. Notable indicators include practices such as mainstreaming in schools and deinstitutionalization of persons with developmental disabilities or psychiatric disorders, laws that identify the needs of and mandate services for persons with a wide range of disabilities (Condelucci, 1990), and research in vocational (Rhoades, 1990), visual (Proteae, 1989), and cognitive areas (Wehman & Kreutzer, 1990).

In the home/community setting, persons with traumatic brain injury can receive clinical services, computer-assisted services, and community reentry services. Most of the traditional clinical services can be provided in the home or in a free-standing office/agency with easy access to the community. Computer-assisted therapy is particularly amenable to the home setting and can be used for process, skill, and functional task training (Engum, Sbordone, & Story, 1987; Story & Sbordone, 1988). Community reentry activities should, by their very nature, be provided in the client's actual community, and may include instruction in activities of daily living, and recreational and vocational services.

Providing these services in the setting in which they will be performed independently increases the likelihood that the ability to perform tasks learned in therapy will carry over into new settings, and that generalization will occur when new tasks that require use of some of the same skills must be learned. Additionally, frequent exposure to family members affords therapists the opportunity to understand better the family's dynamics, expectations, and ability to assist in the rehabilitation process (Story, 1989). Performance in the real world—where clerks ask unexpected questions, where there is no one to provide the cue needed to remember to use a checklist, and where two or three activities require quick and simultaneous processing—provides an opportunity for realistic evaluation of strengths and weaknesses necessary for effective, efficient intervention, and appropriate long-term planning.

This chapter discusses therapeutic intervention in the home/community setting. Included in the definition of the home/community setting is a free-standing clinic with ready access to community services and operating on a nonmedical model. Appropriate clients, types of intervention, use and choice of strategies and devices, and setting up a home program are addressed. References to case studies are included throughout the chapter to illustrate the topics discussed.

APPROPRIATE CLIENTS

Traumatically brain-injured persons of all ages, and all cognitive and physical levels are discharged to home from acute care and rehabilitation facilities. Reasons for discharge include: "reached potential," "inappropriate for program," "family wants him [her] at home," "depleted funds," and the like. Discharge, for many clients, is not the end. Rather, it is frequently the beginning of a long journey. A new and altered person must now learn how to deal with the changed expectations, and dreams of a former lifestyle. This section addresses home/community intervention across different ages, and different cognitive and physical levels.

Age

Clients of all ages can be served in their homes. In particular, working with infants and young children in their homes is ideal. Suddenly removed from everything familiar, subjected to strange and frightening procedures in unfamiliar environments, infants and toddlers cannot help but be frightened and confused at a rehabilitation center. Even outpatient services impose the strain of travel and an unfamiliar environment on an already impaired system. Therapy in the home permits the child to focus energy on the therapy task, not on adapting to the sights and sounds of a new environment.

In addition to using a stable, familiar environment, services in the home provide a forum for modeling approaches to learning and behavior control. The frequent opportunity to observe child-therapist interactions provides parents with a model for daily interactions. The presence of the therapist in the home facilitates discussion of problems and planning. It provides the therapist with the opportunity to explain how the unstructured activities of a birthday party at a pizza parlor can precipitate behavior problems, and to give suggestions for preventing future disruptions. Once families become accustomed to therapists in their homes, they become open about problems and about asking for help. The therapist becomes a person with whom they do not have to pretend that everything is all right.

A therapist's work with adults in the home setting helps families to develop a more realistic picture of abilities and sheds light on the "it can be done at home" myths. Everyone working in rehabilitation has heard "But that's not the way we do it at home," or "She can do it at home." Sometimes the family is seeing the world through rose-colored glasses; sometimes the client can do it at home, but is getting maximum assistance; sometimes cooking a meal is fixing a peanut-butter sandwich; and sometimes the client really can do it. The only way to dispel these myths is for the therapist to be in the home. It may be that the client can cook because someone does all of the preparation and cues him or her. It may be that the noise in the clinic is too distracting. It may be that the client can do it, but that it takes 4 hours to complete a 30-minute task. By working in the home, therapists are better able to determine if there really are myths and are then able to use that information for future planning.

A therapist who observes family dynamics in their natural setting develops insight as to why a client may not appear motivated to learn a new skill or use a specific strategy. Teaching meal planning and "from scratch" food preparation is not going to be meaningful if the family eats fast food, pot pies, and packaged foods. Teaching use of a hygiene routine that includes daily baths is not going to succeed if the rest of the family bathes only twice a week. Trying to establish good work habits and routines is not going to work in a family where finessing the welfare system is considered a talent. Teaching skills for independence may be undermined if a family member receives insurance reimbursement for care and supervision. Working in the home makes it possible to establish goals that the family can support.

Cognitive Level

Traumatically brain-injured clients functioning at Levels II–VIII of the Rancho Los Amigos Scale of Cognitive Functioning (Hagen, Malkmus, & Durham, 1979) can benefit from services provided in the home/community setting (see Table 19.1). Adequate medical and attendant care is necessary at the lower levels. Feeding and sensory stimulation programs can be structured for caregivers, and monitored using checklists. Although home-based therapy at Levels II–V may not generally be the intervention course of choice, there are times when it is necessary and appropriate. Financial resources may be exhausted, family members may not be able to deal with institutionalization, or there may be special factors—as was the case with G.G., where staffing inconsistencies and her extreme sensitivity to sound and environmental changes were too stimulating.

G.G. received a severe head injury in a car-pedestrian accident approximately 2 years prior to referral. She remained at the original acute care hospital for postacute rehabilitation for approximately 9 months. Over the next 15 months, she was in three postacute/transitional programs for periods of up to 3 months each, with interim intervention provided by home health agencies. An occupational therapist was the only professional to see her consistently during this 15-month period.

G.G. was functioning at Level V of the Rancho Los Amigos Scale (Hagen et at., 1979). She had been noted to have 30 agitated spells during a single session at the last facility. In addition to her cognitive deficits, G.G. had spastic paraplegia, and had a nonfunctional left hand and a moderately ataxic right hand. Varying performance on all standardized measures was reported (e.g., Reading Comprehension Battery for Aphasia [La Pointe & Horner, 1984], Minnesota Test for the Differential Diagnosis of Aphasia [Schuell, 1965], Wechsler Adult Intelli-

Table 19.1. Descriptive summary of levels of the Rancho Los Amigos Scale of Cognitive Functioning (Hagen, Malkmus, & Durham, 1979)

Level	Description
I	No response: Client does not respond to external stimuli and appears to be asleep.
II	Generalized response: Client reacts to external stimuli in nonspecific, inconsistent, and nonpurposeful manner with stereotypic and limited responses.
III	Localized response: Client responds specifically and inconsistently with delays to stimuli, but may follow simple commands for motor action.
IV	Confused, agitated: Client exhibits bizarre, nonpurposeful, incoherent or inappropriate behaviors; has no short-term recall; and attention is short and nonselective.
V	Confused, inappropriate, nonagitated: Client gives random, fragmented, and nonpurposeful responses to complex or unstructured stimuli. Simple commands are followed consistently, memory and selective attention are impaired, and new information is not retained.
VI	Confused, appropriate: Client gives context-appropriate, goal-directed responses; dependent upon external input for direction. There is carry-over for relearned tasks, but not for new tasks; recent memory problems persist.
VII	Automatic, appropriate: Client behaves appropriately in familiar settings, performs daily routines automatically, and shows carry-over for new learning at lower than normal rates. Client initiates social interactions, but judgment remains impaired.
VIII	Purposeful, appropriate: Client orients and responds to the environment, but language and abstract reasoning abilities are decreased relative to premorbid levels.

From Wiig, E.H., Alexander, E.W., & Secord, W. (1988). Linguistic competence and levels of cognitive functioning in adults with traumatic closed head injury. In H.A. Whitaker (Ed.), *Neuropsychological studies of nonfocal brain damage* (p. 189). New York: Springer-Verlag; used with permission.

gence Scale–Revised [Wechsler, 1981]). On initial contact, G.G.'s accuracy to the question "Is your name _____?" was approximately 60%, with both false-negative and false-positive responses. Her ability to inhibit was severely reduced: She would try to pry a block out of the therapist's hand before given a command, and responses to pointing tasks occurred almost before the command. Her attentional processes were impaired: A person walking on the carpet 15 feet behind her during therapy could distract her.

Initial intervention with G.G. consisted of shaping a reliable response using successive approximation, structuring tasks to control for impulsivity, and controlling for environmental distraction. A format of "Listen," command, "Think," "Do it" was used. Monthly team meetings were held and included a speech-language pathologist, occupational and physical therapists, the case manager, and G.G.'s mother. The family was counseled to maintain a consistent schedule and a low-stimulation environment. During the first 6 months, there was a decrease in overall agitation and impulsivity and an increase in reliability of responses. At the end of 6 months, G.G.'s ability to inhibit responses and focus attention had increased, as demonstrated by her ability to pick up two of four pictures with 80% accuracy with a 4-second delay between the first and second command. Frequency and intensity of agitation decreased and the occupational and physical therapists reported greater ability to inhibit as well as less impulsivity.

The long-term goal for G.G. is placement in a foster care or nursing facility that specializes in head injury. This case study illustrates that although home services may not ordinarily be considered appropriate for clients functioning at lower cognitive levels, they can, in some circumstances, be quite appropriate and even necessary.

Physical Level

Traumatically brain-injured persons at all levels of physical recovery can be served in the home or community, ranging from persons such as S.S., who has quadriplegia and is dependent on a ventilator, to persons with no physical impairments, such as T.D. and W.D. Therapy for physical impairments resulting from neurological damage generally does not require most of the expensive and bulky equipment found in physical therapy departments. Frequently, intervention can be provided at home using a mat and other inexpensive equipment. Endurance can be maintained or increased through the use of community facilities such as health clubs and community centers, and through participation in teams and leagues. Exercise equipment is readily available and inexpensive, and its purchase is cost-effective when used to extend therapeutic time.

TYPES OF INTERVENTION

Clinical, community reentry, and computer-assisted interventions are all suitable for the home/community setting. Familiarity with the person-injury-environment-outcome (PIEO) interaction paradigm (Sbordone, 1987) is helpful when determining types of intervention. This paradigm requires one to recognize that each client is unique. Intervention must be planned in light of complex interactions involving the preinjury self (physical, emotional, behavioral, intellectual), the constellation of deficits resulting from the injury, the varied and changing environmental demands, and the outcomes (failures, loss of friends, reduced vocational potential) that occur during the recovery period. The following sections discuss types of intervention, using case examples to illustrate the combination of types and methods of therapy available to meet the unique needs of individual clients.

Clinical Services

Clinical services are delivered using traditional, process-oriented, and simulation methods. In the traditional method, therapy uses materials from workbooks and kits and is directed toward improving identified deficits in areas such as sequencing, categorizing, and deductive thinking. An example of this approach would be the use of Mind Benders (Harnadek, 1979), which requires the elimination of possible choices until only one remains (Adamovich, Henderson, & Auerbach, 1985).

In the process method, the focus is on remediation of the underlying cognitive process. Examples can be found in the work of Bracy

(1986) and Sohlberg and Mateer (1989). Activities might include having a client listen for the letter "d" followed by the letter "a," to improve attention. This method draws heavily on the brain behavior model postulated by Luria (1973, 1980) and requires knowledge of the dynamic relationship between the cognitive processes and brain structures.

In a simulation approach, the environment and task demands of real-life jobs and activities are re-created. Using behavior modification techniques of shaping and progressive approximation, skills such as checkbook maintenance, typing, photocopying, and more complex secretarial tasks can be established. Sbordone (1989) reported use of an elaborate simulator for retraining truck drivers in the Soviet Union. Glisky and Schacter (1987) trained a densely amnestic person to perform complicated data entry tasks through simulation. The types of activities for which the simulation method can be used are limited by time, space, and cost. Preparation of materials and monitoring of progress can be time-consuming.

All of these approaches can be used in home and community settings. It is not necessary, and probably not wise, to use only one approach. To obtain desirable outcomes, several methods are frequently combined. A therapist's creativity and understanding of the PIEO interaction are often limiting factors. The following case study illustrates such a combination of clinical methods and types of intervention.

Teaching banking skills to D.T.—who, in addition to tunnel vision and visuoperceptual problems, had severe cognitive and memory problems—involved the use of all types of intervention. In D.T.'s initial attempts to write a check, she consistently failed to fill in various portions of the check and was unable to enter information in a check register on the correct lines or to perform the mathematical operations necessary to keep a running balance. The first time she went to the bank, she attempted to enter the building through the terminal where money card transactions are made. Once inside the bank, she was unable to locate the teller's window and, when it was pointed out, was unable to navigate the roped-off area unassisted.

Clinical intervention involved both traditional and process techniques. Visual scanning, mental manipulation, and shifting attention were addressed with both computer programs and paper-and-pencil tasks. The traditional technique of using workbook sheets to practice check writing was used. Practice was structured in three sequentially more difficult steps: transaction entry; entry and calculation of new balance; and entry, calculation, and transaction identification. Once D.T. could consistently enter transactions on single worksheets, she was given 5–10 single transactions (checks, deposits, withdrawals, bank fees) to enter each therapy session. At the end of a session, she calculated and checked her balance to see if errors had occurred and she then made the necessary corrections. The final step required D.T. to determine the type of transaction by giving her statements such as: "Your paycheck is for $50. You need to keep $10 to pay for food, and the bank has charged you $5 for writing a bad check."

As part of her community program, D.T. went to the bank, post office, and other businesses with similar settings. She worked on scanning the building from afar to find the entrance, stopping once she entered the bank to find the lines, scanning the tellers and listening for auditory cues that it was her turn to move forward, completing her transactions with prefilled forms, finding her way out of the building, and finding her car in the parking lot. Future financial goals involve developing a method for budgeting and an awareness of costs associated with independent living. It is anticipated that she will be able to use a simple computer program for budgeting. Introduction of the budgeting process that includes unexpected expenditures can be provided using a computer simulation. Development of an awareness of costs will be introduced by going to view apartments for rent.

In addressing D.T.'s check-writing and financial management skills, all types of intervention were used. It became clear that just teaching D.T. to write a check or keep a check register would not be sufficient. It was necessary to involve many other areas and skills to get to the final goal. The ideal setting for this interweaving and crossing of processes, goals, and disciplines that must occur to reach the ultimate goal of maximum functioning and independence is the community in which a person has lived and will continue to live.

Community Reentry Activities

Community reentry includes daily living, vocational, and recreational activities. Each is now discussed.

Daily Living

Daily living activities are performed in the home and community and include feeding, dressing, hygiene, writing, phone use, money management, time management, homemaking, driving, and transportation (McNeny, 1990). The therapist needs to observe the client in the client's own home in order to create useful daily routines and strategies. Otherwise, it is possible to anticipate neither the idiosyncrasies of a person's environment, nor the family dynamics that influence the ability to carry over and to generalize new skills. After observing a person perform a task —for example, a morning routine—a therapist can devise appropriate strategies (ones that meet physical-motoric demands and the client's and family's ability to implement them). A therapist who is in the home and in regular contact with the family is better able to predict what will and will not work.

Vocational

Vocational activities can be performed in the home or community; can be volunteer or paid; and can be sheltered, supported, or competitive (Wehman & Moon, 1988). The limiting factors are the therapist's creativity and knowledge of the traumatically brain-injured client's abilities. When told a vocational counselor would determine if a client was employable, a case manager recently replied, "Everyone is employable, it's just finding the right job." To find the right job, the counselor must know the client and scour the community. Traditional placement procedures and training may not find that special employer who is willing to give the client a chance.

Both knowledge of the client's abilities and creativity of the therapist were demonstrated in the case of R.D., a man with spastic quadriplegia with very high-level cognitive deficits, the most debilitating of which was decreased executive functioning as evidenced by a lack of motivation, an inability to initiate, and an inability to change behavior based on feedback. R.D. had been a successful farmer until he sustained a severe head injury in an auto accident approximately 10 years ago. He remained at Level II–III of the Rancho Los Amigos Scale (Hagen et al., 1979) for almost 1 year until shunted. Since that time, he has made slow but steady progress. After the initial year in the hospital, he lived at home until moving to an adult foster care home for persons with head injury 2 years ago. R.D. lived in a small farm community with a limited number of vocational options. To obtain a position for him, the vocational counselor started at one end of town and went to all businesses, churches, and any establishments that might be able to use volunteers. She explained that she was looking for a job that a person in a wheelchair who had severe motor and speech impairments could perform. She assured prospective "employers" that R.D. would have as much support as he needed, for as long as necessary.

Initial placement was in a church office, folding and stuffing bulletins. The speech-language pathologist who had worked with R.D. in the past provided the employer with information as to what could be expected from R.D. and advised of potential pitfalls. She also analyzed cognitive aspects of the task and provided R.D. with instructions and a checklist to use for work. Since the therapist was the member of the rehabilitation team closest to R.D., she also provided support when transportation and scheduling problems occurred. Support involved only a few hours of her time for 1 month.

Because R.D. needed to be occupied in a meaningful way for more hours a week than the church job provided, the vocational counselor continued to look for additional volunteer work. After several months, placement in a grocery store was added. Responsibilities in this setting involved scanning shelves for items that were misshelved, and sorting and crushing aluminum and steel cans returned for recycling. For this job, the occupational therapist was called upon to analyze motoric demands, and the speech-language pathologist once again looked at the cognitive demands, served as a liaison with the employer, provided some preplacement training for sequencing techniques, and monitored performance through direct observation and telephone contact. R.D. performed so well on this job that his hours were increased and the employer offered to pay for his services.

S.S., a man who was ventilator dependent and had quadriplegia with very minor cognitive deficits, illustrates a very different set of intervention needs. S.S.'s employer wanted him to return to his job as a patent agent. His rehabilitation team consisted of a case manager and a vocational specialist from a medical management company, and a speech-language pathologist with experience in cognitive rehabilitation and augmentative systems. Over a period of 1 year, the speech-language pathologist investigated eye gaze, voice recognition, and keyboard emulators operated with a bite switch. A keyboard emulator and a voice recognition system were each leased for 2–3 months, to permit S.S. time first to learn to use them and then to make comparisons. His employer provided both the software that S.S. had used premorbidly and actual projects with deadlines. The employer also provided technical support to assure that S.S.'s computer system would be 100% compatible with the company's system.

During the trial periods, the speech-language pathologist provided training on the use of the systems, technical support, and evaluations of the systems based on factors such as percentage of hits and speed. Due to reduced lung capacity, S.S. fatigued rapidly with the voice system and made more errors. He chose the less technologically sophisticated keyboard emulator. Without the opportunity to preview these systems in the environment where he would be working—in this case, his home—S.S. may not have had enough time to discover the effect of fatigue when using the voice system. He may have incorrectly assumed that the fatigue was a result of the efforts involved in traveling to a center. The opportunity to perform in the work environment prevented what could have been a costly error not only in dollars but in the loss of S.S.'s full potential for vocational success. Thus, by pro-

viding therapeutic intervention in the environment where the job or activity is to be performed, the chance of success is maximized.

Recreational

While in a rehabilitation center, a person can develop the physical and intellectual skills needed for recreational activities. Once that person returns home, sources or resources to continue these activities still must be provided. Even a client with severe impairment can participate in recreational activities in some manner. Rehabilitation team members are responsible for identifying activities and locating groups and facilities available in the client's community. If the client has not developed recreational skills and interests, he or she should be helped to do so. Once recreational outlets have been established, compensatory strategies should be used to assure that long-term scheduling and follow through will occur.

Computer-Assisted Interventions

The technology of the space age has given us a powerful therapeutic tool: the computer. The question of whether we should use computers has given way to asking how we should use computers. When answering this question, the following guidelines must be taken into consideration:

Clinicians must know how to operate the system.

Intervention must be based on theoretically grounded goals.

Computer-assisted intervention must be part of a total rehabilitation program.

Software must be matched to the client.

Usage must be ethical.

There are many advantages to using computers (Table 19.2), and a wide array of applications:

1. Drill and practice
2. Remediation
3. Tutorial
4. Testing
5. Simulation
6. Problem solving
7. Exploratory discovery

Table 19.2.   Advantages of using computers

Computers can:
Allow for stimulus control
  Duration
  Display constance
  Random presentation
Provide immediate feedback
Be reinforcing
Provide repetition
Enable efficient data collection and analysis
Be cost-effective
Serve as an expansion of intervention time
Facilitate independence
Serve as teaching assessment tools
Be interactive
Allow for unlimited gradations of difficulty and
  stimulus control
Increase motivation and self-esteem
Provide vocational applications
Serve as an organizer for financial and daily
  tasks

One of the major advantages of using computers in a home setting is the cost-effective expansion of intervention time. Software selection should be based on a careful evaluation of the client's cognitive profile, the demands of the program, and where the computer program fits into the total rehabilitation plan at a particular time and place. For a person located in an isolated area, computer-assisted therapy can provide organized, structured stimulation and skill practice on a daily basis. Progress can be monitored through client-completed performance records, disk-stored data, and print-outs. Assistance in operating the system and modifying the instruction sheets can be provided by caregivers, with minimal instructions from the therapist.

Computers should be used with the same care and planning as any other tool or technique. Computer-assisted therapy should be used only as part of a total rehabilitation plan based on a careful analysis of a client's needs, goals, and priorities. It should reflect the theoretical bias of the therapy team, be it restoration, compensation, or a combination of the two. When considering the use of computers, rather than only asking *how* to use them, one should also ask: *Who* should use them? *What* should they be used for? *When* should they be used? *Why* should they be used? Only after considering all of these questions should computer-assisted therapy or any

other techniques be a part of cognitive rehabilitation. (For a more in-depth discussion of computer-assisted therapy, the reader is referred to Chapter 13, this volume.)

M.L. provides an example of integrating computer-assisted therapy with the traditional approach in a home/community setting. Prior to the car accident in which he became a paraplegic and sustained a closed head injury, M.L. taught junior high school, coached track, and hunted with his friends. After the accident, he was confined to a wheelchair and had problems with attention, memory, and higher cognitive processing. Following acute hospitalization, M.L., who was a private and quiet man, chose to receive his therapies at home rather than at a rehabilitation center. The case manager arranged for a therapist experienced in computer-assisted intervention to set up a program to supplement traditional intervention. During the first year, there was one computer-assisted session a month, with additional contacts by telephone. Intervention was coordinated, with speech-language and occupational therapy providing traditional activities. In addition to software addressing cognitive process deficits, software to supplement the traditional speech-language and occupational therapy activities was provided.

At the end of the first year postinjury, M.L. resumed coaching track with moderate assistance and support from a fellow teacher. After a 2-month summer break, M.L. requested that the sessions to direct the computer-assisted portion of his program be increased to weekly, as he felt it was the most helpful intervention at that time. Weekly sessions were designed to review records from the past week, observe performance in order to modify the program, teach new programs and implement process training, and teach the use of strategies. Areas addressed using the computer were attention, speed of verbal and visual processing, mental manipulation, information processing, organization, sequencing, reasoning, problem solving, receptive and expressive language skills, word finding, and word processing. M.L. spent 1–2 hours each day on these activities. During this time, M.L. was encouraged to become responsible for his personal and home care and to participate in community and school activities. He also began using a day planner system to organize his schedule and compensate for memory problems.

Two years postinjury, M.L. coached track without special support. Two and one-half years postinjury, he returned to full-time teaching and coached track in the spring. Prior to returning to the classroom, M.L. was assisted in organizing lesson plans and developing strategies for remembering names. Classroom observations, videotaping, and consultations with school administrators were planned to facilitate reintegration.

The next fall, 3 years post injury, M.L. added the position of head football coach to his full teaching load. Although M.L. has returned to his prior level of employment, he still has times when, as his wife says, "he is very head injured." When he becomes fatigued or ill, his flexibility decreases, word-finding problems occur, and his processes and problem-solving abilities decrease.

USE OF COMPENSATORY AIDS

In accordance with the definition of "rehabilitate" in *Webster's Ninth New Collegiate Dictionary,* regardless of our theoretical bias, we must use every possible resource "to bring or restore someone to a condition of health or useful and constructive activity" (1986, p. 993). In the home/community setting, this includes the use of compensatory aids to assure that the client is performing at the highest level possible commensurate with his or her abilities. There are a large number of compensatory aids (electronic, paper, and mental) that can be used. This section reviews some general types of compensatory aids, discusses and provides case examples for some aids that are particularly useful in the home/community setting, and discusses the need to choose them carefully.

Strategies, Techniques, and Devices

Compensatory aids being used by traumatically brain-injured clients to lead useful and constructive lives include:

1. Checklists
2. Thinking and problem-solving strategies
3. Electronic devices

4. Mnemonics
5. Visual imagery
6. Preview, question, read, state, and test (PQRST) approach (Wilson, 1984, 1987) *or* Survey, question, read, recall, and review (SQR³) approach (Davidson, 1986)
7. Computers
8. Day planners

Checklists can be used to aid organization and memory, and to establish procedural memory for daily routines. They can be used by anyone to bypass the need to remember procedures, lists, and sequences. It is beneficial to use checklists after a brain injury because previously automatic acts (walking, talking, thinking) now demand large amounts of cognitive effort, leaving the client with decreased resources to use for other tasks.

Checklists must be developed on an individual basis. A generic checklist for morning hygiene will probably be ineffective because it does not account for previously established sequences, or for physical and social factors. W.D., a high school student with moderate memory problems, was always forgetting parts of his morning routine. Therapy was provided in his home prior to the beginning of his reduced school day. Often, W.D. was not ready when the therapist arrived. The therapist observed the physical layout and the family dynamics, talked to his mother, and with W.D. developed a very detailed checklist. Over a period of several months, the checklist was reduced to a few cue words and then eventually discarded as W.D. learned to perform the routine without cues.

W.D.'s next experience provides a vivid example of the need to individualize checklists. After graduation, W.D. began to work in the clubhouse of the family's recently purchased golf course. Among his duties was maintaining the bathrooms. Creating a workable checklist for this activity required several revisions. The instruction "Check bathrooms" was on the initial list. Because W.D. is easily distractible, he would check the men's but forget the women's bathroom if someone asked a question while he was going from one to the other. It was also discovered that, although he would check the bathrooms, he did not do anything about the dirty sink, depleted toilet paper, or the like. After several revisions, the final checklist contained specific statements such as, "Clean sink in men's bathroom with Zud."

In W.D.'s case, the checklists were used to condition procedural memory. Checklists are also used to lead a person through a novel event such as getting ready for a wedding, or events where places and items may change. However, the general procedure remains the same. An example of a list for variable items is a transportation checklist in which a person answers specific questions prior to initiation of the event (Figure 19.1). The form can be completed independently or with assistance. It can be used as a checklist during the trip or can be kept in a notebook or pocket for emergencies, if the client has sufficient metacognition to remember to use it. Developing and using checklists are important steps on the road to self-sufficiency.

The structured thinking form (Ylvisaker, 1987) is an expanded checklist that provides structure for analyzing and organizing activities. It should be modified to meet an individual's cognitive profile. The modified structured thinking form in Figure 19.2 was developed for D.T. The layout was reorganized to compensate for scanning deficits and specific questions were added to compensate for reduced executive functioning. Initially, the form was filled in by the therapist prior to a session, to be used as a checklist during cooking and secretarial tasks. As D.T. developed the requisite skills, she was trained to complete sections of the form independently. It is important to note that independent use of the form was dependent on the task. Although D.T. can now use the form for cooking and other familiar tasks, she is unable to perform the necessary task analysis to determine the steps for novel activities. As a result of reduced executive functioning, D.T. seldom generates additional questions for the evaluation section. (For more in-depth discussion of strategies and procedures for improving reasoning and problem solving the reader is referred to Ylvisaker, 1985, 1987.)

The technological advances that are responsible for the increased survival rate after brain injury have also provided low-cost electronic aids. Watches, timers, calendars, tape recorders, dictation devices, digital diaries, telephone dialers, car rings, and car locaters are a few of the readily available products (Parenté & Anderson-Parenté, 1990). These can be used to compensate for problems with organization, information processing, and prospective memory. They can save time, reduce frustration, and increase safety. For clients with reduced information processing abilities because of linguistic or speed of processing deficits, the use of a tape recorder is highly recommended.

T.T., a 22-year-old college student, sustained a severe brain injury and was in a coma for several days after stepping in front of a car. When she attempted to return to her college classes a few months after the accident, she experienced difficulty planning and organizing her study schedule, finding her way around the campus, taking notes in classes, and learning new material at the rate required to pass her classes. T.T. used tape recordings of her classes in conjunction with a day planner and techniques for improving learning to complete her degree.

N.G. had problems with speed of processing for auditory information and interpreting ambiguous and abstract language. As she frequently became upset because she misinterpreted her doctors' recommendations, N.G. learned to record staffings and meetings with professionals. After the meetings, she would listen to the tapes several times. If she was still confused or upset, she would take the tape to a therapist for help with interpretation. Stress was reduced because she did not have to worry about missing information, and fewer calls were made to clarify meeting outcomes and recommendations.

The use of mnemonics and visual imagery is of limited value. To be functional, they require the ability to identify the application, to create the mnemonic, and then to remember it when the information is needed. This is a very complex task for a person with impaired cognition to perform. PQRST (Wilson, 1984, 1987) and SQR[3] (Davidson, 1986) are approaches for learning new material. When using these techniques, people preview or survey the material, then formulate questions based on the survey. They then read, recall, and review or test themselves.

COMMUNITY OUTING FORM

1) **WHERE are you going?**

   Place: _____

   Address: _____

   Phone Number: _____

2) **WHY are you going?**

   _____

   _____

3) **WHEN is this happening?**

   Day of Week: _____

   Date: _____

4) **How much MONEY ($) do you need?**

   _____

   _____

5) **What ITEMS do you need TO BRING?** (library card, shopping list, $, etc.)

   A. _____

   B. _____

   C. _____

6) **TIME information**

   Time of leaving: _____

   Time of return: _____

7) **TRANSPORTATION source** (feet, Dial-A-Ride, bus, private, etc.)

   _____

   _____

8) **Time CONFLICT?** (Check appointment book)

   _____

Cognitive Rehabilitation - November/December 1985   *Developed by Sandra B. Milton*

Figure 19.1.   Example of a community outing form. (From Milton, S.B. [1985]. Compensatory, memory, strategy training: A practical approach for managing persisting memory problems. *Cognitive Rehabilitation, 3*[6], p. 10; Copyright © 1985 by NeuroScience Publishers; reprinted by permission.)

These techniques, taught in speed reading and study skills courses, can serve as an organizational procedure for high-level-functioning clients in high school and college.

Computers can be used not only as a supplement to traditional clinical intervention, as discussed earlier, but also to facilitate graphic expression, to organize finances, to supplement

TASK: _____

Materials: ·—————————————————————————————— □
—————————————————————————————— □
—————————————————————————————— □
—————————————————————————————— □
—————————————————————————————— □
—————————————————————————————— □
—————————————————————————————— □

Time Estimate ——————————

Questions?? Do I understand what I am to do? □
Do I have all of the information I need? □

Plan

Steps

1 _____ □
2 _____ □
3 _____ □
4 _____ □
5 _____ □
6 _____ □
7 _____ □
8 _____ □
9 _____ □
10 _____ □

Review

Are steps correct? yes or no ———————➤ IF NO Make corrections
or
Ask for help
Are materials correct? yes or no

DO IT

Evaluation

1. Was it finished on time?

2. Did you put all materials away?

3. Did you check each step off completely?

4. Is my work acceptable ? (Neat and in order?)

5._____

6.—————————————————————

Figure 19.2.   Example of a modified structured thinking form. (Adapted from Ylvisaker, 1987).

education, and for recreation. Ease of reorganization and increased verbal expression are benefits of word processing. The availability of spelling and grammar checkers and thesauruses makes more polished letters and reports possible. Programs for monitoring finances and balancing checkbooks are available and easy to use. The wide variety of software available makes it possible to find compensatory applications appropriate to the needs of clients of all ages and levels.

At the other end of the technological spectrum from computers, but no less sophisticated, is the Franklin Day Planner (FDP). This planner is an excellent organizer and memory aid for clients with traumatic brain injury. It can be used for planning, organizing, time management, and prospective memory. It is intended for use by executives and professionals with heavy demands for long-term organization and time management. Multinational corporations provide day-long seminars on its use for middle and upper level management. The core of the system consists of a one-page monthly calendar, a daily task list and schedule, note pages, and a daily planning session during which information is transferred from the previous day's notes to the appropriate section. The monthly pages are used for noting appointments where physical presence is required. The daily task list is to be arranged by numbering in order of priority. Items can be placed on this list up to 12 months in advance. The daily schedule is completed by transferring appointments from the monthly page and scheduling time for items from the task list. The note page is used to record any information from conversations, telephone calls, and so forth that will be needed in the future. This information is then indexed in a monthly index or transferred to the task list for the appropriate day (e.g., "telephone Sue to check on 12/1/90 status of registrations" would appear on the 12/1 task list as "T/C Sue (6/20)," to tell the individual to look at notes on 6/20 for the reason for the call). The daily page also has a section of noting expenses. Additional sections for phone numbers, addresses, key and financial information, meeting planning, menu planning and shopping, and the like are available. Binders made from vinyl to full-grain leather are available, making the daily planner's appearance socially acceptable for most people.

The FDP can be used at many levels. Two clients discussed earlier in this chapter—D.T., who was severely impaired, and C.G., who exhibited only high-level cognitive deficits—are good examples of the different uses and methods of establishing use. D.T. had previously used a memory log and did not see the need for a memory aid because "who needs to recall what they had for breakfast." Her initial use of the FDP involved noting doctor and therapy appointments on the monthly calendar. This took many months to establish, including encouraging the family to reinforce its use rather than keeping their own schedules. During this time, D.T. was also asked to fill in her daily therapy schedule. At the beginning of each day, she was given a list of all the therapy modules and approximate completion times. She then planned the order and filled in the daily schedule section. In addition to establishing use of the FDP through consistent practice, this addressed planning, time-management and estimation, and visuospatial problems, and gave D.T. a sense of control and participation. When D.T. progressed to a volunteer job, she kept directions for word processing, structured thinking forms, and checklists in special sections. She also used the notes section for recording oral directions. Establishing use of the FDP as a memory and organizational aid took place over several years, with changes in its use paralleling D.T.'s level of functioning.

For C.G., use of the FDP was established in only a few sessions. C.G., a widow who was managing her household, had notes on dozens of little pieces of paper in books, purses, and drawers. Her receipts and important papers were everywhere from a small safe to brown paper bags. After setting up an organizational system for receipts and papers, C.G. was given an FDP. It took only two sessions to explain the use of the monthly calendar and task list, although she did not initially prioritize the tasks. Over a period of a few months, C.G. incorporated the use of most sections of the planner, including telephone, financial, and key information. She did need encouragement to prioritize tasks and incorporate them in her daily schedule. C.G. independently obtained "frills" for her system, such as compartments to hold receipts, pencils, credit cards, and calculators. She carries her FDP with her at all times, placing it in a backpack together with her purse and other important papers and items in order to free one hand for a cane. Her success with this system is indicated by the vocational counselor's comment that C.G. was able to find any information she did not remember by looking in her planner. It is obvious that C.G. is clearly aware of her problems, and she has sufficient executive functioning to allow her to use the system to its fullest.

Choosing

Determining what compensatory strategies, techniques, or devices to use with specific clients requires careful consideration of the following variables:

Cognitive
Behavioral
Emotional
Physical
Social
Educational
Executive

Both the client and the strategy/technique/device must be profiled using these variables. The client's strengths must be matched with the demands of the strategy/technique/device, making sure that skills the client does not possess are not required.

Failure to consider any one of these variables can result in a client's learning to do something that never gets used in the real world or not learning something that is necessary to function in the real world. R.D., a man with severe dysarthria, appears to be an excellent candidate for an augmentative communication system. He possesses the cognitive, behavioral, physical, and educational skills needed. However, due to his lack of social awareness, he does not perceive the need for an augmentative system. Also, reduced executive functioning causes him not to realize or care that his speech is extremely difficult for people to understand. A degree of intact executive functioning is essential for the effective use of any strategy, technique, or device that

requires a person to make a judgment as to when it needs to be used. Simply put, knowing how to do something is of no value if you do not know when you need to do it.

When choosing strategies, devices, and techniques the therapist must ask:

Is it functional?
Will it be used?

To answer these questions, the therapist should consider the PIEO interaction:

Person: Is it meaningful to him or her?
Injury: Does he or she possess the skills to use or execute it?
Environment: Does it support or encourage its use?
Outcome: Does he or she get something he or she wants from it?

HOME PROGRAM

The entire spectrum of sequelae of brain injury is represented by clients living at home and in the community. They have varied backgrounds, aspirations, and support systems. A set protocol of exercises and activities for reintegration would be difficult to develop, and could not possibly be responsive to the uniqueness of the individual's person-injury-environment-outcome interaction. There are three basic phases in developing an individualized intervention plan: researching, planning, and implementing. Although the phases occur in this order initially, the order is not static and there are many times during the course of recovery that a phase needs to be repeated because of changes in conditions or in the individual.

In the research or exploration phase, therapists must develop a profile of the client, determine available finances and services, and be sensitive to expectations and ambitions. A good understanding of cognitive, behavioral, emotional, social, educational, physical, and executive functioning is necessary for a good profile. The therapist needs to know at what stage the client is in recovery, and what services and approaches have already been attempted. This can be done through a review of records, an interview of client and family, and administration of selected diagnostic tests to fill in the missing information.

Identification of sources of funding is a crucial factor. If resources are severely limited, a therapist must choose the interventions that will result in the greatest *functional* gains in the least time. This can be difficult when one knows that more rigorous intervention could result in greater long-term gains—but, as a house with walls and no roof will offer no protection from a Northern winter, a person who can remember a list of 16 items during therapy will not be helped if he or she cannot remember to turn off the water when the phone rings. In exploring services, the therapist must consider not only the resources available in the therapist's own clinic, but also all resources available in public and private agencies for fee and free. Consideration of how these can be coordinated must be made. Another major consideration when looking at services is the potential provider's knowledge of and experience with brain injury. Lack of experience can be offset by creativeness and a willingness to seek out information. It is possible to provide coordinated interdisciplinary therapy with common goals using therapists and counselors from different agencies if the professionals involved are willing to communicate and compromise when necessary.

Sensitivity to a client's expectations requires the therapist to ask, "Where is it the client wants to go?" rather than, "Where do I think the client can or should go?" It is frequently difficult to blend the client's desires with his or her abilities. Community experiences and discussion help develop awareness of ability.

Once the profile of abilities, financial resources, services, and expectations is established, it is time to design an individualized plan—the second phase. To do this, the therapist must generate both functional long-term goals, identifying both the deficits that will block their attainment and the strengths that will help accomplish them, and initial short-term objectives necessary to work toward the long-term goals.

The third phase is implementation. Of vital importance at this point is an ongoing analysis of what is happening and why. There is a constant movement between planning and implementing, with both occurring at times. As short-term objectives are met, the strategies and processes needed to reach the long-term goals are frequently altered, requiring a reassessment of what the next step needs to be. During this procedure, it is important to consider using all of the types of intervention, strategies, and techniques discussed earlier. It is also important during this phase to keep the family and significant others involved, because their understanding and agreement can make or break a program. Their support by both action and words is crucial. They can provide the therapist with information as to why something is not working and how it might be improved.

SUMMARY AND CONCLUSIONS

Therapeutic intervention in the home/community setting following brain injury is a strong alternative to the traditional medical model. By providing services in the home/community setting, the clinician is better able to assess the PIEO factors and their influence on the client's performance, an essential assessment for planning appropriate, effective intervention.

There are wide ranges in the ages, and cognitive and physical levels of those for whom appropriate intervention can be devised. Clinical, community reentry, and computer-assisted interventions should be integrated in order to meet the unique demands of each client's PIEO interaction. The use of compensatory aids to provide the maximum possible level of independence is essential for a good outcome.

Providing rehabilitation services in the home and community is an exciting and humbling experience. To design solutions to the real-life problems faced by persons with brain injury, therapists must improvise, integrate, and adapt their techniques, devices, and strategies for each individual based on his or her needs.

The final judgment as to the value of cognitive rehabilitation should not be based on performance on tests, or the ability to perform in clinical, sheltered, or contrived settings. It should be based on the ability to successfully meet the challenges found in the setting in which one lives one's life. To maximize success, cognitive rehabilitation services should be provided in this same setting—the head-injured person's home and community.

REFERENCES

Adamovich, B., Henderson, J., & Auerbach, S. (1985). *Cognitive rehabilitation of head injured patients*. Boston: Little, Brown.

Bigler, E.D. (1990). Introduction. In E.D. Bigler (Ed.), *Traumatic brain injury* (pp. 1–9). Austin, TX: PRO-ED.

Bracy, O.L. (1986). Cognitive rehabilitation: A process approach. *Cognitive Rehabilitation, 4*(2), 10–17.

Condelucci, A. (1990). Community factors and successful work reentry. In P. Wehman & J. Kreutzer (Eds.), *Vocational rehabilitation for persons with traumatic brain injury* (pp. 307–321). Rockville, MD: Aspen.

Condelucci, A., Cooperman, S., & Seif, B. (1987). In M. Ylvisaker & E.M. Gobble (Eds.), *Community re-entry for head injured adults* (pp. 301–347). Boston: College-Hill Press.

Davidson, J. (1986). *How to study for success*. Torrance, CA: Davidson & Associates.

Engum, E., Sbordone, R., & Story, T. (1987). Hard talk about software. *Cognitive Rehabilitation, 4*(2), 8–16.

Glisky, E.L., & Schacter, D.L. (1987). Acquisition of domain-specific knowledge in organic amnesia: A training for computer-related work. *Neuropsychologia, 25,* 893–906.

Hagen, C., Malkmus, D., & Durham, P. (1979). Levels of cognitive functioning. In *Rehabilitation of the head injured adult: Comprehensive physical management* (pp. 8–11). Downey, CA: Professional Staff Association of Rancho Los Amigos Hospital.

Harnadek, A. (1979). *Deductive thinking skills*. Pacific Grove, CA: Midwest.

La Pointe, L., & Horner, J. (1984). *Reading Comprehension, Battery for Aphasia*. Tigard, OR: C.C. Publications.

Luria, A.R. (1973). *The working brain: An introduction to neuropsychology*. New York: Basic Books.

Luria, A.R. (1980). *Higher cortical functions in man* (2nd ed.). New York: Basic Books.

McNeny, R. (1990). Daily living skills: The foundation of community living. In J.S. Kreutzer & P. Wehman (Eds.), *Community integration following traumatic brain injury* (pp. 105–113). Baltimore: Paul H. Brookes Publishing Co.

Milton, S.B. (1985). Compensatory memory strategy training: A practical approach for managing persisting memory problems. *Cognitive Rehabilitation, 3*(6), 8–16.

Parenté, R., & Anderson-Parenté, J.K. (1990). Vocational memory training. In J.S. Kreutzer & P. Wehman (Eds.), *Community integration following trau-matic brain injury* (pp. 157–169). Baltimore: Paul H. Brookes Publishing Co.

Proteae, L. (1989). *A sensorimotor basis for motor learning: Evidence indicating specificity of practice*. Manuscript submitted for publication.

Rhoades, D. (1990, April). *Behavior management: A team approach including the TBI person and the family*. Paper presented at Workshops in Traumatic Brain Injury Rehabilitation, Williamsburg, VA.

Sbordone, R.J. (1987). A conceptual model of neuropsychologically based cognitive rehabilitation. In J.M. Williams & C.J. Long (Eds.), *The rehabilitation of cognitive disabilities* (pp. 1–25). New York: Plenum.

Sbordone, R.J. (1989, April). *Recent advances in head injury*. Paper presented at Staff Conference of Head Injury Therapy Services, Midland MI.

Schuell, H. (1965). *Minnesota Test for the Differential Diagnosis of Aphasia*. Minneapolis: University of Minnesota Press.

Sohlberg, M.M., & Mateer, C.A. (1989). *Introduction to cognitive rehabilitation: Theory and practice*. New York: Guilford Press.

Story, T. (1989, June). *Computers as therapeutic tools*. Paper presented in the 13th Annual Post Graduate Course on Rehabilitation of Brain Injured Adults and Children, Williamsburg, VA.

Story, T., & Sbordone, R. (1988). The use of microcomputers in the treatment of cognitive-communicative impairments. *Journal of Head Trauma Rehabilitation, 3*(2), 45–54.

Webster's ninth new collegiate dictionary. (1986). Springfield, MA: Merriam-Webster.

Wechsler, D. (1981). *Wechsler Adult Intelligence Scale–Revised*. New York: Psychological Corporation.

Wehman, P., & Goodall, P. (1990). Return to work: Critical issues in employment. In P. Wehman & J. Kreutzer (Eds.), *Vocational rehabilitation for persons with traumatic brain injury* (pp. 1–17). Rockville, MD: Aspen.

Wehman, P., & Kreutzer, J. (Eds.). (1990). *Vocational rehabilitation for persons with traumatic brain injury*. Rockville, MD: Aspen.

Wehman, P., & Moon, M.S. (Eds.). (1988). *Vocational rehabilitation and supported employment*. Baltimore: Paul H. Brookes Publishing Co.

Wiig, E.H., Alexander, E.W., & Secord, W. (1988). Linguistic competence and levels of cognitive functioning in adults with traumatic closed head injury. In H.A. Whitaker (Ed.), *Neuropsychological studies of nonfocal brain damage* (pp. 186–201). New York: Springer-Verlag.

Wilson, B. (1984). Memory therapy in practice. In B. Wilson & N. Moffat (Eds.), *Clinical management of memory problems* (pp. 89–111). Rockville, MD: Aspen.

Wilson, B. (1987). *Rehabilitation of memory.* New York: Guilford Press.

Ylvisaker, M. (Ed.). (1985). *Head injury rehabilitation: Children and adults.* San Diego: College-Hill Press.

Ylvisaker, M. (1987). A framework for cognitive rehabilitation therapy. In M. Ylvisaker & E.M. Gobble (Eds.), *Community re-entry for head injured adults* (pp. 87–136). San Diego: College-Hill Press.

Zola, I.K. (1986). The medicalization of aging and disability: Problems and prospects. In C. Mahoney, C. Estes, & J. Heumann (Eds.), *Toward a unified agenda.* Berkeley, CA: World Institute in Disability.

CHAPTER 20

Cognitive Rehabilitation in the Workplace

PAUL H. WEHMAN

Traumatic brain injury is rapidly becoming recognized as a problem of epidemic proportions. Annually, in the United States, approximately 400,000 to 500,000 individuals sustain a brain injury of sufficient degree to require intervention, with anywhere from 44,000 to 90,000 sustaining injury that will result in severe, chronic, debilitating impairments (Frankowski, 1986). Persons with severe brain injury typically exhibit cognitive, physical, and/or psychosocial impairments that will inhibit employment and other activities of daily living and adversely affect their quality of life (Klonoff, Costa, & Snow, 1986).

Advanced medical technology has decreased mortality rates and increased life expectancies for persons with severe head injury. Because a significant proportion of these individuals are young adults who are either just beginning or yet to begin their careers, brain injury frequently results in long-term economic hardship on the individuals, their families, and, ultimately, to society (McMordie & Barker, 1988). At each of these levels, the costs of traumatic brain injury are staggering: Recent estimates place the total financial burden in the United States at $6 billion for direct costs such as acute medical care and rehabilitation, and $22 billion for indirect costs, such as lost productivity and wages, ongoing income and health maintenance, and long-term care (Stonnington, 1986).

A significant proportion of the costs of traumatic brain injury can be directly linked to discouraging rates of postinjury employment. Estimates of the percentage of persons with traumatic brain injury who will enter or reenter the competitive work force have generally fallen below 30% (Brooks, McKinlay, Symington, Beat-

tie, & Campsie, 1987). Moreover, estimating the employability of persons with head injury is much more complicated than simply calculating the percentage of those who become employed postinjury. Recent research has indicated that many individuals who return to work do so in less demanding or menial positions, in sheltered employment or volunteer work, or for benevolent employers in positions having no specified duties or accountability (Wehman, Kreutzer, et al., 1989). Some researchers have reported that many who returned to work were not able to maintain employment for any substantial length of time. One study found that individuals who returned to work frequently required assistance from co-workers in performing their duties (Wehman, West, et al., 1989). These findings underscore the difficulties that individuals with severe brain injury experience in attempting to return to productive lives.

A prospective study of vocational outcomes concluded that an individual's ultimate vocational status will be achieved 6 months from the date of injury. Thus, there is a need to enable persons with brain injury to achieve a higher vocational potential. Cognitive rehabilitation in the workplace—by way of supported employment—is a viable means to that end.

SUPPORTED EMPLOYMENT FOR PERSONS WITH TRAUMATIC BRAIN INJURY

Traditional vocational rehabilitation services are time-limited; that is, intervention efforts are concentrated prior to and immediately following job placement. Yet individuals with severe traumatic brain injury frequently fail to maintain employment due to the episodic and unpredictable nature of their impairment, with problems in vocational or social functioning arising days, months, or years following job placement. Recently, a service strategy known as *supported employment,* first conceptualized for individuals with mental retardation and other developmental disabilities, has been utilized with persons with severe traumatic brain injury.

Supported employment became a vocational rehabilitation service option by way of the 1986 Amendments to the Rehabilitation Act (Federal Register, 1987). In those amendments, supported employment is defined as "paid work in a variety of settings, particularly regular work sites, especially designed for handicapped individuals: (1) for whom competitive employment has not traditionally occurred, and (2) who, because of their disability, need intensive ongoing support to perform in a work setting" (p. 30550). This commitment to both time-limited training and long-term support services distinguishes supported employment from traditional vocational placement models. Supported employment is unique in that professional staff provide training and support at the job site once the person is hired and for as long as is necessary. Outcome reports from supported employment projects for persons with severe traumatic brain injury have been cautiously optimistic. These reports have generally indicated that participants have achieved employment earnings and work hours comparable to their preinjury status. Moreover, despite frequent work-related problems, participants have generally maintained stability on the job, and have become reemployed rapidly in the event of job loss (Wehman et al., in press).

It is the purpose of this chapter to discuss how cognitive interventions can occur in the workplace. The use of a job coach can be a very effective means of delivery of cognitive rehabilitation in an individualized fashion for workers with traumatic brain injury. The bulk of this chapter comprises case study descriptions. The chapter concludes with a discussion on public policy and long-term funding issues.

COGNITIVE INTERVENTIONS AT THE JOB SITE

Clearly, cognitive rehabilitation has been a major aspect of services usually provided for persons with traumatic brain injury. Most persons with traumatic brain injury present some form of significant cognitive deficits in memory, planning, thinking, organizing, and/or sequencing. These characteristics are usually critical to some form of successful work reentry.

Traditionally, clients with traumatic brain injury receive medical services for a number of weeks and months postinjury. Eventually, the client is referred to an occupational therapist or psychologist for cognitive retraining. It is during this time that a cognitive retraining program may be provided. Usually, clients come to a clinic or hospital-type setting and receive instruction using computers, workbooks, or other classroom aids. The purpose is to improve cognitive function by stimulating the brain. The advent of personal computers has influenced the direction of many cognitive retraining programs.

Most rehabilitation programs that serve persons with traumatic brain injury offer cognitive retraining programs. Indeed, much of this book is about these very types of programs. Some centers, however, are beginning to question the efficacy of exclusively using clinic-based programs; increasingly, there seems to be a move to provide services in natural environments such as the home, community, and workplace. While many professionals agree that this type of service delivery would enhance the quality and outcome of cognitive retraining, there is usually difficulty in getting staff to these sites. Administratively, it is typically not very convenient for cognitive therapists to drive all over a community. Also, this approach truly necessitates an individualized approach depending on the clients' needs within the particular environment.

The use of a job coach in a supported employment model is a superb means of delivering highly specific cognitive intervention based on the work needs and demands of the job site. Since the job coach is at the work site with the person during employment, the supervisor can call if there is a problem, and cognitive rehabilitation strategies can be crafted directly to the needs of the person and the work environment. Assessment of the work environment, which is described in the next sections, is important in determining what interventions are necessary.

Within this book, ample strategies for cognitive retraining have been delineated. What this chapter does, however, is to show applications of these techniques in a case study format. Several clients with traumatic brain injury who are working in supported employment and who are benefiting from this type of job-coach services are described. The compensatory techniques are also identified.

ASSESSMENT OF JOB REQUIREMENTS IN THE WORK ENVIRONMENT

The job inventory is perhaps the most important aspect of employment evaluation, yet it is one that is rarely conducted thoroughly in most rehabilitation evaluation centers. Table 20.1 provides an outline how to conduct a job inventory for a position as a dishwasher in a community drugstore or restaurant.

There are many types of competitive jobs for clients with traumatic brain injury. Two examples of entry-level positions in food service utility and landscaping are dishwasher and groundskeeper, respectively. An overview of a job inventory for each is provided next.

Dishwasher

The dishwasher's main duty is a sequence of rinsing and stacking dishes, placing them in racks, running them through the dishwashing machine, catching them when they come out, and putting them in the proper places. He or she must work quickly during peak serving times to supply the servers with dishes. Because the dishwasher's work is busy at times, he or she usually works with one or two other people in the dishroom; therefore, he or she must be able to work in a group. Sometimes the dishwasher has to run dishes out to the serving line. This brings the

Table 20.1. Outline for conducting a job inventory for a dishwasher position in a community drugstore or restaurant

I. General Information
  A. Reasons why persons with traumatic brain injury or other severe handicaps are considered for this job
  B. General description of the job
  C. General description of the work setting
  D. General description of the social environment
    1. Information related to fellow workers
    2. Information related to supervision
    3. Information related to special contingencies of the employer

II. Specific skill requirements of the job
  A. Listing of the basic physical/sensory motor skills required
  B. Listing of the basic interpersonal skills required
  C. Listing of the basic language skills (verbal and nonverbal) required
  D. Listing of the basic functional academic skills required
  E. Listing of the basic machine and tool skills required
  F. Listing of the basic hygienic skills required

III. Supportive skills and other information useful
  A. Transportation skills required
  B. Skills related to work preparation
  C. Basic money-management skills useful
  D. Time-telling and time-judgment skills useful
  E. Health code requirements
  F. Informed consent and legal requirements

Note: The above job inventory could be used for a number of different positions (e.g., groundskeeper, stock clerk, packager).

dishwasher into contact with more people, demanding a cheerful attitude. He or she must understand commands because servers or supervisors may ask for certain dishes or silverware that are needed immediately. A quick response is essential.

Groundskeeper

The groundskeeper has to become familiar with a large area of space. His or her primary tasks are sweeping outside, cleaning bathrooms, and picking up trash. The groundskeeper may come into contact with different people, so he or she needs to be polite and have a pleasant attitude. His or her appearance is also important for the same reason.

The groundskeeper works independently and may be given instructions to do something outside the normal routine. He or she must be able to carry out the duty without constant supervision. He or she must be able to recognize signs on doors since the groundskeeper has to enter restrooms and janitorial closets, and may be asked to clean up a particular room such as the auditorium. On occasion, there may be large jobs that require teamwork for completion. The groundskeeper must be willing to accept a break in the routine in order to give extra help when needed.

EVALUATING SOCIAL AND PHYSICAL FEATURES OF THE WORK ENVIRONMENT

After completing an observation and subsequent write-up of a particular job, an evaluator can begin to identify requirements for successful job completion. The next step is to conduct a similar analysis and write-up of the work environment. This will yield information about co-workers, employers, consumers, and the physical layout of the area. Thus, the goal of a viable assessment process is to match the client's competence on a behavioral checklist of general work skills to the requirements from the work environment analysis.

Role of Co-workers

As assessment of the co-workers in the client's work environment must be undertaken. Co-workers play a very significant role—one that cannot be taken lightly—in the long-term job retention of clients with traumatic brain injury. For example, several complaints to the supervisor from co-workers may well influence the supervisor's perception of the client's work performance. Also, co-workers can provide advocacy efforts on behalf of a client, if they choose to do so. They can be good models and/or teachers for how to perform new or complex tasks.

Evaluators and other instructional personnel must ask the following questions in visits to a potential work environment:

1. How many co-workers are in the vicinity of where the client would be?
2. How often do the co-workers interact?
3. What is the rate of co-worker turnover?
4. What is the co-workers' attitude toward management?
5. Are there any other employees with disabilities working there?
6. What is the predominant age of the co-workers?
7. What is the predominant gender of the co-workers?
8. What is the predominant race of the co-workers?
9. Do the co-workers belong to any union organization?

The answers to these questions will not only help in identifying an appropriate placement, but will also provide insight to staff who might be involved in an on-the-job intervention program.

Employer Perceptions

If the employer is not willing to hire an employee with brain injury, then this evaluation need go no further, at least for the time being. However, in most cases, if a job is available and the client is qualified, it is unlikely that a blanket rejection will be forthcoming.

Whether the employer will follow through with promises of employment or back out when the time actually comes to hire must be evaluated. Also, the degree of employer support that will be provided for the client in the initial stages of employment must be determined. Although these two areas are not easy to assess, local rehabilitation counselors can usually provide some information as to how selected employers (or at least industries) react to employees with disabilities. Some employers may be willing to sign short-term contracts on trial employment for workers with traumatic brain injury. This is usually a fairly good indicator of commitment.

A third area that requires assessment is how many supervisors there will be and how their styles differ, if at all. Different requirements for the same job can confuse some workers with brain injury and interfere with performance. Determining which supervisor really has the power in the organization is no easy task, but it is of critical importance to meet with the specific individual who can hire or fire the client.

Physical Layout of Work Environment

The physical design of the work area will play an important part in deciding to make a placement. Narrow doorways, inappropriately designed toilets, or other physical barriers may prohibit persons in wheelchairs from working—despite assurances from the resolutions of the Rehabilitation Act Amendments of 1986 and the passage of the Americans with Disabilities Act in July 1990.

Mobility and orientation requirements for completion of the job should be evaluated at an early point in the work environment analysis. For example, in a groundskeeping position on a college campus it is necessary to be able to find one's way around without getting lost. Although this is a skill often taken for granted, many persons with traumatic brain injury lack it. The ability to maneuver around a work area independently is best taught through an on-the-job training model, since no two work environments are likely to be laid out in the same way.

COMPONENTS OF EFFECTIVE JOB-SITE TRAINING PROGRAM

There are several integral components in successful vocational programs for clients with traumatic brain injury. These elements are briefly outlined and discussed next.

1. Task analysis and compensatory strategies are instrumental in making the job easier for the worker, thus increasing the probability of success. Breaking a social skill or work task into smaller, logically sequenced increments allows the individual to absorb the information more easily. The small increments of behavior are gradually chained together through reinforcement, and thus develop the whole skill. In vocational programming with brain-injured clients, work tasks should be task analyzed by the

teachers before training sessions begin. Eventually, a program notebook of task analyses can be completed and prescribed for each worker.

2. A high degree of structure in the vocational setting and consistency in the approach of job coaches in the initial stages are necessary for optimal performance. Instructions must be consistent and there should be little variation in the methods of presentation and criteria for reinforcement. Initially, the physical environment should be a setting with few distractions. Reinforcers must be individualized for each worker, and it must be clear that they are instrumental in increasing behavior. Often it is difficult to discern what reinforcers will influence work behavior. The job coach must test out different reinforcers and evaluate the effect of each on work performance. Presenting a variety of functional reinforcers initially, on a continuous schedule of reinforcement, and gradually on a more intermittent schedule, will result in acquisition of the desired vocational behavior.

3. Job-site programs that utilize carefully gathered data of workers' performance are most effective in helping to make program modifications and decisions. Workers with traumatic brain injury may make behavioral gains slowly, and the evaluation of program methods is usually subjective and not carefully documented. There are several steps involved in implementing an effective data-based approach to programming: 1) gaining an accurate pretreatment index of the degree (frequency) of behavior; 2) clearly defining the behavior, which must be discrete and observable; 3) charting and graphing gradual improvements, thus providing positive feedback to staff and parents; 4) precisely identifying length of treatment, as well as the effects of treatment on behavior; and 5) gaining an objective index of accountability with parents and administrators.

4. Methods that facilitate the transfer of training and response maintenance must be planned and developed within the overall program. It cannot be expected to occur spontaneously. Persons with traumatic brain injury frequently do not generalize across settings or tasks readily. Methods for enhancing generalization include: 1) varying the stimulus conditions of

training (i.e., using different job coaches and materials); 2) including different co-workers in training; 3) gradually fading reinforcement contingencies and substituting naturally occurring reinforcers, such as attention from co-workers; 4) training skills that have a high probability of being performed daily by the worker and are meaningful in content; and 5) developing self-control techniques (i.e., letting the trainee reinforce himself or herself).

5. Use of color coding, easy-to-hard sequencing, and other learning variables that minimize failure are important in helping workers with traumatic brain injury learn complex tasks. The job coach must take the responsibility for the worker's inability to demonstrate proficiency on the job by making the task easier initially.

With these guidelines in mind, a series of case studies is presented of persons with traumatic brain injury who have been placed competitively through the Medical College of Virginia's supported employment program.

Case Study #1: P.R.

Background Information

P.R. is a 33-year-old male who sustained a severe head injury in an alcohol-related automobile accident in 1975, which resulted in his becoming traumatically brain injured. Prior to his injury, P.R. had no physically related medical problems. As a result of some psychological problems, he had been an inpatient at a psychiatric hospital for 2 weeks. As reported by P.R., this was because he and his parents had not been getting along. He also stated that his parents had put him there to get him off drugs. Reportedly, P.R. was a heavy alcohol and drug abuser. He had had many difficulties with the authorities and had been arrested for being drunk in public, stealing gasoline, using fake IDs, and assaulting a police officer. All of these instances happened while P.R. was a juvenile. As far as educational goals and expectations of himself, P.R. had none. He had dropped out of high school in the 9th grade, and stated that he could not see the value of continuing his education. He had found numerous jobs such as bricklayer's and carpenter's assistant, but had been unable to maintain these jobs for more than a few weeks at a time.

At the time of his injury, P.R. was 18. He remained in a coma for 4 months and continued to be hospitalized for 3 more months. Both physical and cognitive deficits were noted postinjury. His physical deficits included: functional blindness in his left eye and left-field cut in his right eye; left hemiparesis in his arm and leg, which was greater in his arm than in his leg; significant trunk deformity with spinal curvature; no sense of smell; and an unbalanced gait, which was compounded by his obesity. His cognitive deficits included: inattention, lack of concentration, poor organizational skills, short-term memory loss, lack of reasoning abilities, and inappropriate interpersonal skills.

At age 20, a vocational evaluation was administered to P.R. by the state center for rehabilitation. A vocational evaluation was requested to see if he had the potential to be prepared for competitive employment. The evaluation indicated that P.R. needed a sheltered employment-type placement. This was thought to be able to help him improve his work behaviors and awareness of work demands. The evaluation indicated that he would not be a good candidate for competitive job training or placement. Because of this, P.R. participated in a sheltered workshop for 2 months and then was referred for a neuropsychological evaluation.

A neuropsychological evaluation was not done until 12 years later—on March 20, 1989, by the Department of Rehabilitation Medicine at the Medical College of Virginia. The purpose of the evaluation was to determine P.R.'s emotional status and the effects of his cognitive deficits on his vocational potential. The results of his emotional status evaluation showed that P.R. displays no evidence of significant depression or anxiety. However, he is still at risk for depression if awareness of his deficits increases. Vocationally, P.R.'s problems with sustained attention and concentration, learning, memory, and motor/speed dexterity are felt to influence his work performance. Because of these deficits, the evaluations suggested that he will take more time to complete tasks, have problems learning and retaining information, and have difficulty focusing on tasks requiring sustained attention.

No psychiatric or psychological problems appeared evident. However, P.R. does display inappropriate behaviors at times. The behaviors include inappropriate verbalizations, invading physical space, and inappropriate touching.

P.R.'s only addictive behavior postinjury is that he is a heavy cigarette smoker. He no longer uses illegal drugs or alcohol. His family is very supportive of him. However, P.R.'s grandfather, who is his legal guardian, plays a much more active role in P.R.'s life. His mother and father are divorced and his father lives out of state. His mother speaks with him biweekly via phone but does not play an active role in his affairs.

P.R. is currently living independently in an apartment and is working through the local supported employment program. He has been working part time (3½ hours per day) since July 12, 1989, as a dining room attendant in a fast-food restaurant. His duties include wiping tables, emptying trash, cleaning lunch trays, stocking condiments, maintaining the upkeep of the bathrooms, and general maintenance of the dining area. He was given more responsibilities along with more hours on October 23, 1989, and now his duties also include stocking and maintaining the cold and hot food bars. He is now working a total of 5½ hours per day. His rate of pay is $4.25 per hour. He does not receive benefits from the company except for one free meal per day. The company also provides him with a uniform.

This position was chosen for P.R. because he is very sociable and outgoing, but mainly because this job can be structured to compensate for his poor organizational skills and short-term memory.

P.R. is currently receiving Social Security Disability Insurance (SSDI) benefits along with his biweekly earnings. He has not verbalized any higher aspirations and appears content with his life at the present. P.R. has stated more than once that he is better off now (postinjury) than before (preinjury). He says that if he had not been injured, he would probably be in jail or dead!

Job Training

Initial job training began July 12, 1989. The employment specialist was completing 60% of P.R.'s job and he was completing 40%. After 6 weeks, P.R. increased his percentage to 75%. By August 20, 1989, P.R. could perform tasks independently with one prompt. The employment specialist was finding that she could fade during some tasks and return when he was finished. P.R. did not know what to do next until she gave him the next prompt. The employment specialist made a schedule for him to follow and posted it where it was accessible to him. P.R. liked the idea of the schedule and used it daily. Problems arose with the schedule because as P.R. performed tasks regularly, he increased his speed; therefore, when he looked at his schedule, he was ahead of time. He went to the next duty but was more confused as time went on. A new strategy needed to be implemented. The employment specialist then made a pocket schedule that had one task on each page. It had no times on it—just a number on the bottom corner so he would know what direction to turn the page after he completed a task. He was trained not to turn the page until he was finished with the task at hand. This pocket schedule was the answer to P.R.'s inability to organize himself. He no longer needed prompts to go to the next task. With the pocket schedule, he could now do it independently.

Another problem area for P.R. was that when cleaning the dining room area, he would skip tables because he would jump from one row to another. What P.R. needed was to establish a set pattern. A specific route for him to follow was devised. He found that if he followed this route, he improved his accuracy and speed because he did not have to go back and wipe the missed tables. Another adaptation that was added to his route was the use of a caddy. In this caddy, he could put his cleaning supplies on one side and the small trash he picked up on the other. This made him more efficient because he did not have to stop his cleaning to throw a piece of trash away. He could just put it in the caddy and go on to the next table.

Another job duty—stocking the condiment stand—presented two obstacles for P.R. The first problem was that P.R. did not know when it needed to be stocked. This was easily resolved by putting red tape with the name of the item imprinted on it and attaching it to the inside of the bin. When the item needed restocking, P.R. would see the red tape. If he did not see the tape, the item was adequately stocked.

The other obstacle regarding the condiment stand was stocking it quickly. The supplies were stored in the stockroom, which meant that P.R. had to walk to the stockroom, get the needed item, and replace it on the stand. This was not a problem, except when he needed seven or eight items. Because of his left upper extremity paralysis, he could not carry everything. A small cart was purchased and he was taught to stock it with everything he needed for the day, and to push it out to the stand, filling all bins and placing leftover supplies under the counter for later use in the day. This adaptation increased his efficiency and speed.

Due to the increase in job duties, P.R.'s inappropriate behaviors, and a changeover in management, the employment specialist could not begin a set fading schedule until October 9, 1989. She began fading for the first hour and has since faded for the first hour and a half. She checks in on him to see if he is on schedule. If he is on schedule, she leaves for another hour and then returns. At that time, he should be cleaning the dining room and the lunch rush should be over. The employment specialist watches to make sure he stays on task and gets his work completed. During this time, P.R. has displayed inappropriate behaviors such as talking too much to customers, joking too much with co-workers, and neglecting his job duties. A behavioral contract was drawn up; when P.R. displayed any of these behaviors, he was reminded of the contract and its consequences. The managers of the restaurant have gotten very good at redirecting P.R. and getting him back on task.

Although training is not yet completed, P.R. has shown an increase in skill acquisition and has expressed that the job has helped to increase his self-esteem and self-image. He recently received his 3-month supervisor's evaluation; from his ratings and the comments made by the manager, P.R. is on his way to becoming a valued employee.

Case Study #2: C.M.

Background Information

C.M. is a 32-year-old male who experienced a severe traumatic brain injury in October 1981, as a result of his falling asleep in his car while driving at night. C.M.'s automobile hit a tree and he

was not discovered for nearly 12 hours. He was in a coma for 21 days and remained hospitalized for 5 months.

Prior to his injury, C.M. had graduated from college with a degree in journalism and had worked as a sportswriter for two major newspapers. He attempted to return to work as a sportswriter 9 months postinjury, but he was terminated due to his inability to meet story deadlines. As a client of the Department of Rehabilitative Services (DRS), C.M. then attended a state residential center for 2½ years and received certification as an office aide. He was placed by DRS in a mail processing position, but left the job 1 month later because he could not meet productivity standards. C.M. was unable to locate employment on his own and had been working as a volunteer at an outpatient rehabilitation center, as a physical therapy aide, when he was referred for supported employment services by his state rehabilitation counselor.

At the time of referral, neuropsychological evaluation results revealed strengths in verbal skills (e.g., written and spoken communication), and his greatest areas of weakness included visual perception, visual-motor integration, and memory functioning. Vocational recommendations suggested jobs that required communication skills, with minimal demands placed on visual skills, motor skills, and new learning. C.M. was found to have good social skills, and would likely get along well with co-workers. Also, because C.M. was distractible, he would likely function best in environments with little extraneous noise or background confusion. The neuropsychological evaluation also reported that C.M. would most likely be dissatisfied with exclusively repetitive work. Further, consumer assessment activities revealed that C.M. wanted to work "helping people" and in a part-time position, so his Social Security benefits would not be jeopardized.

Eight months after being referred to the supported employment program, C.M. was placed in a position as an activities aide at a convalescent center. The job duties involved one-to-one visitations with roombound residents documentation of visits on a patient interaction report, and assisting the activities director in the planning and implementation of the activities programs. This part-time job (20 hours per week) paid $3.55 per hour.

C.M.'s good communication skills, his preference for nonrepetitive work in the human services field, and his desire for part-time employment made him a good candidate for the position. In addition, the position would place minimal demands on visuomotor skills and the working environment was fairly quiet, which would increase C.M.'s ability to concentrate and perform his job duties.

Job Training

After the interview and 3 days prior to C.M.'s first day at work, the assistant activities director telephoned the employment specialist with concerns about placing an individual with traumatic brain injury in the position. She stated that they needed someone who had common sense, was capable of thinking for himself, and was a quick thinker. The assistant activities director also stated that she was afraid for C.M. to have one-to-one contact with residents. The week before, a resident with Alzheimer's disease had wheeled himself down the stairs and she questioned how C.M. would have responded if faced with such a situation. The employment specialist reassured the employer that she would be there 100% of the time to train C.M. and that if C.M. failed to meet the job requirements independently, the program would seek a more suitable job placement for him. The employment specialist also reemphasized C.M.'s strengths and reiterated why he was the "man for the job." Next, the director of activities called the employment specialist and stated that she, too, had concerns. The director vacillated between choosing not to hire C.M. and to hire him for 3 days. Finally, the activities director agreed to give C.M. an opportunity to be employed at this job.

One of the areas with which C.M. had difficulty was memory functioning. The employment specialist structured and organized the visitation and documentation procedures. Also, books with daily reading were purchased to enable C.M. not to have to keep track of the previous day's readings. Reducing C.M.'s distractibility and poor concentration were areas of concern during training, too. The employment specialist trained C.M. to create a "quiet environment" during a visit by always asking the resident whether or not he could lower the volume of the TV or radio and by shutting the door during his visit. Modeling was a strategy used during training. The employment specialist modeled appropriate ways to interact with residents during room visits and provided C.M. with feedback on his performance. Table 20.2 describes these and other adaptations and strategies that were introduced at the job site to assist C.M. in reaching skill acquisition and production standards.

At the time of writing this case study, total staff intervention time totaled approximately 290 hours. The employment specialist contacts C.M. and/or the employer at least twice a month to ensure that the job is being completed to the employer's satisfaction. C.M., the employment specialist, and the activities director meet quarterly to update the visitation schedule. C.M. has been employed for 29 months. He has earned over $8,300 in wages and has paid over $1,900 in taxes. C.M. expresses a strong desire to continue working in this field and hopes to obtain a full-time position in the future.

Case Study #3: H.N.

Background Information

H.N. is a 25-year-old single white male who is currently residing with his family in his parent's home. His family consists of his parents, and his sister and brother-in-law and their five children. He has a brother and three other sisters who live on their own. He states that he frequently used drugs and alcohol before his head injuries but abstains from using such substances now. He claims that his brother is a heavy substance abuser. H.N. attended high school but dropped out in the 9th grade due to low grades and lack of interest. H.N. reports his best subject in school to have been math. Prior to his head injuries, H.N. worked as a carpenter at $3.50 per hour for 4 months, as a service station attendant at $4.50 per hour for 6 months, as an automobile mechanic at $3.35 per hour for 8 months, and at a car dealership doing odd jobs at $3.35 per hour for 1 month. He also helped his dad load bakery

Table 20.2.   Adaptations and compensatory strategies for C.M.

Situation	Strategy
Forgetting to punch in and out on a daily time card	Introduced use of Casio 3 alarm watch. C.M. was insulted and refused to use the watch, but never forgot to punch out again.
Organizing daily visits	Purchased two notebooks: divided residents into one visit per week, two visits per week, or three visits per week; and by floor numbers. Implemented use of daily note sheets. Divided patient interaction reports according to number of visits per week and by floor numbers. Established time limits for visits.
Stories C.M. was reading were too long and he could not remember what materials he had already read to the residents	Purchased books that have daily readings.
Sloppiness and not following correct documentation procedures	The employment specialist would identify sloppy and incorrect documentation and C.M. would rewrite it.
Smoking in inappropriate areas	The employer designated specific times and places to smoke.

trucks for a local bakery without pay for an extended period of time. H.N.'s goals before and after his head injuries was to become a mechanic. H.N. was convicted of a misdemeanor as a youth, for vandalizing a boat, and had to pay a fine.

H.N. had his first head injury in a car accident at age 16 on July 5, 1980. Alcohol was involved. He sustained his second head injury on July 20, 1985, after falling 35 feet from a train trestle. Drugs and alcohol were involved in this accident also. It is unknown how long he was in a coma after his first accident. After his second accident, he was in a coma for 3 days. Length of hospitalization is unknown for each injury. H.N. gives as the account for his first injury that his friend was driving his cousin's car when they hit a tombstone. He states that he was blamed for the accident and that the police say that H.N. was the one driving. H.N. states that he sustained his second head injury after hanging around with friends on a bridge. He was climbing down a rope when a friend cut the rope, causing his fall.

H.N. was on the Department of Rehabilitative Services caseload from 1981 to 1984 after his first accident. After his second injury, H.N. received physical therapy and speech therapy.

These services were discontinued in 1986 because neither H.N. nor his family thought they were helping him. He continued to have regular meetings with the psychiatrist and to get yearly neuropsychiatric evaluations. Physical handicaps attributed to his injury include motor slowness, lower toleration to frustration resulting in loss of temper, and dysarthric speech. H.N. does not bend his knees to walk. He claims he gets tired more easily when he does.

H.N. is currently taking no medications. He has exhibited suicidal tendencies occasionally since his injuries, but further evaluations have found denied suicidal intent. Major sources of H.N.'s depression have been dissatisfaction with living arrangements, dependency on others for transportation, lack of friends, and lack of employment. H.N. has not passed the written driving evaluation on a number of tries and is medically restricted from driving. Results of these evaluations show H.N. to have poor reflexes, reaction time, and depth perception.

H.N. scored in the average range on his neuropsychological evaluation on tests measuring word finding, oral fluency, auditory comprehension, and visuoperceptual skills. H.N. scored low average to borderline impaired on tests of math reasoning, handwriting accuracy, immediate and sustained attention and concentration, remote memory, common sense, judgment of safety reasoning, bilateral coordination, and visuoconstructional skills. Significant deficits were found on tests of math computation, immediate attention and concentration, spelling, reading accuracy and comprehension, immediate and delayed auditory memory, immediate visual memory, auditory and visuomotor learning, bilateral motor speed/dexterity, logical deductive reasoning, and hypothesis testing.

H.N. reports that he does not get along well with his brother or brother-in-law. H.N.'s dad has been very supportive of H.N. since his accident. He and H.N. go nearly everywhere together. H.N.'s family situation at the present has proven to be very stressful for him, with complaints of lack of privacy and lack of sleep. His brother was also living at home but was kicked out and is now living with H.N.'s grandmother.

Preemployment, H.N. received $260 a month in Social Security Insurance (SSI) payments, and $36 a month in SSDI. Postemployment, H.N. earns too much to continue receiving SSI. H.N. is also ineligible for services from DRS because his household income is too high.

H.N. had been on a supported employment referral list since 1986, and was insistent that the only job in which he was interested was that of a mechanic. After much persuasion by the physician and the employment specialist, H.N. agreed to try something else, since the employment specialist found it very difficult to locate a garage or dealership that needed a mechanic's helper who could not drive and could not work quickly. H.N.'s major concern about getting a job was being able to retain his Medicaid benefits.

H.N. was taken to Bowl America several times to consider a maintenance position. Finally, he agreed to meet with the manager about a day porter position that was available. On September 11, 1989, H.N. was hired as the day porter at Bowl America. He earns $5.25 an hour and works from 9:00 A.M. to 3:00 P.M., Monday through Friday. Since he works less than 40 hours per week, he is ineligible for benefits or profit sharing. His duties as the day porter include cleaning windows and display cases, wiping down computer consoles and ball returns,

sweeping the proshop two times a week, sweeping around the video games and the front desk, busing tables two times a week, picking up trash in the parking lot when other duties are done, wiping down tables in the afternoons, vacuuming the nursery three times a week, checking the restrooms for trash and toilet paper daily before leaving, and wiping off the railing three times a week. This position was chosen because it is 6 miles from his house; the schedule does not conflict with his father's, so his dad can transport him; and quality of work is more important than speed.

Job Training

Initial training lasted from September 11 until November 13, 1989, with the employment specialist fading gradually after this period. H.N. had many problems during initial training. His biggest problem was with remembering the duties in his routine and finding the most comfortable and most efficient way to do these duties. Because of H.N.'s motor slowness, the employment specialist grouped all related duties together to save time and steps between duties. H.N. tended to be very dependent on the job coach, constantly asking, "How's this/that look?" and "Did I do this already?" It was discovered that H.N. did much better if the job coach forced him to make his own decisions and use his own judgment by increasing the distance between H.N. and the job coach and decreasing the number of given answers to these questions. H.N.'s attitude had always been, "I can't win for losing," and "I have very poor judgment." This has been improved by H.N.'s using a checklist. H.N. also began using physical reminders of what was next on his agenda after breaks and lunch by placing a piece of equipment for his next task nearby during his break. H.N.'s dependency also extends to his co-workers. He frequently asked co-workers to do something for him to make his job easier by allowing him not to have to take extra steps. This dependency has gradually decreased from a few times a day to a few times a week.

Another problem during initial training was the speed or amount of time it took H.N. to do each duty. This was a problem mostly because

H.N. had great difficulty finishing his tasks before 3:00 P.M., when his father arrived to pick him up. A time study was done and since Bowl America has no standard times to complete each duty, H.N. was instructed in ways to beat his record of the previous week's averages. H.N. has improved greatly in time spent on some duties, while occasionally backsliding in time spent on other areas. H.N. wants everything to be perfectly spotless before he will end a task. It is this that has prevented him from finishing some tasks in a more timely manner. H.N. also wanted to go back over something already done if he saw that a customer had messed it up. This was discouraged because it made H.N. frustrated and once the job was done he could mentally mark it off his checklist and move on to the next task. H.N. is now aware of when he is working too slow at whatever task. He tries to adjust his speed on the next task in order to catch up.

Another problem during initial training was with H.N.'s being "insubordinate." The job coach defined this as not doing what he had been asked, not responding when spoken to, telling the job coach he was going to do what he wanted to do, talking back, yelling, and losing his temper. H.N. had many incidents of insubordination between September 18 and September 28, and between October 11 and October 20, 1989. Most of these incidents stemmed from H.N.'s low tolerance for frustration involving everyday problems that popped up and from not being allowed to take a break before sweeping due to his inability to finish his work in a timely manner.

He lost his temper over not being able to clean windows without leaving streaks and lint from the paper towel. The employment specialist got him a squeegee but he did not have the balance to drag it across the glass without leaving streaks. He tried using a rag and found that to work better than paper towels or the squeegee. It also enabled him to work a little faster as it did not require as much control. H.N. also lost his temper when he thought too much about not being allowed to drive. The employment specialist talked about leaving problems at home and only thinking about work while at work. H.N. talks a lot about the past and his inability to

drive. He has gained more control over his temper around these issues because he is practicing not thinking about other problems while he is at work. H.N. has also lost his temper over not being able to get everything up while sweeping, vacuuming, picking up trash in the parking lot, cleaning ashtrays, and taking out boxes.

H.N. and the employment specialist have discussed talking to people when upset to let them know he does not want to talk about *why* he is upset until he has calmed down. H.N.'s temper accelerates when someone tries to talk to him about why he is mad. Usually when H.N. loses his temper, he raises his voice, does not listen to what others are saying, curses, and says he hates his job. The last time H.N. lost his temper (October 20, 1989), the manager talked with him about the importance of going outside, away from customers, and not cursing around the customers. Since then, H.N. has gone outside when he is upset and has practiced dealing with the things that anger him in an appropriate manner.

H.N. frequently had difficulty remembering to put away and get his supplies for different duties. The employment specialist purchased a caddy for him to keep stocked with all supplies related to similar duties and after a few days he no longer had a problem remembering what to do with supplies. He also keeps an extra checklist in his caddy. H.N. uses a cart to stock supplies needed for busing and wiping tables. Other memory problems were forgetting which windows he had cleaned, forgetting what areas he had already swept, and forgetting where he had already vacuumed in the nursery. The employment specialist, with H.N.'s assistance, established patterns for him to follow for each of these tasks and incorporated following the patterns into his original task analysis form. He was remembering and following the patterns regularly 1 month after his training began.

H.N. was very awkward in the ways he maneuvered his body to clean, sweep, and vacuum. He used to fight against the equipment he was using in order to keep his balance. He has since learned to move with the equipment, and cleans, sweeps, and vacuums in a more flowing, easier fashion. When his body was in an awkward position, he would start shaking. During H.N.'s first 2 weeks, the employment specialist redirected his movements and demonstrated how much easier it was to reach things if he avoided stretching excessively and standing in one spot to clean an entire area. H.N. still does not bend his knees very much, but he had learned to comfortably work around this.

Transportation has also been an issue with H.N. and his father. During H.N.'s second week of working, his father was frequently very late coming to pick H.N. up from work and H.N. would have to call to remind him. His father previously had said he did not mind providing transportation, but has since changed his mind. He agreed to provide transportation until other arrangements could be made. So far, the employment specialist has had no luck finding coworkers who live near H.N. or in utilizing Ridefinders. Hence, this problem continues to be an impediment to long-term employment stability, and is a challenge to the employment specialist.

H.N. had been working for 9 weeks, at the time of writing this case study. He has earned approximately $1,417 in gross wages, and has paid approximately $326 in taxes. A total of 304.35 intervention hours have been spent. On H.N.'s 1-month supervisor evaluation, the manager stated that H.N. needs to improve in areas of work speed and communication. He is "satisfied" to "very satisfied" with all other areas. He is concerned that H.N. will lose his temper if he is asked to do something extra. H.N. has begun to show initiative to do extra work and he does not complain because he knows that he chose to do the extra work. H.N. now is feeling a sense of pride at what he does and always endeavors to do the best he can. He feels he is a valued employee at Bowl America and tries harder to project an image of pleasantness to the customers.

Case Study #4: H.D.

Background Information

H.D. is a single 33-year-old male who sustained a severe closed head injury in December 1986. He was 29 when he sustained his head injury. This non-alcohol-related injury occurred while H.D. was washing second-story windows at a private residence, at which time he fell approximately 15 feet from the ladder. H.D. and some of his co-workers operated a window-washing business in their spare time. His co-workers transported him to the nearest rescue squad who, in turn, brought him to Medical College of Virginia (MCV) Hospital in Richmond, Virginia. H.D., who reportedly was comatose for nearly 7 weeks, was diagnosed to have suffered a right subdural hematoma. He progressed steadily until 3–4 months after his injury, when medical personnel noted that H.D. appeared somewhat "slower and lethargic." A computerized axial tomography (CT) scan was performed, which showed progressive ventricular dilation consistent with communicating hydrocephalus. Subsequently, a right ventriculo-peritoneal shunt was introduced. H.D. was discharged from MCV in May 1987, 6 months after admission. He was then referred to a local day treatment program for 3½ months, where he progressed considerably in the areas of mobility, standing balance, coordination, and postural awareness. Improvement was still to be made in physical strength. Tegretol (500 mg.) was the only medication prescribed at this time.

There were no psychological, psychiatric, or addictive problems postinjury. Posthospitalization, H.D. returned to his own home under his mother's care, which caused considerable conflict due to his mother's overprotectiveness. He received an $800 per month Social Security payment to cover his living expenses. After completing classes at the day rehabilitation program, H.D. was unable to find employment on his own and, subsequently, he hund around his house all day becoming bored and frustrated. His mother expressed concern regarding her son's inactivity and apparent lack of feelings of self-worth. She reported that he fatigued easily, experienced dizziness, and had gained a great deal of weight. Furthermore, she reported her son to be increasingly depressed, irritable, and apathetic, and that he frequently made socially inappropriate comments.

Prior to his injury, H.D. had been a firefighter for 9 years and earned approximately $23,000 annually. He was very satisfied with the vocation and had planned to continue with this career. In his first year with the fire department, he was awarded "Rookie of the Year." H.D. was, therefore, very motivated to return to his position as a firefighter.

Two weeks after being discharged from the day rehabilitation program, H.D. underwent a 5-day work capacity evaluation. Recommendations from this evaluation indicated placement in a sheltered workshop followed by on-the-job training with continuous job coach involvement for work adjustment and behavioral management. As a result, H.D.'s hopes of returning to his job as a firefighter were diminished.

Twelve months following this initial evaluation, a second work capacity evaluation was conducted. Specifically, this 3-day evaluation was undertaken to determine if H.D. was able to resume his duties with the fire department. Unfortunately, it was determined that H.D.'s capabilities were not compatible with the job demands of a firefighter. The evaluators recommended supported employment services with special considerations given to employment possibilities where H.D. could perform structured, routine activities. He was subsequently referred for neuropsychological evaluation by his doctor.

The initial neuropsychological evaluation reported a significant degree of residual cortical dysfunction attributable to his head injury, resulting in his experiencing difficulties across a wide range of functional areas. Performance on measures of substance concentration and information processing fell in the defective range. Furthermore, his scores suffered on tasks requiring quick visuomotor responses. Finally, the evaluation reported that H.D. demonstrated poor self-awareness with his frequent inappropriate behavior.

Due to his significant memory problems, positions requiring regular communication with customers were not recommended. It was recommended that he work at a job where accuracy rather than speed was important, due to his impaired visuomotor abilities. Furthermore, a job in which the tasks were highly structured, in a distraction-free environment, with close supervision or co-worker participation was desirable.

Job development strategies were focused on H.D.'s excellent recognition, memory, and reading comprehension skills; vocational interests compatible with his previous occupation; and his need for a well-developed benefit package.

Job Training

In April 1989, a full-time forklift operator's position at a small paper distribution company was located. The job included a $5.50 per hour wage, plus health benefits available at the end of 3 months. The job consisted of two major tasks: 1) unloading trucks with a hydraulic pallet jack, and 2) putting up stock with the use of a hydraulic forklift. The initial training lasted approximately 3 months, or 380 staff hours. During these initial months, H.D. did not miss any days of work nor was he tardy. Also, he always dressed appropriately for the job site.

H.D. reached skill acquisition unloading the truck with the pallet jack approximately 1 month after placement. Skill acquisition was technically never reached using the forklift due to recurring mistakes in stock identification. However, it should be noted that H.D. was proficient in mechanical operation of the forklift. Fading began on May 17, 1989, in an effort to investigate H.D.'s initiative to work independently of the job coach. Due to production complications, a consistent fading schedule could not be developed. Almost full-time intervention was a necessity.

During the first 2 months of H.D.'s employment, other problems occurred concerning: disorientation in the warehouse, equipment maintenance, sequencing and prioritizing job tasks, and understanding the warehouse's bin-location system. The following job modifications and cognitive strategies were used to assist in these problems:

1. $4'' \times 6''$ letters signifying aisle location were posted at the end of each aisle to assist in problems with disorientation in the warehouse.
2. Visual cues were used to have H.D. properly maintain/hook up equipment.

3. A pocket index card listing job task priorities was implemented.
4. Instruction and modeling were used to help H.D. understand the bin-location system.

H.D. was separated from his job at the paper distribution company in August 1989, approximately 3 months after the initial placement. He had rejected the presence of the job coach on site throughout the last month of his placement. The reason for the separation was due to a slow production rate, advocacy problems, and too many errors on his job performance. Positive results were: the development of H.D.'s stamina to tolerate an 8-hour work day, a clearer understanding of how to deal with co-workers and upper management, awareness of his need for memory and orientation aids, and technical mastery of the hydraulic equipment.

Less than a month after termination from the paper distribution company, H.D. was placed at an area hospital, as a distribution clerk in the purchasing department. His job duties dealt with stocking the hospital units with standard nursing supplies. This job required that H.D. restock the hospital supply carts daily and then transport these carts to the appropriate unit where the carts are switched with the cart from the previous day. He was also responsible for taking daily inventory of certain stock items that are kept on the unit, replacing them as needed. In addition to the above duties, H.D. was responsible for placing charge stickers on all personal care items used by the patients. When screening the job, the job coach was told by the department supervisor that it usually took a person about 1 month before becoming proficient at this job.

Initially, H.D. was responsible for stocking seven units daily. For the first 2 weeks, he worked alongside the job coach, learning to identify the different items and their proper locations. He had little difficulty reaching a skill-acquisition level that allowed him to work semi-independently. After 3 weeks, he was able to stock a cart, switch it out, and take floor inventory unassisted. When errors were made, they were usually of an "absent-minded nature" caused by distractions. He reached skill acquisition at an acceptable rate but his production rate was extremely low. It took him approximately 6 hours to complete one unit. After 1 month, this time was decreased by 50% and H.D. was stabilized at this rate for another month. Ideally, on the larger floors, a completion time of no more than 1½ hours was necessary if the day's production standard was to be met. During this period, H.D. was able to complete no more than two units daily, and the production level was kept on par by the job coach.

To date, the majority of intervention hours have been devoted to meeting production standards, and the development and implementation of interventions for behaviors that appear to stand in the way of meeting production standards and that if ignored, could jeopardize H.D.'s position. Because H.D. tends to be resentful of needing a job coach, he often resists instructional training and constructive suggestions made by the job coach. He often becomes defensive, as though he were being personally attacked. Because of this, the job coach frequently uses H.D.'s supervisor to address issues and set necessary limits. This has been an effective strategy in developing behavioral interventions. Table 20.3 describes adaptations and compensatory strategies used to assist H.D. in meeting skill acquisition and production standards.

After almost 2 months of employment, a new female supervisor assumed responsibility for the purchasing department. H.D.'s former supervisor was subsequently assigned a subordinate role in the department. H.D.'s reaction to the new supervisor and the subsequent "demotion" of his previous supervisor, with whom H.D. had good rapport, demonstrated that he had some difficulty accepting this new supervisor. On at least two occasions, he became very angry at her, refusing to speak for days at a time. The employment specialist spent a great deal of time advocating for H.D. and attempted to identify possible methods of dealing with the resistance to the new supervisor.

As with most businesses after a change in management, there have been many procedural changes initiated in the purchasing department. In many ways, H.D.'s job appeared to have been

Table 20.3.   Adaptations and compensatory strategies for H.D.

Situation	Strategy
Frequent confusion as to the sequences of tasks and performing tasks that were not part of job description	Typed list of all job duties in 30 sequences. List also included duties and behaviors that should be limited, and tasks that should be performed in spare time. This list is attached to H.D.'s clipboard for easy reference.
Job required numerous trips to shelves in stockroom to get supplies when stocking cart	To reduce number of walks between carts and stockroom shelves, a hand shopping basket was introduced so many items could be picked up at one time.
Difficulty locating stock items on sheet and learning proper location of items on stock cart and stock room	Stock sheets were revised so stock items were listed in the sequence in which they appear on the cart. Uniformed containers with labels were added to the cart shelves for easier identification of items and stockroom location of items were listed on stock sheet.
Continual difficulty meeting an adequate production rate	After consultation with supervisor, it was decided that position needed restructuring so as to make job more manageable for H.D. Job now requires H.D. to complete three units instead of seven.
Wasting a lot of time constantly looking for rubber bands to use when stocking carts and while doing inventory	Supervisor agreed to keep a supply of rubber bands within H.D.'s access.
Resistance to intervention from job coach	Job coach frequently informed supervisor of issues that needed to be discussed. Supervisor's comments to H.D. are often originated from the employment specialist.
Off-task behavior on units and making a "pest of himself" by annoying staff on units	Was not allowed to perform job duties independently. Had to be accompanied by job coach for suitable period of time.
Excessive "fooling around" with co-workers, subsequently not completing all of his tasks	A production sheet was designed that outlined each task and the time expected to complete each task. As a way of keeping him conscious of time, H.D. was asked after completing each task to record the actual time it took to perform the task.
Rude and inappropriate remarks to female employees	Conference with job coach and male supervisor
Wasting time with compulsive and unnecessary neatness while stocking carts	The supervisor and job coach would reshuffle and rearrange materials that H.D. had organized, demonstrating to him that his excessive neatness was unnecessary because of the time factor.

redesigned into an entirely new position, requiring the job coach to relearn the job in order to retrain H.D. The employment specialist recognized that learning new skills and improving work speed would require intensive training. At this point, the employment specialist determined that it was necessary to make sure the new supervisor fully understood the practice of supported employment and was committed to continuing to work with the program.

H.D. has fared better than expected in dealing with all of the changes. After retraining, several error checks by the job coach have shown skill acquisition to be at a satisfactory level. There have been significant changes in H.D.'s job description that have had a positive effect. One of these changes occurred as a result of several discussions between the job coach and the new supervisor. Ultimately, it was decided that H.D.'s job responsibilities were too much for one person to perform effectively. His job was restructured so that now he is responsible for restocking three units daily, as opposed to seven. Responsibility for the other floors are now divided among other staff in the purchasing department. H.D. is now expected to complete his duties within a 6-hour period, with the remaining 2 hours of the day set aside for stocking the shelves, putting patient charge stickers on medical supplies, and performing errands. It should be noted that although H.D. now has less work and therefore more time to complete the job, the new supervisor is less concerned with production and places a greater emphasis on detail, thoroughness, and a less flexible working environment.

Thirteen months after his date of hire, he had received a total of 579 hours of employment specialist intervention on his job site. He earns $5.00 per hour, and receives full benefits. H.D. occasionally has difficulties with consistently meeting production standards as a result of distractions in the environment. At the time of this writing, he received two to three job-site visits per month.

MAJOR OBSTACLES

1. *Perceptions of Rehabilitation Potential* Rehabilitation counselors may be reluctant to offer services to individuals with severe brain injury because of a historical pessimism regarding their rehabilitation potential. Indeed, some researchers found an inverse relationship between severity of injury and the likelihood of receiving significant levels of rehabilitative services, and other investigators have found that few persons with severe brain injury are enrolled in work retraining, sheltered workshop, or volunteer activities (Wehman & Kreutzer, 1990).

2. *Perceptions of Vocational Rehabilitation Services* The enduring concept of vocational rehabilitation services is that they are time limited and purely vocational, and this continues to be the focus of state programs. Many professionals agree that the vocational rehabilitation service system can be beneficial to individuals who have sustained a mild injury who can make a successful transition from medical rehabilitation to their home community without specialized services. Persons with severe traumatic brain injury will generally have more complex, varied, and multifaceted deficits and needs that require long-term service obligations. Moreover, the service process (i.e., vocational evaluation) presupposes that clients can remember and build upon their experiences during service phases and generalize their training to actual work environments—abilities that are frequently impaired as a result of severe head injury. Finally, the time-limited nature of vocational rehabilitation services does not address the episodic occurrences of emotional/behavioral impairments that frequently accompany severe traumatic brain injury.

3. *Funding Sources for Extended Services* The coordination of funding from time-limited to extended services has often been problematic for agencies serving persons with traumatic brain injury, who do not fall under the traditional mental health/mental retardation funding umbrella. For example, a group of researchers found that of the 27 states that awarded system change grants in 1986–1987 to develop supported employment as a service option, only 5 had identified funding sources for extended services for this population, and then only for those individuals who also met the additional criteria of the state mental health, mental retardation, or developmental disability agency (Wehman, Kugel, & Shafer, 1989). Table 20.4 lists ten additional sources of funding for extended services for brain-injured clients.

4. *Problems with the Service System* Limited funding sources for extended employment services appears to be symptomatic of disjointed, complicated, restrictive, limited, or absent systems of long-term support services for individuals with traumatic brain injury and their families. One study discovered that only a few states have developed approaches to address the

Table 20.4. Funding sources for extended services for persons with traumatic brain injury

1. Social Security funds (e.g., Impairment task-related expenses)
2. Private foundations
3. United Way
4. Vocational Education Act funds
5. Job Training Partnership Act (JTPA) monies
6. Federal/state requests for proposals (RFPs) (i.e., state developmental disabilities councils)
7. Fee for Services
8. Interagency funding coalitions
9. Third-party payers (e.g., Blue Cross)
10. Private rehabilitation companies and brokers

long-term comprehensive rehabilitation needs of this population.

5. *Types and Availability of Services* Although there has been progress within recent years in developing services for persons with traumatic brain injury, the majority of programs continue to focus on acute medical care and acute rehabilitation, according to the National Head Injury Foundation (1990). Specialized post-acute vocational, neurobehavioral, and independent living services are limited in number, and demand for services far exceeds availability. These services also tend to be very expensive, and are therefore beyond the means of most persons with head injury and their families, and beyond the willingness of most public and private funding sources to pay.

RESEARCH NEEDS

The issues discussed in this chapter underscore both the paucity of knowledge regarding employment for persons with severe traumatic brain injury, and the limited commitment of public expenditures (time, effort, and money) to resolve the problems that persons with traumatic brain injury experience in attempting to enter or reenter the work force. These issues also suggest directions in the research and public policy arenas for improving the vocational outlook for these individuals.

The literature has noted that it is very difficult to predict which persons with traumatic brain injury will become employed and which will not (Wehman & Kreutzer, 1990). Available research is contradictory and has typically not included individuals involved in intensive interventions (Kreutzer & Wehman, 1990). Research is needed that addresses the following areas:

1. There is a need for a better understanding of the reasons why some members of this population fail to achieve long-term employment success, even within a program of supported employment. For example, Sale and his associates have analyzed data that show that once clients with traumatic brain injury stay employed at least 6–9 months, their long-term vocational stability improves (Sale, West, Sherron, & Banks, in press). The high-risk time period is in the first several months of employment.

2. There is also a need to examine the types of interventions that are most effective in addressing specific vocational and social deficits, including job placement strategies, employer/co-worker preparation, compensatory strategies, crisis interventions, and the effective use of counseling, medical, neuropsychological, behavioral, respite, and other support services. More specifically, what is the most efficient and cost-effective way of arranging these services?

3. Research on the impact of rehabilitation efforts is confounded by the difficulty in determining, retrospectively, the types of rehabilitation services that individuals have received and the effects of specific services. Traumatic brain injury program outcome research must attempt to identify and address the effects of prior services, and the effects of spontaneous recovery over time through the brain's natural recovery and compensation process.

4. Research-and-demonstration efforts are also needed on the efficacy of using group models or modifications of individual supported employment, such as enclaves or clustered placements, for members of this client group. Are these viable alternatives for individuals whose need for monitoring and intervention are relatively permanent, and who repeatedly fail to achieve stabilization in individual placement? If so, how can group models be designed and im-

plemented so as to achieve maximum integration and earnings while minimizing stigma?

5. There is virtually no information on the costs and benefits of providing necessary interventions that allow individuals with severe traumatic brain injury to become employed and stay employed, or cost-effectiveness comparisons across various return-to-work methods. Likewise, there is limited information on the costs of *not* providing vocational services as well, including alternative day support services, permanent income maintenance, and the loss of contributions to the tax base from both the person with brain injury and family members who must forego or limit their own employment to provide daily care for their loved one who is injured. West et al. (1991) reported that 291 hours of staff intervention time were necessary for each person placed, with costs to stabilization averaging $6,896 and the annual costs of extended services averaging $2,476. However, this report stated nothing about the benefits accrued for clients with traumatic brain injury.

Addressing these research needs should serve not only to improve services to persons with traumatic brain injury and their families, but to encourage expenditures of vocational rehabilitation case service dollars and access to vocational services as well. The research data collected in areas such as those just described will lead directly into beginning to address public policy needs in this area.

PUBLIC POLICY NEEDS

Integrated, community-based services are still in infancy stages for persons with severe traumatic brain injury. There are a number of steps that state and federal agencies can take to spur development of services. While research provides an important foundation, public policy issues are critical in establishing long-term systems change.

1. First and foremost, state and federal funding agencies should being the arduous process of developing a comprehensive, coordinated system of services for persons with severe brain injury, from the acute medical stage, through acute rehabilitation, to long-term ser-

vices. Funding dollars should be earmarked specifically for programs to meet the unique needs of these persons, and should include supported and independent living, respite care and other family supports, behavioral and crisis intervention, counseling, case management, and social/recreational development, as well as extended supported employment services.

2. Research-and-demonstration grants should be expanded in number and scope to develop a firm knowledge base of models, methods, and activities for improving vocational rehabilitation services to persons with traumatic brain injury. More multicenter efforts need to be performed in a systematic way for replication.

3. Vocational rehabilitation counselor training and education should present a clear and unbiased picture of the needs and abilities of persons with severe traumatic brain injury. State programs should encourage the investment of case service dollars for employment services, as well as for other acute and postacute services that might promote future employment, such as physical therapy, occupational therapy, speech-language and communication therapy, cognitive rehabilitation, supervised housing and independent living services, and personal and family counseling.

4. Finally, efforts must be made to bring public and private programs within the reach of more families of persons with severe traumatic brain injury.

The long-term funding problems that affect employment services for individuals with traumatic brain injury are not unique to this group of clients. However, individuals with traumatic brain injury are unique in that their long-term needs encompass medical, psychological, residential, and social services, as well as vocational services. In short, funding for extended employment services cannot be provided in a vacuum apart from funding for other services.

SUMMARY AND CONCLUSIONS

The purpose of this chapter has been to describe how supported employment can be utilized as a means of providing cognitive rehabilitation to clients with traumatic brain injury in the workplace. Several case studies were presented, along with tables that described cognitive strategies. Several research and public policy issues were also developed.

The key aspect of cognitive rehabilitation in the workplace is to individualize what the client needs, based on the work requirements associ-

ated with the job. Only when service delivery arrangements are modified to allow for cognitive interventions to be provided on the job site will workers with traumatic brain injury maximize their capabilities. Cognitive rehabilitation holds great potential—but it must be delivered in a more functional way.

REFERENCES

Brooks, D.N., McKinlay, W., Symington, C., Beattie, A., & Campsie, L. (1987). Return to work within the first seven years of severe head injury. *Brain Injury, 1*, 5–19.

Federal Register. (1987, August 14). 1986 Amendments to the Rehabilitation Act.

Frankowski, R. (1986). Descriptive epidemiologic studies of head injury in the United States: 1974–1984. In L. Karger & R. Basel, Trauma treatment in practice: The head injured patient. *Advanced Psychosomatic Medicine, 16*, 152–172.

Klonoff, P.S., Costa, L.D., & Snow, W.G. (1986). Predictors and indicators of quality of life in patients with closed-head injury. *Journal of Clinical and Experimental Neuropsychology, 8*, 469–485.

Kreutzer, J.S., & Wehman, P. (1990). *Community integration following traumatic brain injury.* Baltimore: Paul H. Brookes Publishing Co.

McMordie, W.R., & Barker, S.L. (1988). The financial trauma of head injury. *Brain Injury, 2*, 357–364.

National Head Injury Foundation. (1990, November). *Managing psychosocial dysfunction for optimal employability.* Paper presented at the national meeting of the National Head Injury Foundation, New Orleans.

Sale, P., West, M., Sherron, P., & Banks, D. (in press). An analysis of why employees with traumatic brain injury leave employment. *Journal of Head Trauma Rehabilitation.*

Stonnington, H. (1986). Traumatic brain injury rehabili-

tation. *American Rehabilitation, 22* (4,5), 19–20.

Wehman, P., & Kreutzer, J. (1990). *Vocational rehabilitation of persons with traumatic brain injury.* Rockville, MD: Aspen.

Wehman, P., Kreutzer, J., West, M., Sherron, P., Diambra, J., Fry, R., Groah, C., Sale, P., & Killam, S. (1989). Employment outcomes of persons following traumatic brain injury: Pre-injury, post-injury, and supported employment. *Brain Injury, 3*, 397–412.

Wehman, P., Kreutzer, J., West, M., Sherron, P., Zasler, N., Groah, C., Stonnington, H., Burns, C., & Sale, P. (in press). Return to work for persons with traumatic brain injury: A supported employment approach. *Archives of Physical Medicine and Rehabilitation.*

Wehman, P., Kugel, M., & Shafer, J. (1989). *A study of supported employment in 27 states.* Richmond: Virginia Commonwealth University, Rehabilitation Research and Training Center.

Wehman, P., West, M., Fry, R., Sherron, P., Groah, C., Kreutzer, J., & Sale, P. (1989). Effect of supported employment on the vocational outcomes of persons with traumatic brain injury. *Journal of Applied Behavior Analysis, 22*(4), 395–405.

West, M., Wehman, P., Kregel, J., Kreutzer, J., Sherron, P., & Zasler, N. (1991, February). Costs of operating a supported employment program for clients with traumatic brain injury. *Archives of Physical Medicine and Rehabilitation, 72*, 127–131.

Index